The Chinese HEART in a Cognitive Perspective

Applications of Cognitive Linguistics
12

Editors
Gitte Kristiansen
Michel Achard
René Dirven
Francisco J. Ruiz de Mendoza Ibáñez

Mouton de Gruyter
Berlin · New York

The Chinese HEART in a Cognitive Perspective

Culture, Body, and Language

by
Ning Yu

Mouton de Gruyter
Berlin · New York

Mouton de Gruyter (formerly Mouton, The Hague)
is a Division of Walter de Gruyter GmbH & Co. KG, Berlin

♾ Printed on acid-free paper
which falls within
the guidelines of the ANSI
to ensure permanence and durability.

Library of Congress Cataloging-in-Publication Data

Yu, Ning, 1954–
The Chinese heart in a cognitive perspective : culture, body, and language / by Ning Yu.
p. cm. – (Applications of cognitive linguistics ; 12)
Includes bibliographical references and index.
ISBN 978-3-11-020516-9 (hardcover : alk. paper)
1. Xin (The Chinese word) 2. Heart – Symbolic aspects – China. I. Title.
PL1315.X56Y8 2009
495.1'81–dc22
2008046424

Bibliographic information published by the Deutsche Nationalbibliothek

The Deutsche Nationalbibliothek lists this publication in the Deutsche Nationalbibliografie; detailed bibliographic data are available in the Internet at http://dnb.d-nb.de.

ISBN 978-3-11-020516-9

ISSN 1861-4078

Printed in Germany

Preface

This book project on the Chinese HEART started in the autumn of 2003 when I was on a one-semester sabbatical leave. For a few years before that, I had been exploring the role of the body in human understanding and meaning. I had studied some Chinese body-part terms with regard to their metonymic and metaphoric extension into more abstract domains as cases of the embodied nature of human cognition (Yu 2000, 2001, 2002, 2003a, 2003c, 2004). For apparent reasons, the conceptualization of internal body parts displays more cultural variation than that of external ones. For instance, that the internal organ *dan* 'gallbladder' is involved in the understanding of courage in Chinese is very culture-specific and can be traced back to its cultural roots in traditional Chinese medicine, where the gallbladder is said to have a function in making judgments and decisions and in determining one's degree of courage (Yu 2003a). I decided that I should focus next on the much more challenging task of studying the Chinese cultural conceptualization of the heart, although previously I had already touched upon the topic when I studied Chinese expressions of talking about feelings (Yu 1995, 1998, 2002) and thinking (Yu 2003d). It was obvious to me that this study should be a book-length project; after the necessary search for the cultural roots in ancient Chinese philosophy and traditional Chinese medicine, and a desired, though perhaps doomed to be limited comparison with Western cultures and the English language, the amount of linguistic data collected was simply too vast to consider publishing anything other than a book. In the past few years, this book project has been intermittent due to other academic, teaching and service commitments at my university and beyond. I am very pleased that the time has come to assemble the various parts together into one final work.

In the meantime, I have also written three articles that are related to the topic of, and share some content with, this book. The first, titled "The Chinese conceptualization of the heart and its cultural context: Implications for second language learning", appeared in Farzad Sharifian and Gary Palmer (eds.), *Applied Cultural Linguistics: Implications for Second Language Learning and Intercultural Communication* (Amsterdam and Philadelphia: John Benjamins, 2007, pp. 65–85). The second, "Heart and cognition in ancient Chinese philosophy", came out in *Journal of Cognition and Culture* (2007, 1/2, pp. 27–47). The third one, "The Chinese heart as the central faculty of cognition", will be forthcoming in Farzad Sharifian, René Dirven,

Ning Yu, and Susanne Niemeier (eds.), *Culture, Body, and Language: Conceptualizations of Internal Body Organs across Cultures and Languages* (Berlin and New York: Mouton de Gruyter, 2008).

In the past decade, I have learned and benefited enormously from many scholars, too many to list them all here, but I want especially to extend my heartfelt gratitude to Eugene H. Casad, Marcelo Dascal, René Dirven, Charles Forceville, Roslyn Frank, Raymond Gibbs, Zoltán Kövecses, George Lakoff, Ronald Langacker, Susanne Niemeier, Jan Nuyts, Gary Palmer, Günter Radden, and Farzad Sharifian. My interaction with them and my benefiting from their scholarly works have inspired my research and shaped my academic career.

I also want to take this opportunity to express my sincere and hearty thanks to the reviewers for their invaluable and helpful comments and suggestions, and to the series editors of "Applications of Cognitive Linguistics", Gitte Kristiansen, Michel Achard, René Dirven, and Francisco J. Ruiz de Mendoza Ibáñez, as well as the editor-in-chief Anke Beck, the managing editor Birgit Sievert, and the production editor Monika Wendland at Mouton de Gruyter, for their editorial guidance and assistance during the preparation of this book manuscript. My special thanks go to René Dirven for sharing with me his profound insight and knowledge.

Finally, I want to thank my parents, parents-in-law, wife, and son, for their affection and support. My "whole-hearted" concentration on this "heart" book project has taken away much of my time that I should have spent with my wife and son. I greatly appreciate their understanding and unfailing love. I am especially grateful to my wife, who has always been behind me with all the support crucial to the completion of this book project.

Table of contents

Chapter 1
Introduction: Heart, body and mind

1.1. Object and goal: Chinese concept of *xin* 'heart'

This book focuses on a single concept, the concept of "heart" in Chinese, encoded in the Chinese character 心 *xin* (pronounced close to *shin*). For me, however, working on this research project is akin to drilling the earth for oil: On the surface there is only a very small hole, but once the drill reaches a certain depth, it encounters an immense reservoir of resources.

The term "heart" may seem susceptible to a straightforward definition, perhaps as the internal organ that pumps blood for circulation inside the body. However, that is a scientific definition of the "physical heart", which, in terms of its bodily functions, should be the same among all human beings, regardless of their cultural or ethnical background. What I want to concentrate on in this book instead is the cultural conception of the "mental heart", which may vary distinctly across different cultures or even within one culture across different periods of its history (see, e.g., Doueihi 1997; Erickson 1997; Høystad 2007; Jager 2001; Sharifian et al. 2008a; Wierzbicka 1989, 1992). Behind the Chinese word *xin* 'heart' there is a long and rich cultural history through which the Chinese concept of "heart" has been formed. Reflecting this long and rich cultural history is an enormous amount of linguistic data in the Chinese language that manifest the Chinese conceptualization of the heart. But this conceptualization of the heart, the cultural models underlying it, and the linguistic usages manifesting it, as far as I know, have never been studied in a systematic manner. For this study, therefore, my goal is twofold: Using the analytical tools of Cognitive Semantics I will, first, delineate the Chinese conceptualization of the heart in its historical and cultural context and, secondly, make a semantic analysis of the linguistic data that reflect the conceptual network centered on the *xin* 'heart'. In other words, I will characterize the Chinese conceptualization of the heart as exhibited in Chinese culture and manifested in the Chinese language. I will also compare it with Western conceptions of the heart, especially those manifested in English.

In Chinese, the word *xin* that primarily denotes the heart organ may also refer to it as the "organ for thinking" and the "seat of thought and emotions". This fact is displayed clearly in the unique ideographic writing system of Chinese. Thus, many Chinese characters for words related to thought and feeling contain the "heart" radical as their semantic component. Here are a few examples pertaining to thinking or thought: 思 *si* 'think; consider; deliberate; think of; long for; thought; thinking', 想 *xiang* 'think; ponder; think back; try to remember; recall; recollect; consider; miss', 虑 *lü* 'consider; ponder; think over; concern; worry', and 念 *nian* 'think of; miss; thought; idea'. The following are two common characters representing words for feeling: 感 *gan* 'feel; sense; feeling' and 情 *qing* 'feeling; affection; sentiment; passion'. Two things about Chinese are worth mentioning in passing. First, the "heart" radical has two variants. The canonical one, which looks the same as the character 心 *xin* 'heart', often occurs at the bottom of a character, as in 思 *si*, 想 *xiang*, 虑 *lü*, 念 *nian*, and 感 *gan*. The other one, usually called the "vertical heart radical", stands on the left side of a character, as in 情 *qing*. Second, the single-character words often combine with others to form so-called compound words in modern Chinese. For instance, the preceding single-character words can form the following compounds: 思想 *sixiang* 'thought; thinking; idea; ideology', 思虑 *silü* 'consider; contemplate; deliberate', 思念 *sinian* 'think of; long for; miss', 感情 *ganqing* 'emotion; feeling; sentiment; affection', and 情感 *qinggan* 'emotion; feeling'. As suggested by the ideographic characters and meanings of the words they encode, or the connection between form and meaning, the heart represents a person's intellectual and affective center and locus of mental and emotional life. It is, therefore, traditionally regarded as the central faculty of cognition in Chinese culture (Yu 2007a, 2007b, 2008c).

In this way, the Chinese word *xin* 'heart' covers the meanings of both "heart" and "mind" as understood in English, which, like various other European languages, upholds a heart-head dichotomy. According to the Western view, the heart is seen as the center of emotions and the head (the locus of the brain with which the mind is associated) as the center of thought. In contrast to this Western dualism, Chinese takes on a more holistic view that sees the heart as the center of both emotions and thought. This contrast is an important one, characterizing two groups of cultural traditions that have developed distinctive conceptualizations of the person, the self, and the cognitive agent (see, e.g., Wierzbicka 2005).

Before I move on, however, I want to digress from Chinese briefly for the purpose of establishing an external reference point in English, which is also the working language, for my study. I need to point out that the English word *mind*, as much as the Chinese word *xin* 'heart', represents a culture-specific concept constructed in the Anglo-Saxon context (see Wierzbicka 1989, 1992). What it means has also changed over time, interacting with the concepts encoded by other English words such as *spirit*, *soul*, and *heart*. In the older stratum of English, *mind* was closer to the present-day *spirit*, and was linked with both emotions and moral values. The present-day *mind*, however, is basically free of emotions, which are now normally linked with *heart*, and is morally neutral. That is to say, the older *mind* had spiritual and psychological dimensions, whereas the current *mind* has the predominantly intellectual and rational orientation, with a modern emphasis on thinking and knowing, not on feeling, wanting, or any other nonbodily processes. Therefore, present-day *minds* are no longer described as "happy" or "fiery" (emotional), or "noble" or "ignoble" (moral) as in older English, but instead as "inquisitive" or "inquiring" (seeking knowledge), "brilliant" (good at thinking), "keen" (active in thinking and seeking to know), and so on. A "good mind" nowadays has unambiguously intellectual implications just as a "good heart" has emotional and moral ones (see Wierzbicka 1989: 48–50). Thus, as Wierzbicka (1989: 49) summarizes, in the history of semantic change *mind* "shed its spiritual connotations, lost its links with values and emotions, and became a concept focused on the intellect, more or less to the exclusion of any other aspects of a person's 'inner' life". This change reflects the modern emphasis on rationalistic, intellectual, and scientific orientation of mainstream Western culture. It is worth noting that dualism in English has changed over history from the soul-body to mind-body dichotomy (Wierzbicka 1989: 50):

> The *soul* used to be a very comprehensive concept, combining religious, psychological, and moral aspects, seen as one and jointly opposed to the material body. In the course of its history, however, *soul* became restricted to the purely religious sphere. A concomitant change affected *mind*, which replaced *soul* as a word referring to the psychological aspect of the human person and as the dominant counterpart of the *body* in modern Anglo-Saxon thinking. This victory of *mind* over *soul*, combined with the shift in the meaning of *mind*, attests to the birth of a new kind of dualism in English "ordinary ways of thinking", a dualism devoid of religious and moral connotations and reflecting the supreme value placed on rational thinking and knowing, rather than on other aspects of the human person. To put it rather crudely, a human being used to be thought of as composed of a body and a transcendental, moral, emotional, "inscrutable" soul; and now it tends to be thought of as composed of a body and an intellect.

This quotation captures, rather succinctly, the nature and essence of "the decline and fall of the word *soul*, and the ascendancy of the word *mind*" in English (p. 56). The significance of such a lexical analysis lies, however, in the fact that it testifies to the change of the conceptual landscape in the corresponding cultural history and prevailing ethnophilosophy, as Wierzbicka (1989, 1992) claims.

This is also the intended significance of my in-depth study of the Chinese word *xin* 'heart' to be presented in this book. For the present study, I will use the English word *mind*, as in the title of this chapter, as a shorthand term referring to such mental aspects and functions as thinking and knowing of a person. Other English words representing culturally constructed notions (especially in Ch. 4) should be read and interpreted in a similar way.

This book intends to look into the cultural models underlying the Chinese conceptualization of the heart. According to Quinn and Holland (1987: 4), "*Cultural models* are presupposed, taken-for-granted models of the world that are widely shared ... by the members of a society and that play an enormous role in their understanding of that world and their behavior in it" (see also Holland and Quinn 1987). In the light of this definition, my book presents a study of Chinese cultural models pertaining to the heart by tracing conceptions to their roots in ancient Chinese philosophy (Ch. 2) and traditional Chinese medicine (Ch. 3). The diachronic study is followed by a systematic analysis of the relevant linguistic evidence in present-day Chinese that reveals the Chinese conceptualization of the heart as the central faculty of cognition (Ch. 4). The study of conventionalized linguistic expressions is then complemented and supplemented by an analysis of the Chinese conceptualization of the heart as surfacing in modern Chinese discourse, both prosaic and poetic (Ch. 5).

To prepare the ground for cross-cultural comparisons (Ch. 6), I present a brief survey of the Western history of conceptions of the heart and the brain from classical antiquity to early modernity. The Western story unfolds itself in the interaction of "cardiocentrism" and "cerebrocentrism" (or "cephalocentrism", "encephalocentrism") (see, e.g., Clarke and O'Malley 1968; Crivellato and Ribatti 2007; Foolen 2008; Sharifian et al. 2008b; Ch. 6 of this book). The English word *heart* reflects the early dominance of cardiocentrism, which eventually gives way to the modern dominance of cerebrocentrism with the mind/brain as the perceived center of the human body; that is, the perceived center of the body has moved up from the heart to the head (Jager 2001). I also compare two cultural systems of internal bodily forces relating or corresponding to the functions of the heart and other organs. These are the theory of the four humors developed in ancient

Greek medicine and the theory of the five elements or phases developed in ancient Chinese philosophy and traditional Chinese medicine.[1]

It must be pointed out from the outset that the Chinese word *xin* is polysemous, as is its English counterpart *heart*,[2] with a number of distinct but related meanings ranging from the most concrete meaning, i.e. "the heart organ", to the more abstract meanings such as the "seats" of mental and emotional states, processes, and activities, and the "workings" of the "heart" and/or the "mind" which are both intellectual and affective in nature. The various distinct but related meanings form a radial structure (see, e.g., Lakoff 1987a), of which the center is the basic meaning of "heart organ". Other meanings radiate from the center along a variety of dimensions and are linked to the central meaning by propositions, usually representing cultural beliefs (e.g. HEART AS THINKING ORGAN), metonymies (e.g. HEART AS CONTAINER FOR EMOTIONS AS CONTENTS), and metaphors (e.g. HEART AS CONTAINER, which is a metaphor with a robust metonymic basis). The closer a particular meaning is to the central point, the stronger its link is to the central meaning; and conversely, a meaning further away from the center has a weaker tie to it. For instance, the following chain with a number of links extends from the central to the peripheral meanings: heart organ → center of the human body → center of something concrete (e.g. *the heart of the city*) → center of something abstract (e.g. *the heart of the matter*). The conceptualizations of the heart based on such a web-like semantic structure represent cognition at the cultural level, and they are therefore called "cultural conceptualizations" (Sharifian 2003, 2008).[3] They are so named because they are formed through negotiation and renegotiation within societal collectives over generations, and are distributed heterogeneously across speakers in a community. That is, their distribution is uneven and varies across individuals' conceptual systems. This also means that, when indi-

---

1 In this book, I will mainly use "five elements" as the translation of 五行 *wuxing*, which is commonly used in China (e.g. Zhang 2001; H-YCD 1995; H-YDCD 1993). However, some scholars prefer the translation "five phases" because the original term, they argue, refers to the movement and mutation of five entities – wood, fire, earth, metal, and water – rather than the constituents of the material world (see, e.g., Wiseman and Feng 1998: 205–206).

2 Readers are referred to Driven (1985) for a thorough study of the polysemy of the English word *heart*.

3 As defined by Sharifian (2003: 187), cultural conceptualizations "enable the members of a cultural group to think, so to speak, in one mind". However, they "are not equally imprinted in the minds of people but are rather represented in a distributed fashion across the minds in a cultural group".

viduals use the word *xin* 'heart' in any polysemous sense derived via metonymy and/or metaphor, they do not necessarily have the image of the "organ of flesh and blood" in their mind, nor do they have to think of its tie to the central meaning of "heart organ". Nevertheless, such an image can be retrieved and such a tie can be traced, if required by the pragmatic context of a given language use event, because all the links are stored as part of the "cultural sediment" (Yu 2003a: 27) in the collective memory of the cultural group and are deeply entrenched in its cultural models (see Ch. 4).

In the remainder of this chapter, I will review relevant literature for this study. I first show why it is necessary to study the concept of "heart" in the understanding of culture and cognition. I then point out that the study of "heart" is but part of the study of the human body as a source of social and cultural symbolism or a common denominator for human cognition. Following a review of the relationship between body, mind, and culture, I review the embodiment hypothesis as upheld by Cognitive Linguistics in line with Frank et al. (2008) and survey the development of cognitive semantic theories of conceptual metaphor and blending. The chapter ends with an explanation of the structure of the book.

1.2. Heart, culture, and cognition

In his recent book titled *A History of the Heart*, Høystad (2007: 7) points out that "the heart is the main symbol of what it means to be a human being"; however, "there are few specialist books on the heart in world literature". The "restless heart" within our breast, he writes, "has been the great enigma and mystery of human life" since the dawn of human cultural history. The heart "represents something very different in various cultures", and it "may just as well divide as unite people" (p. 9). One telling example is found in *Memories, Dreams, Reflections*, an autobiography dictated by the Swiss psychiatrist Carl Jung, in which he describes his encounter with a Native American chief, "Mountain Lake", in New Mexico in 1932. Their dialogue goes as below when the chief expresses his dislikes of the whites (from Godwin 2001: 17):

> "We do not understand them. We think that they are all mad."
> When Jung asks why he thinks they are all mad, Mountain Lake replies, "They say they think with their heads."
> "Why of course," says Jung. "What do you think with?"
> "We think here," says Chief Mountain Lake, indicating his heart.

As referred to in the previous section, Wierzbicka (1989, 1992) presents cross-linguistic studies comparing some folk concepts encoded in, for example, *soul, mind,* and *heart* in English. The central message of these studies is that the lexical and semantic differences of such concepts, if interpreted properly, can serve as "clues to the different cultural universes associated with different languages", or as "significant evidence for cultural history and for prevailing modern ethnophilosophy" (Wierzbicka 1992: 63). This is what she refers to as the approach to understanding cultures through their key words (Wierzbicka 1997a). Key words are defined as "words which are particularly important and revealing in a given culture … and offer invaluable insight into this culture" (pp. 15–16). They embody and manifest "core cultural values" (p. 15). She argues that "words with special, culture-specific meanings reflect and pass on not only ways of living characteristic of a given society but also ways of thinking" (p. 5). For this reason,

> some words can be studied as focal points around which entire cultural domains are organized. By exploring these focal points in depth we may be able to show the general organizing principles which lend structure and coherence to a cultural domain as a whole, and which often have an explanatory power extending across a number of domains. (Wierzbicka 1997a: 16–17)

The Chinese *xin* 'heart' can be considered to be such a key word, as much as the English *heart.*

In his book about the evolving delineation of the human heart in English narrative and culture of the early modern period, Erickson (1997: xi) argues that the paradoxical nature of the heart being so crucial to us yet so taken for granted by us is due to the fact that it is so central to our selves and to our physiological and symbolic functioning that we are tempted to overlook it. That is why it has received little critical attention until recently. As noted by Erickson (1997), the figurative and symbolic values of the heart arise from its physical centrality to the life forces and processes of the body. In human beings, and other creatures, "the heart is the first organ to live and the last to die" and "its location in the middle of the body is the most honorable place" (p. 12). "Because the human heart as a physical organ is so fundamental a part of the basic rhythms and forces of life, it has always had a multitude of literal and figurative associations with life processes" (p.12), he asserts. Erickson's observations on English apply to the Chinese language and culture as well.

In Chinese culture, the heart has been traditionally – and still is – regarded as the central organ of the body. The Chinese concept of *xin* 'heart' lies at the core of Chinese thought. This is because the heart is traditionally believed to be the cognitive agent or cognizing subject. Its importance in cognition can be seen in the following famous quotations from two representative figures of the "Learning of the Mind-and-Heart" (心学 *xinxue*), or literally the "Learning of the Heart", a school of Neo-Confucianism lasting from the Song (960–1279) to the Ming (1368–1644) dynasty (see Cai 2000; De Bary 1981):[4]

> 宇宙便是吾心，吾心即是宇宙。《陆九渊集・年谱》(Ji 1995, vol. 50: 2407)
> The universe is my heart, and my heart is the universe. *Collected Writings of Lu Jiuyuan: Chronological Life*

> 人者，天地万物之心也；心者，天地万物之主也。《王阳明集・答季明德》(Ji 1995, vol. 54: 83)
> The human being is the heart of Heaven and Earth and the ten thousand things; the heart is the master of Heaven and Earth and the ten thousand things. *Collected Writings of Wang Yangming: Reply to Ji Mingde.*

Apparently, the heart is the most important thing in the whole universe to these two philosophers. In the first quotation from Lu Jiuyuan (1139–1193), the heart is metaphorically equated to the universe, thus highlighting the unity and correspondence between the macrocosm and the microcosm. That is, the heart as the central faculty of cognition is the "mirror" or "duplicate" of the universe. In the second quotation from Wang Yangming (1472–1529), also known as Wang Shouren, "Heaven and Earth and the ten thousand things", namely "Heaven and Earth and all things in between", is the literal translation of the Chinese phrase that can be interpreted as meaning, again, the "universe". The saying defines the human being metaphorically as the "heart" of the universe, as much as the heart is the cognitive and physiological center of the human being. It is because the heart is conceived of as the cognitive center of the human that it can, by metonymy or synecdoche, stand for the human as the "master" of the universe. As suggested in this saying, the heart is the microcosm of the human being as

---

4 The English translations, here and hereafter, are my own unless otherwise noted. For my translations, however, I referred to various versions of existing translations if such sources are available to me, and made modifications to varying degrees.

much as the human being is the microcosm of the universe.[5] Regardless of what philosophical outlook these sayings manifest, the fact that the heart is regarded as the central faculty of cognition is obvious. The universe will make no sense to us without our heart functioning as the organ for thinking, knowing, understanding, reasoning, as well as feeling. In this sense, the whole universe converges and hinges on the human heart.

In his monograph, Lee (2005: 10–11) summarizes the significance of the concept of *xin* 'heart; mind' and how it distinguishes Chinese philosophy from Western philosophy as the following:

> The notion of *xin* is one of the most important concepts in the history of Chinese philosophy. Generally speaking, while much of Western philosophy can be said to hinge on the notion of a rational agent who can investigate the world and humankind objectively, Chinese philosophy requires an agent who is able to carry out the self-transformative cultivation through which a human being can attain ideal personhood. Considering the overriding concern for self-cultivation in the major philosophical trends of Confucianism, Buddhism, and Daoism, it is not difficult to see the importance of the notion of *xin* for these religious and philosophical schools.

As Lee (2005) points out, for instance, although Buddhism and neo-Confucianism differ widely in their understanding of the world and of the nature of successful living, they both give great weight to the notion of *xin* as an agent for self-cultivation.

The concept of *xin* 'heart' is centrally important in Chinese culture because the heart is taken as fulfilling the functions of both "heart" and "mind" as understood in present-day English. Chinese culture is not alone in this regard. This is true in some of its neighboring cultures as well. At this point, it is especially worth noting a book titled *Heart Talk* (1992) written by Christopher G. Moore, a Canadian novelist and playwright, on the conceptions of *jai* 'heart' in the Thai language and culture. Although it is "not a scholarly book", said the author, it "contains over 330 *Heart Talk* root phrases" and "over 1,000 phrases which are connected with the heart" (Moore 1992: 12–13). Moore starts his introductory chapter with this statement: "Heart or *jai* is a powerful, pervasive, and complex metaphor. In Thai, you can experience and understand heart as black, cool, diamond, dry,

---

5 It is worth mentioning in passing that the idea that the heart is the microcosm of the human being/body, which in turn is the microcosm of the universe, was not specific solely to ancient Chinese philosophy. It existed in Western thinking as well (see sections 1.3 and 6.2).

fast, hot, lost, open, merged, mixed-up, poor, tall, turbulent, wasted, wet or worried" (p. 11). Citing Lakoff and Johnson (1980) that human thought processes are largely metaphorical, he suggests that "If you wish to row in the Thai conceptual boat, an understanding of *jai* is indispensable". "The Thai language has the Thai word for heart in hundreds of different phrases" and the "cumulative force of *Heart Talk* will help increase your awareness of how consciousness is shaped and defined in the Kingdom of Thailand" (p. 11).

Noting that Thai is "a language in which notion of 'heart' and 'mind' were never separated" and the Thais "look, evaluate, decide, react, and judge as if their heart and mind were one" (p. 16), Moore makes a keen observation, from a Western viewpoint, on the difference between the more holistic Thai view of *jai* and the English, or Western at large, dualism between heart and mind, which I would like to quote below at length (pp. 13–14):

> To understand the importance of "heart" provides access to the Thai way of looking at themselves and life. *Jai* in Thai means both "heart" and "mind". In the English language, these two perspectives heart and mind have become accepted as two categories. In English, either one employs words which suggest to the listener he or she is invoking the rational, logical mind to perceive the world or self, or one's words suggest the speaker has resorted to his or her emotional, nonrational side. Since the Age of Reason, English speakers have become accustomed to viewing heart and mind as different. In English it is common to think of left brain and right brain "thinking" as an explanation for conduct and vocabulary. In Thailand, the consequences of the post-Enlightenment tradition did not split mind and heart into separate orbits of perception.
>
> Thus to comprehend the world with your "heart" in Thai often overlaps into many different contexts which a native English speaker would not associate with heart but only with the "intellect". The Thai language also is concerned with the intellect but the emphasis that the emotive way of seeing and feeling is not separate from intellect is an essential and important feature of understanding the Thai language, culture and people. The Thai is rarely at a loss for an exact "heart" phrase to express a feeling or idea.
>
> Have we in the west lost our range of communicating feelings? What would it be like to have a language where hundreds of phrases are about treating the state of our heart and mind as one? … You may discover some aspect of yourself that has been surrendered, forgotten or neglected in English. That realization may bring a smile or a tear. *Heart Talk* may open up the vast possibility of feelings that lie beneath the surface of our rational, logical, empirical world.

> ......
>
> With this emphasis on feelings in Thai culture, the language of the heart assumes a place of central importance. ... In English the "heart" connotes a sense of romance or medical science. We fall in love with our hearts or have heart transplants. The word "heart" in English, though of importance, occupies a secondary position to the logical or analytical path. Or at least it appears so when compared with the diverse uses of "*jai*" in the Thai language.

Here, Moore's penetrating observation points to a fundamental difference in understanding the cognizing subject and the self characteristic of distinctive cultures.

Similar conceptualization of mental life is also found in Newar culture of Nepal, another neighboring country of China. In his study of "Newar concepts of mind" Parish (1991: 315–316) notes that in Newar culture such mental states and processes as indicated by the English words *desire*, *feeling*, *emotion*, *thought*, and *memory* "are located in the chest, since for Newars the mind is in the heart, not the head". Although some informants mentioned the head and brain as involved in mental processes, especially thinking, Parish (1991: 347) is not sure to what extent this idea "reflects culture change and a 'modern' viewpoint influenced by outside conceptions", but dispositions, attitudes, and more enduring thoughts seem to be located in the "heart". Newars believe that a god inhabiting the "heart" (*nuga:*) animates the mind. That is, the "heart god", or "god who dwells in the heart", makes possible, or empowers, perception and cognition (p. 316). In addition to being "the seat of cognition, memory, and perception", the Newar heart "is also the locus of emotional experience" and "moral qualities" (pp. 317–318). In Parish's words (p. 318):

> the Newar "heart" is a multiplex, metonymic sign – a sign of the self. The part stands for the whole; but the whole has many facets – it encloses a range of ways of being and knowing. Thus, talk of the heart helps Newars know themselves, by providing ways to formulate and evaluate experience and relationship.

Thus, the language of the heart is the language of emotional experience and the discourse of the heart helps mediate self-awareness and self-identity.

Matisoff's (1986) article titled "Hearts and minds in Southeast Asian languages and English" presents a cross-linguistic study that examines examples from a number of languages in the region, including Thai, Tibetan, Burmese, Lahu, Jingpho, Chinese, with a comparative perspective from

English. Matisoff (1986: 8) points out that many languages of East and Southeast Asia tend to treat the semantic area of psychological phenomena (i.e. mental activities, qualities, and processes) with an overt mention of the bodily organs, such as the heart and liver, perceived as "the *receptacle* or *arena* where the psychological phenomenon unfolds". He notes that Chinese makes extensive use of body-part terms for "heart", "liver" and so on in psycho-collocations, just as any other language of the region. What is "unique about Chinese is the fact that its logographic writing system has a means of phenotypically marking individual morphemes as having psychological reference – the use of the *heart-radical*" (p. 9; see, also, Ots 1990).

In short, the study of conceptions of the heart and other bodily organs based on linguistic analysis can add to the general understanding of human cognition in diverse cultures, especially with regard to cultural changes and cultural differences in viewing how the mind is related to the body, and provide "an intriguing glimpse of how different cultures believe the body and the mind work" (Small 1997: 131; see, also, Sharifian et al. 2008a, 2008b; sections 1.4 and 6.2).

1.3. Body, society, and cognition

The study of conceptions of the heart is only a part, though a central part, of the study of conceptions of the body. The notion of "body" has been a most fundamental one in the social sciences and humanities ever since the "corporeal turn" in twentieth-century thinking (see, e.g., Foolen 2008; Violi 2004, 2008). As Johnson (1987, 1989a, 1989b, 1999, 2007) argues, the fact that every human being has a body bears directly on the nature of human cognition. To be human is to be embodied: "What we can experience, what it can mean to us, how we understand that experience, and how we reason about it are all integrally tied up with our bodily being" (Johnson 1989a: 109). Exploring the deepest and most profound bodily sources of human meaning and understanding, Johnson (2007: ix) argues that "meaning grows from our visceral connections to life and the bodily conditions of life". That is, our embodied experience in and with the world sets out the contours of what is meaningful to us and determines the ways of our understanding. This is because our "conceptual structure has everything to do with one's body and with how one interacts as part of one's physical environment" (Lakoff 1994: 42). In short, our mind is embodied in the profound sense that the very structure of our thoughts comes from the nature of our body (Lakoff and Johnson 1999).

The notion of "body", however, is by no means a self-evident one; on the contrary, it is a multifaceted concept, socially and culturally, as well as biologically and phenomenologically, constructed. Highly polysemous, "body" means quite different things across cultures, or even within cultures. Speaking from a Western viewpoint of the plurality and multiplicity in the meaning of the human body, or "body social", Synnott (1993: 3–4) points out:

> The body, …with all its organs, attributes, functions, states and senses, is not so much a biological given as a social creation of immense complexity, and almost limitless variability, richness and power. The creation and learning of the body as a social phenomenon varies from culture to culture, however; and even within "our own" culture, which we can perhaps broadly describe as Greco-Roman and Judaeo-Christian, many different creations persist.
>
> Our task here is to explore this body social in some of its many variations and dynamics. The body social is many things: the prime symbol of the self, but also of the society; it is something we have, yet also what we are; it is both subject and object at the same time; it is individual and personal, as unique as a fingerprint or odor-plume, yet it is also common to all humanity with all its systems, and taught in schools. The body is both an individual creation, physically and phenomenologically, and a cultural product; it is personal, and also state property.

Synnott (1993: 2), therefore, calls for efforts "to restore the body to its central place in personal and social life".

"Body" also means quite different things across the broad range of disciplines in the social sciences and humanities that are interested in this construct. The present widespread use of the notions of "body" and "embodiment" across different fields and with different meanings makes it particularly important to develop a better understanding and clarification of these two notions (Violi 2008). In what follows, I briefly survey the rich output resulting from the research into broader notions of "body" and "embodiment" in the social sciences and humanities, in order to situate my study in the larger academic context or, so to speak, to locate the "heart" inside the "body". It is hoped that this brief survey will lead to glimpses of the sociocultural nature of the body, as well as the embodied nature of societal and cultural situations, in line with linguists' and cognitive scientists' growing interest in the "sociocultural situatedness" of embodiment from a wider cognitive perspective (see, e.g., Frank et al. 2008; Ziemke, Zlatev, and Frank 2007).

Metaphorically speaking, the human body is a kaleidoscope capable of producing amazingly diversified and ever-changing colorful patterns of view. As pointed out nicely by Armstrong ([1987] 2004: 111), "The body is what it is perceived to be; it could be otherwise if perception were different. The question is not therefore concerned with the nature of the body but with the perceiving process which allows the body's nature to be apprehended". Synnott (1993: 37) summarizes the wide range of meanings, metaphorical and otherwise, which the body carries, as follows:

> In sum, the body has been, and still is, constructed in almost as many ways as there are individuals; it seems to be all things to all people. Thus the body is defined as good or bad; tomb or temple; machine or garden; cloak or prison; sacred or secular; friend or enemy; cosmic or mystical; one with mind and soul or separate; private or public; personal or the property of the state; clock or car; to varying degrees plastic, bionic, communal; selected from a catalogue or engineered; material or spiritual; a corpse of the self.

French author and symbolist poet Paul Valéry once said that the body is commonly used to refer to a wide variety of things. It is the privileged object we possess, although our knowledge of it may be extremely variable and subject to illusions. We speak of it as a thing that belongs to us; but for us it is not entirely a thing; and it belongs to us a little less than we belong to it (see Kuriyama 2002: 13–14). As Kuriyama (2002: 14) suggests, "The body is unfathomable and breeds astonishingly diverse perspectives precisely because it is a basic and intimate reality. The task of discovering the truth of the body is inseparable from the challenge of discovering the truth about people". The body is "never just a purely biological entity but one which has social and cultural dimensions too" (Blaikie et al. 2004b: 20), being influenced by social and cultural forces which shape or attempt to shape it in their own image.

In the past decades, the human body has become an object of extensive critical scrutiny, attracting considerable scholarly attention in a wide range of disciplines of social sciences and humanities.[6] For instance, the "history

---

6 See, e.g., Berdayes, Esposito, and Murphy (2004), Blacking (1977a), Blaikie et al. (2004a, vols. 1–5), Featherstone, Hepworth, and Turner (1991), Feher, Naddaff and Tazi (1989, vols. 1–3), Forth and Crozier (2005), Gallagher (2005), Hillman and Mazzio (1997a), Johnson (2007), Kirby (1997), Kuriyama (2002), Lingis (1994), Lyons (2006), O'Neill (1985), Stafford (1991), Strathern (1996), Synnott (1993), Young (1997). Interestingly, Berthelot ([1986] 2004) complained about a negative impact even two decades ago,

of the human body", as Feher (1989) points out, studies the changes undergone by the body. Only when a historical perspective on the body is adopted can what is new about it be appreciated and what will become of it be predicted based on what transformations it has already gone through. The "historiography of the body" demonstrates that the body is not a transhistorical entity, but rather deeply fragmented and fundamentally situated in different sociocultural contexts (Forth and Crozier 2005). Thus, back in history, the reason for resorting to a metaphor or an organic model of the body and its organs "is essentially to naturalize a political institution, a social hierarchy or a moral principle" (Feher 1989: 16):

> This is the case when the sovereignty of the Pope or of royalty seeks legitimacy in the fact that a State needs a "head", or that a society needs a "heart". This is the case when the necessity for man's domination of woman is ascribed to the superiority of sperm, with its formative power, over the merely nourishing qualities of female milk and blood.[7]

The rise of the feminist movement led to the study of "the politics of women's bodies" as an essential part of the study of sexual or gender equality (Canto [1986] 2004; Currie and Raoul [1992] 2004). The studies of "ideology of the body" and "politicalization of the body" led to the realization that the judgment of humans' superiority or inferiority in terms of their bodily differentiation is the basis of racism (Synnott 1993: 31–32; see also Young [1995] 2004).

The "sociology of the body", stressing the interconnections between social, cultural, and biological factors in the constitution of the body and the diverse and heterogeneous nature of bodies, sees "each body's existence as socially mediated, and thus as profoundly enveloped by social mores and cultural forms" (Blaikie et al. 2004b: 1). It is therefore called for sociologists to "put the body into sociology" and to "bring society into the

---

which came with the rise of "corporealism" in the 1970s that yielded an enormous amount of references to the body in the human and social sciences without much real significance: "The body would appear to be everywhere and…many researchers, who, in fact, don't deal with the topic in their work refer to it implicitly on every page" (p. 121). It is suggested that the current attention accorded to the body and an excessive use of the term "body" are "perhaps indicative of a fashion or even an intellectual movement which does not necessarily involve a step forward in knowledge" (p. 121).

7 See section 6.2 for more of the head-heart discussions in the Greek-Roman antiquity and the Middle Ages.

body" (Freund [1988] 2004). Indeed, the body "is not a 'given', but a social category with different meanings imposed and developed by every age, and by different sectors of the populations" (Synnott 1993: 1). It is found that "people have also conceived the relation between their individual lives and the institutions of society in terms of the imagery of the human body" and "there is an embodied logic of society" (O'Neill 1985: 48–49). Just as they "think society with their bodies", they also "think their bodies with society" (p. 51). Within "social bodies", the imagery of the "body politic" recurs in political community and imposes a fundamental structure on political and economic life (pp. 67–90). It seems that "one can hardly escape falling back upon the human body as an image for the development of a balanced social and world order" (p. 117). In sociology, as is concluded, "the body has been variously a resource for broadening the parameters of traditional sociological thought deriving from the nineteenth century, and for over-turning that paradigm and fundamentally reorienting the assumptions and concepts of sociological thinking" (Howson and Inglis [2001] 2004: 284).[8]

The "anthropology of the body", assuming that society is also a biological phenomenon with shared somatic states, studies "the extensions of the body in culture" by gaining "an understanding of the limitations and possibilities of individual and social bodies" (Blacking 1977b: 24–25). It raises the argument that "the body is a productive starting point for analyzing culture and self" (Csordas 1990: 39). It investigates the workings of the human body as a "complex" and "universal symbol system" with "its organization, its spatial arrangement, and its priorities of needs". This investigation would help gain insights into "the total pattern of self-understanding of the society, such as its perception of its own workings, its organization, its power structure, and its cosmology" (Isenberg and Owen 1977: 3). Anthropomorphism sets upon us a task to understand how we can rethink social institutions with our bodies, which are "the permeable ground of all social behavior" and "the very flesh of society" (O'Neill 1985: 18–23). That is, "the human body is an intelligent and critical resource in the anthropomorphic production of those small and larger orders that underlie our social, political, and economic institutions" (p. 16). The anthropomorphic view of social structures reflects a more fundamental worldview in cosmography where "the human body is the bridge for all microcosmic and macrocosmic exchanges" with "the parallels of wholeness between the planets, the stars, and the human body" (p. 38). "The cosmos may in some

---

8 Readers are especially referred to Blaikie et al. (2004a), which consists of five volumes that collect a total of 89 articles on or in "the sociology of the body".

cases be regarded as a vast human body; in other belief systems, visible parts of the body may be taken to portray invisible faculties such as reason, passion, wisdom and so on; in others again, the different parts of the social order are arrayed in terms of a human anatomical paradigm" (Turner 1970, quoted in Young 1997: 9). That is, the "physical body is a microcosm of society" and "is polarized conceptually against the social body"; also, the "social body constrains the way the physical body is perceived. The physical experience of the body, always modified by the social categories through which it is known, sustains a particular view of society" (Douglas 1973, quoted in Young 1997: 9–10).

The "phenomenology of the body", interested in the ontological and epistemological status of the human body, views it as the locus of the self, the site of experiences, the fulcrum of movements, and the source of perspectives (Young 1997: 1). Thus, as embodied knowers, human beings "think nature and society with their bodies" and "think the world and society as one giant body" (O'Neill 1985: 28). That is, with an embodied logic, they interpret the divisions of the world and of society in terms of the divisions of the body. This embodied way of thinking and knowing served as "the very foundation on which later, abstract and rationalized modes of categorization could be developed in both the human and the natural sciences" (p. 28).

Some cultural studies examine the "extent to which aspects of culture were imagined to reside in, on, and about individual parts of the body" (Hillman and Mazzio 1997b: xi), trying to arrive at "an image of the corporeal whole" by "assessing the state of the parts" (Forth and Crozier 2005: 2–3). They characterize bodies and body parts as "loaded with cultural symbolism, public and private, positive and negative, political and economic, sexual, moral and often controversial" (Synnott 1993: 1). Other cultural studies, interested in the "body symbols", examine the body as "the source as well as the site of symbolic understandings" in order to understand how the "intelligibility of the world is constituted corporeally" and how "animate bodies are potential semantic templates" (Young 1997: 9; see also Sheets-Johnstone 1990, 1992; Feher, Naddaff, and Tazi 1989, vol. 3). Still others, attempting to interpret "body symbols" of "the symbolic body", analyze the ways in which "cultural inscriptions become visible in the body" and "corporeal inscriptions become visible in culture" (Young 1997: 10; see also Hillman and Mazzio 1997a; Feher, Naddaff, and Tazi 1989, vol. 3). Studies of popular culture also look at the "government of the body" or "modification of the body" via dietary control or plastic surgery, weight watching or body building, tattooing or piercing, with regard to current fashion, individual identity, social value, and cultural significance (e.g., Davis [1995] 2004; Sweetman [1999] 2004; Turner [1982] 2004; Tyler and Abbott [1998] 2004). Religious studies analyze how the notions of "body" and "embodiment" play central roles in religious knowledge about the self, the universe, and deities, and also about religious institutions and practices, underlying religious visions, beliefs, and rituals, or religious cognition at large, of various kinds of religion in the world, such as Buddhism, Daoism, Hinduism, and Christianity (Barsalow et al. 2005).

In the arts, images of the body, among others, are analyzed for their persisting significance and value in terms of "body metaphors" derived from aesthetic and medical practices in a visually centered culture (Stafford 1991). As bodies and their parts are "scattered throughout the literary and cultural texts" (Hillman and Mazzio 1997b: xi), literary studies scrutinize the body as "both source and site of discourse of the self", and analyze stories as "corporeal acts", in an effort to understand how "the body gives rise to narratives" and how "stories give rise to the body" (Young 1997: 141). Focused on the domain of the human body as an ideal focus for semantic typology and human experience, linguistic studies analyze the semantics of body-part terms in order to understand cross-linguistic categorization of the body (Majid, Enfield, and van Staden 2006; Wierzbicka 2007) and the role of the body in description of emotion (Enfield and Wierzbicka 2002a). Realizing that human meaning and understanding are rooted in bodily experience in a crucial fashion, linguistics also analyzes evidence in language and beyond that shows how the body makes linguistic and nonlinguistic signs meaningful and how it imbues objects and events with meaning (Johnson 1987, 2007; Kövecses 2006).

In the realm of medicine, which falls beyond social sciences and humanities, the body is "rendered an object", "inspected, palpated, poked into, cut open"; it is thus "transformed into an object of scrutiny" and inscribed into "a discourse of objectivity" (Young 1997: 1; see also Blaikie et al. 2004b: 15).[9] Nevertheless, even in medical science, the body cannot escape or transcend the nature of human subjectivity. It is instead a construal, so much so that different medical practices in different cultures construe as

---

9 It is worth mentioning in passing, however, that such notions as "lived body" and "subject body" have gained increasing importance in Western clinical practice and medical theory as medical and philosophical researchers call for attention to "alternative medicines" in other cultures and exploration of new directions for medicine. See, e.g., Gadow ([1980] 2004), Leder ([1984] 2004), Mauss ([1973] 2004).

many different bodies as there are cultures (Violi 2008). In exploring the fundamental question of how perceptions of something as basic and intimate as the body can differ so much, which is a "riddle" that "lies at the heart of the history of medicine", Kuriyama observes in his *The Expressiveness of the Body and the Divergence of Greek and Chinese Medicine* (2002: 8):

> The true structure and workings of the human body are, we casually assume, everywhere the same, a universal reality. But then we look into history, and our sense of reality wavers. ...accounts of the body in diverse medical traditions frequently appear to describe mutually alien, almost unrelated worlds.

After all, from an anthropological point of view, "medicine is a culture with its own language, gestures, customs, rituals, spaces, costumes, and practices. Within medical culture, the body becomes the locus that corporealizes culture, enculturates bodiliness" (Young 1997: 2).

In sum, as Synnott (1993: 1) argues, the body "is not just skin and bones, an assemblage of parts, a medical marvel", but is "socially constructed, in various ways by different populations, as are the various organs, processes and attributes of the body". The real challenge is "to demonstrate how the body is constructed, and why, and also why these constructions vary and change" (p. 1).

1.4. Body, mind, and culture

For the overall goal of this study, it is relevant to explore the conceptions of the body not only because the heart is a critical organ and a central part of the body, but also because there seems to be a broad spectrum of diverse conceptualizations of how the "mind" (or "soul") is related to the body across cultures or within cultures over history. More generally, there exist different "ethnotheories of the person" across cultures in the world (see, e.g., Goddard 2003; Wierzbicka 1992, 2005)

As mentioned previously, the conceptualization of the heart in the body has to do with the understanding of "mind", which, including perceptual, emotional and intellectual operations in its broad sense (Robinson 1998) and generally conceived in metaphorical terms (Sternberg 1990; see also

Robinson 1998),[10] figures prominently in the concepts of self and person. The person consists of both social and corporeal entities (Fajans 1985). Certain parts of the physical body are socially and culturally elevated to stand for the person. For instance, the human face, which is the most distinctive part of the body, is socially accepted as the focus of interpersonal interaction and relationship and even culturally constructed as the locus of dignity and prestige of a person (Yu 2001). Therefore, the face stands for the person as a social being.[11] While the reason for the face standing for the person in social life seems obvious (see Yu 2001), the part of the body that takes the central role in a person's mental life has been historically less so. Thus, there is need to "look for the mind inside the body" across various cultures, which vary with the location of emotionality, mentality, rationality, and morality in certain parts of the body (Sharifian et al. 2008b).

The central aim of Sharifian et al. (2008a) is "to contribute to the knowledge of various cultures' conceptualizations of the heart and other internal body organs, and in particular how feeling, thinking and knowing are related to internal body organs in different cultures, as they are reflected in the respective languages" (Sharifian et al. 2008b: 3). The volume studies "the synchronic variation and the diachronic development of 'heart' conceptions in various languages" including Kuuk Thaayorre, Indonesian, Malay, Basque, Chinese, Japanese, Korean, Persian, Northeastern Neo-Aramaic, English, Dutch, and Tunisian Arabic. The articles of the volume are divided into three sections depending on whether the languages they study show abdomen-centering, heart-centering, and/or head-centering conceptualizations of the mind. As the co-editors explain (Sharifian et al. 2008b: 3–4):

---

10 In Snell's (1953: vi) words, "We cannot speak about the mind or the intellect at all without falling back on metaphor". According to Sternberg (1990), who sees metaphors as foundations for theories of intelligence, the mind, or intelligence in particular, is understood in numerous metaphorical terms including the geographic, computational, biological, epistemological, anthropological, and sociological. Various metaphorical terms give rise, apparently, to different understandings of the mind within and across cultural boundaries.

11 It is interesting to note that the recent medical case where a woman had had the face transplant surgery in France triggered off moral concern over the identity of this person: Is she still the same person when she has obtained the face of another person? There is no similar concern over, say, a heart transplant.

> Both cultural models of the mind and more scientific approaches in philosophy and/or medicine have in various cultures invoked central parts of the human body as the locus of the mind. The major loci have been the abdomen region, the heart region and the head region or, more particularly, the brain region. These three types of conceptualizations can be labeled "abdominocentrism", "cardiocentrism", and "cerebrocentrism" (or "cephalocentrism"), respectively.[12]

This quotation characterizes the study of conceptions of the heart and delineates its place within the larger context of "cultures' search for the locus of the mind" (Sharifian et al. 2008b: 3). That is, in certain cultures such as Chinese, Thai and Newar, the heart is conceptualized as the locus of the mind (see section 1.2 above), and the study of its conceptions contributes to the understanding of the "cognizing subject" or "cognitive agent" and the concept of the self in these cultures (Varela, Thompson, and Rosch 1991). Even in cerebrocentric cultures, such as English-speaking and other Western cultures today, the heart is still the "seat" of feelings and emotions in contrast with the head/brain as the "center" of intellect and thought within the conceptual framework of dualism. In other words, the heart is regarded as one part of the dichotomy that is characteristic of the cognitive landscape in these cultures. Tracing back the history of these cultures, furthermore, one finds that present-day dualism is preceded, most of the time, by the dominance of cardiocentrism over cerebrocentrism.[13]

Examples of divergence in cultural beliefs regarding the functions attributed to particular organs are also found in Howes (1991), which collects studies showing how different cultures and societies use and combine the senses of the body in different ways and to different ends. Howes and Classen (1991: 283–284) cite various sources to demonstrate how cultures may differ in conceptualizing and localizing the "soul" or "mind" within the body. Thus, the "soul" may be associated with the breath and the lungs, as well as with the heart or head (the ancient Greeks), or placed in the eye (the Mehinaku of Brazil) or the blood (the Zinacanteco of Mexico). More globally speaking, the "mind" is thought as residing in the head in the West,

---

12 As the co-editors point out, these three labels only intend to capture the idea that the region in question is the main center of the body, which does not exclude a similar role for body parts in other regions.

13 Readers are referred to section 6.2 of this book for a more detailed survey of the historical change resulting from the interaction between cardiocentrism and cerebrocentrism in the West from Greek antiquity to early modernity.

whereas it is located in the stomach by the Uduk of the Sudan. The Aguaruna of the Amazon would defend a cardiocentric folk theory as follows:

> The people who say that we think with our heads are wrong because we think with our hearts. The heart is connected to the veins, which carry the thoughts in the blood through the entire body. The brain is only connected to the spinal column, isn't it? So if we thought with our brains, we would only be able to move the thought as far as our anus. (Howes and Classen 1991: 284)

Besides, both Indonesian and Malay, two related languages, display the abdomen-centering view in that they localize feelings and thought in the *hati* 'liver' (Goddard 2008; Siahaan 2008). In contrast, Tsou, a language spoken in Southwest Taiwan, shows a head-centering conceptualization as it connects thinking and feeling to the *koyu* 'ear', which is "the seat of Tsou emotion and mentation" (Huang 2002: 172). It is interesting to note that Kuuk Thaayorre, a Paman language of Cape York Peninsula, displays a much more diversified picture in terms of what mental functions are connected with what body parts or organs. In this language, the primary site of emotion, spirit and life force is the *ngeengk* 'belly' although other internal organs, such as the *thip* 'liver', *man* 'throat' and *man-ngeengk* 'heart', are also linked with these mental functions; the intellect, however, is situated primarily in the *kaal* 'ear' and secondarily in the *meer* 'eye' and *paant-thuur* 'brain' (Gaby 2008). All these instances illustrate how cultural models may be widely different with respect to the mind-body problem.[14]

For further examples, we turn to Asian philosophical traditions. In a study of the classical Chinese conception of the body, Ames ([1984] 2004) makes a distinction between dualism and polarism: Dualism divides the world into dichotomies of discrete "things" whereas polarism views the world as composed of interconnected "processes". He claims that "mind and body are polar rather than dualistic concepts" in classical Chinese philosophy (p. 270). By "polarism" he refers to "a symbiosis: the unity of two organismic processes which require each other as a necessary condition for being what they are" (p. 271). A significant implication of this dualism versus polarism distinction lies in the perceived relationship between mind and

---

[14] See Sharifian et al. (2008a) for further examples that illustrate different cultural models of the mind centering around the abdomen, the heart, and the head/brain. See also Chapter 6, especially section 6.2, of this book for a historical survey of cardiocentric, cerebrocentric, and dualistic views in Western cultures.

body. The mind/body problem did not exist in the polar metaphysics of the classical Chinese tradition because there "'person' was seen holistically as a psychosomatic process" (p. 275). That is, body and mind form one "whole human process" (p. 276).

Now let us shift our attention eastward to Japan. Kasulis ([1993] 2004) investigates the traditional Japanese conception of the body and notes that, very much akin to the Chinese, "the Japanese do not recognize the mind-body problem at all" (p. 99) because to them there is only one "mind-body complex". The traditional Japanese categories are generally framed so that the mental and physical are interdependent facets of a single phenomenon, rather than two separate phenomena in an external relation to each other. Thus, instead of asking how the mind and body are "related", they ask how they are "interrelated" within a single complex (p. 100). Similar observation has been made from the perspective of India in South Asia. According to the Indian philosophical tradition, Koller ([1993] 2004: 288) notes, "the human body is viewed as a living process that integrates a complex variety of mental and physical processes. That is, the human body is really a body-mind, rather than a mere body or a body to which a mind is somehow attached".

> Unlike modern Western philosophy, which draws the line between the mind and the body, regarding them as substantially different, and sometimes exclusive, kinds of entities, Indian philosophers have tended to see the mental and physical as aspects of an integrated process, seeing the body as conscious and consciousness as bodily activity. (Koller 2004: 289)

Apparently, there is much similarity among the three philosophical traditions in Asia, and their shared oriental view of mind-body unity in a holistic framework contrasts with the popular dualistic view of mind-body dichotomy in the West, to which we now turn (see also Feher, Naddaff, and Tazi 1989, vol. 2).

The human body carries a wide range of ever-changing meanings and symbols. Despite its profound significance, social and cultural, literal and metaphorical, it has not always been given its due in the West (Sheets-Johnstone 1992). Back in antiquity, the soul and the mind were already regarded in an influential stream of Greek thought as "being 'above' the body, in the twin sense of being morally superior to it, and of being lodged inside the body only unwillingly and temporarily" (Blaikie et al. 2004b: 3). For example, Socrates (c. 470–399 BC) saw the body as a "prison" when he described the soul as a "helpless prisoner" in the body, compelled to view reality not directly but only through its prison bars. Plato (c. 429–347 BC) considered the body as "no more than a shadow which keeps us company" and as "the grave of the soul" from which only in death is the soul liberated from the desires and evils of the body. During the time of the Roman Empire, the Stoic philosopher Seneca (c. 4 BC–65 AD) stated that "a high-minded and sensible man divorces soul from body" and that "nature has surrounded our soul with the body as its cloak". Epictetus (c. 55–135), another Stoic philosopher, spoke of "two elements mingled in our birth, the body which we share with the animals, and the reason and mind which we share with the gods", and also talked about the body being a "corpse", an "ass", or "clay and corruption". Besides, during the medieval period, some of the Christians who disliked corporeal matter upheld the belief in the evil of the body. For instance, Francis of Assisi (1182–1226) said, "We must hate our bodies with vices and sins". One of his followers, Brother Giles, echoed him by saying "Our flesh is like a hog that runs eagerly into the mud and enjoys being in the mud" (Synnott 1993: 9–16). A medieval divine saint also called the body "nothing but fetid sperm, a bag of manure" (Blaikie et al. 2004b: 3). Thus, "the body remained condemned as an inessential component of the human life in comparison to the mental faculties" (p. 4).

At this point, it is worth discussing the Cartesian dualism, represented by the French philosopher and scientist René Descartes (1596–1650),[15] which has been the dominant view on the mind-body relations in Western philosophy during the past few hundred years. According to the Cartesian mind-body split, the body, which has material properties and follows the law of physics, works like a machine; in contrast, the mind (or soul), which is a nonmaterial entity that does not follow the law of physics but has the capacity to think, controls the body. Descartes postulated an absolute difference in kind between the mind and the body, the former defining selfhood and personhood and having supremacy over the latter; in his words, "I think, therefore I am" and "the mind, by which I am what I am, is entirely distinct from the body" (from Synnott 1993: 22). So postulated,

---

15 In actuality, dualism between soul and body already existed as early as in Greek antiquity when philosophers such as Plato and Aristotle held various forms of it, by which subsequent thinkers such as Augustine and Descartes were influenced (see Synnott 1993: 9–10). Other forms of dualism, such as those between mind and matter (including the body) and between head (as the seat of the intellect) and heart (as the seat of emotions), existed in Western thought as well (Sharifian et al. 2008b).

Cartesianism tends to deprecate the body in favor of the mind, to privilege the mind over the body, or even to describe the body as an enemy to the mind (see, e.g., Strathern 1996: 1–8; Synnott 1993: 1–37). The Cartesian mind is disembodied. "A problem for Descartes, as for all Cartesianists subsequently, is how to account for the intermingling of mind and body, given their absolute difference and separation" even though Descartes gave the mind an ethnolocation and considered the pineal gland in the head as the site for interaction between mind and body (Strathern 1996: 5). In the modern West, however, the self and the person have been largely conceptualized in terms of oppositions between reason, thought and intellect, on the one hand, and emotion, feeling and desire, on the other, all along the Cartesian dualistic line between mind and body. The mind-body dualism is also conceptualized metonymically as a dichotomy between head (LOCATION FOR ACTIVITY) and heart (PART FOR WHOLE).

While Cartesianism has dominated Western thought in the past few hundred years, it has faced some challenges. For instance, Neapolitan philosopher and historian Giambattista Vico (1668–1744) responded to Descartes' mechanism with his own humanism, relying on a complex etymology in classical rhetoric and philology. In his *New Science* (1725) he argued for the evolution of human language and cognition as the extension of bodily experiences through human imagination structured by metaphor and metonymy:

> The human mind is naturally inclined by the senses to see itself externally in the body, and only with great difficulty does it come to understand itself by means of reflection. This axiom gives us the universal principle of etymology in all languages: words are carried over from bodies and from the properties of bodies to signify the institutions of the mind and spirit. (O'Neill 1985: 27)

The magnificent insight is that human language and cognition have evolved with the human mind thinking and knowing on the basis of and with the help of the human body.

In the twentieth century, the Cartesian dualism was first seriously challenged by phenomenology represented by French philosopher Maurice Merleau-Ponty (1908–1961). Merleau-Ponty's philosophy is an explicit attempt to think beyond the dualism of mind and body. Rather than two separate entities, mind and body are "fundamentally interwoven components of an indivisible human whole", a "body-subject" that is simultaneously physical and mental (Blaikie et al. 2004b: 11). In his words, "The body is our general medium for having a world" (from O'Neill 1985: 17) and "It is through my body that I understand other people; just as it is through my body that I perceive 'things'" (from Blacking 1977b: 1). In Merleau-Ponty's work, the body is described not as a material object of nature agitated by stimuli, but as an organism capable of perceiving and activating itself in organized ways, i.e. the body as a structure of perceptual and behavioral competence (Lingis 1994: 4). As Young (1997: 7) observes it, "I am inserted into the world bodily and my experience of the world comes to me through my body". That is, the human being is first and foremost a bodily being and human cognition is achieved through its bodily experience. Human thinking is "a movement of the body", and humans "are moved into thinking" (Blacking 1977b: 20).

The key concept here is *embodiment*, which has stimulated increasingly growing research in cognitive science, an interdisciplinary field where a number of disciplines such as anthropology, artificial intelligence, linguistics, philosophy, psychology converge and overlap for the study of the mind in cognition.[16] As Krois et al. (2007b) point out, the concept of embodiment provides a way to link scientific and humanistic disciplines. Their volume *Embodiment in Cognition and Culture* (Krois et al. 2007a) shows that the notion of embodied cognition, which has transformed the scientific study of intelligence, has the potential to reorient cultural studies as well. The papers included in this volume study embodied cognition in such different fields as art history, literature, history of science, religious studies, philosophy, biology, as well as cognitive science. Looking across disciplines, indeed, we notice that studies have also been done on, for instance, embodied realism, embodied mind, embodied agent, embodied thought, embodied reason, embodied knowledge, embodied language, embodied meaning, embodied experience, embodied being, embodied self, embodied mathematics, embodied robots, to give a list that is far from being exhaustive. As is claimed, "the essence of human existence is embodiment", the self is inseparable from the body, and philosophy can no longer address

---

16 See, e.g., Anderson (2003), Berdayes, Esposito, and Murphy (2004), Clark (1999), Csordas (1990, 1994, 1999), Frank et al. (2008), Gallagher (2005), Gibbs (2003, 2006), Johnson (1987, 1999, 2007), Krois et al. (2007a), Lakoff (1987a), Lakoff and Johnson (1980, 1999), Lakoff and Núñez (2000), Lock and Scheper-Hughes (1987), Strathern (1996), Thompson and Varela (2001), Varela, Thompson, and Rosch (1991), Weiss and Haber (1999), Ziemke, Zlatev, and Frank (2007). It is worth noting that within cognitive science there is a split between the disembodied and embodied paradigms (see, e.g., Lakoff and Johnson 1999, Ch. 6).

problems of mind and consciousness in abstraction from their existential ground, the body (Gadow [1980] 2004: 70). The term *embodiment*, as suggested by the root of the word itself, has to do with the body and the body is actually "the very core of 'embodiment'" (Armstrong [1987] 2004: 117), but it is really about how the body is related to the mind in human experience and cognition. Scholars have already put forward a variety of programmatic theses for the embodiment paradigm: for instance, the body being mindful, the body being in the mind, the body grounding the mind, the body extending the mind, the body enacting the mind, the body informing the mind, the body schematizing the mind, the body shaping the mind. In a general sense, the term *embodiment* "collapses the duality of mind and body...by infusing body with mind" (Strathern 1996: 181) and attributes a more active and constructive role to the body in human cognition.

In the past decades, however, the meaning of the term *embodiment* "has been stretched in different directions" as it has become more popular (Strathern 1996: 196).[17] There exist, therefore, different theories of embodiment, often highly divergent from one another, and sometimes having very little in common (Violi 2004, 2008). In his recent book titled *Embodiment and Cognitive Science*, Gibbs (2006: 9) outlines the "embodiment premise" as follows:

> People's subjective, felt experiences of their bodies in action provide part of the fundamental grounding for language and thought. Cognition is what occurs when the body engages the physical, cultural world and must be studied in terms of the dynamical interactions between people and the environment. Human language and thought emerge from recurring patterns of embodied activity that constrain ongoing intelligent behaviour. We must not assume cognition to be purely internal, symbolic, computational, and disembodied, but seek out the gross and detailed ways that language and thought are inextricably shaped by embodied action.

---

[17] For instance, Violi (2004) discusses various forms of embodiment ranging from the weak to the strong one; Núñez (1999) distinguishes trivial, material, and full embodiment; Wilson (2002) reviews six views of embodied cognition; Rohrer warns against three dogmas of embodiment (2006) and identifies twelve dimensions of embodiment (2007); Maalej (2004) studies, in addition to physiological embodiment, culturally specific and culturally tainted embodiment; Maalej, Sharifian, and Yu (2006) mentions physiological, cultural, neural, and robotic dimensions of embodiment. See, also, Ziemke and Frank (2007).

Gibbs suggests that the key feature here for understanding the embodied nature of human cognition is to "look for possible mind-body and language-body connections" (p. 9) as formed in the interaction between the body and the physical and cultural world.

While embodiment has to do with the physical and biological body, what is embodied, however, "is always some set of meanings, values, tendencies, orientations, that derived from the sociocultural realm" (Strathern 1996: 197). The concentration on the human body as such, therefore, "may cause us to miss the ethnographic point in cultures in which the body is seen as a part of a wider cosmos" (p. 197). In other words, although it is always the same biological and physical body that is said to embody various aspects of human experience, what is embodied is clearly not just the biological and physical but the social and cultural as well. It is socioculturally-situated embodiment, as some cognitive linguists and cognitive scientists would call it (see, e.g., Frank et al. 2008; Krois et al. 2007a; Ziemke, Zlatev, and Frank 2007).

1.5. Cognitive semantic study of metaphor: Embodiment

In this section, I briefly outline Cognitive Semantics, the theoretical background for my book project, as is relevant to the notion of "embodiment". Cognitive Semantics is a branch of Cognitive Linguistics (see Geeraerts 1995, 2006c), and studies language, especially the semantic and conceptual structure underlying it, as a window into the mind and culture.

During the past decades, cognitive science has seriously challenged the fundamental assumption that most of our thinking about the world is literal, directly corresponding to the external reality (see, e.g., Gibbs 2006; Lakoff and Johnson 1999).[18] Against this backdrop, Cognitive Linguistics asserts that the "meaning we construct in and through the language is not a separate and independent module of the mind, but it reflects our overall experi-

---

18 Again, in cognitive science in general and in linguistics in particular, there is a split between the disembodied and embodied paradigms, which distinguishes between the "first generation" and "second generation" cognitive science (Lakoff and Johnson 1999, Ch. 6). Early cognitive science assumed a strict dualism in which the mind is disembodied, "characterized in terms of its formal functions, independent of the body" (p. 76). Second-generation cognitive science is one of the embodied mind, arguing for "the central role of our embodied understanding in all aspects of meaning and in the structure and content of our thought" (p. 78).

ence as human beings" (Geeraerts 2006c: 4–5). There are at least two main aspects to the broad experiential grounding of linguistic meaning in which Cognitive Linguistics is especially interested, as Geeraerts points out (p. 5):

> First, we are embodied beings, not pure minds. Our organic nature influences our experience of the world, and this experience is reflected in the language we use. ... Second, ... we are not just biological entities: we also have a cultural and social identity, and our language may reveal that identity, i.e. languages may embody the historical and cultural experience of groups of speakers (and individuals).

Indeed, the findings of cognitive linguistic studies have shown that human minds are embodied in the cultural world, and human meaning, feeling, and thinking are largely rooted in bodily and sociocultural experiences.[19] It is argued that "all cognition is embodied in cultural situations" (Gibbs 1999b: 156). While manifesting embodied cognition, language is after all a cultural form and should be studied in its social and cultural context, as conceptualizations underlying language and language use are largely formed and informed by cultural systems (Palmer 1996).

As Rohrer (2006) points out, the embodiment hypothesis is especially associated with a particular strand of Cognitive Linguistics, i.e. the cognitive-semantic approach to the study of metaphor and metonymy, which can be traced back to its origin in Lakoff and Johnson's seminal book *Metaphors We Live By* (1980). Over the past two decades, cognitive semantic theory of metaphor, generally known as conceptual metaphor theory, has yielded an enormous number of studies on metaphor, metonymy, and figurative language in general.[20]

---

19 See, e.g., Athanasiadou and Tabakowska (1998), Cuyckens, Dirven, and Taylor (2003), Dirven, Frank, and Pütz (2003), Fauconnier and Turner (2002), Geeraerts (1997, 2006a), Gibbs (1994, 1999a, 2006), Johnson (1987, 2007), Kövecses (2000, 2005, 2006), Lakoff (1987a), Lakoff and Johnson (1980, 1999), Langacker (1987, 1990, 1991, 1999), Niemeier and Dirven (1997), Palmer (1996), Palmer, Goddard, and Lee (2003), Palmer and Occhi (1999), Sweetser (1990), Talmy (2000a, 2000b), Turner (1991). Read, also, Geeraerts (2006b) for an updated guide to readings in Cognitive Linguistics, Kristiansen et al. (2006) for current applications and future perspectives of Cognitive Linguistics, and Ruiz de Mendoza Ibáñez and Peña Cerval (2005a) and Dirven (2005) for the internal dynamics and divergence of Cognitive Linguistics.

20 See, e.g., Barcelona (2000a), Dirven, Frank, and Pütz (2003), Dirven and Pörings (2002), Forceville (1996), Gibbs (1994, 2008), Gibbs and Steen (1999), Goatly (2007), Johnson (1987), Kövecses (2000, 2002, 2005, 2006),

According to conceptual metaphor theory, metaphor is not merely a figure of speech, but also a figure of thought, giving rise to understanding one conceptual domain in terms of another conceptual domain. Conceptual metaphors in people's conceptual systems influence a great deal how they think, understand, reason, and imagine in everyday life, and "many concepts, especially abstract ones, are structured and mentally represented in terms of metaphor" (Gibbs 1999b: 145). In fact, the most sweeping claim of conceptual metaphor theory is that abstract concepts "are defined by systematic mappings from bodily-based sensorimotor source domains onto abstract target domains" (Johnson and Rohrer 2007: 37). It is metaphor that "makes it possible to extend body-based meaning and inference into abstract thought" (Johnson 2007: 176–177).

The cognitive linguistic view of metaphor is a complex theory, where metaphor is seen as involving a variety of components interacting with each other. These components include: (a) source and target domains (or frames), (b) experiential basis, (c) linguistic expressions, (d) mappings, entailments, and blends, and (e) cultural models (Kövecses 2003, 2004, 2005). Specifically, conceptual metaphors, expressed in the formula A IS B, consist of a source and a target domain. The source is generally a more physical domain whereas the target a more abstract one. That is why conceptual metaphors are usually unidirectional, projecting elements from one domain to the other, but not the other way around. The choice of particular pairings of source and target domains is motivated by an experiential basis.

Such pairings of sources and targets, primarily conceptual in nature, give rise to metaphorical linguistic expressions. There are basic conceptual correspondences or mappings between the source and target domains. Very often, however, additional mappings, called entailments or inferences, are also mapped from the source to the target domain. The connection of a source with a target domain can result in blends, that is, conceptual integrations that are new with respect to both the source and the target. Conceptual metaphors converge on, and often structure as well, cultural models, which are, simultaneously cultural and cognitive, culturally specific mental representations of aspects of the world (Kövecses 2003, 2004, 2005).

It is worth stressing that the experiential basis of conceptual metaphors is both bodily and cultural. Cognitive Linguistics maintains that our minds

---

Lakoff (1987a), Lakoff and Johnson (1980, 1999), Lakoff and Núñez (2000), Lakoff and Turner (1989), Panther and Radden (1999a), Panther and Thornburg (2003), Ruiz de Mendoza Ibáñez and Otal Campo (2002), Steen (2007), Sweetser (1990), Turner (1987, 1991, 1996), Yu (1998).

are embodied in such a way that our conceptual systems draw largely upon the peculiarities of our bodies and the specifics of our physical and cultural environments (e.g., Gibbs 1994, 1999b, 2003; Johnson 1987, 1999, 2007; Lakoff 1987a, 1993; Lakoff and Johnson 1980, 1999). In *Metaphors We Live By* (1980), Lakoff and Johnson argue that conceptual metaphors, which structure our conceptual systems to a significant extent, are not arbitrary, but grounded in our physical and cultural experience. While they emphasize the importance of "direct physical experience", or embodied experience, as part of the experiential basis of conceptual metaphors, they also point out that such experience (p. 57):

> is never merely a matter of having a body of a certain sort; rather, *every* experience takes place within a vast background of cultural presuppositions. ... Cultural assumptions, values, and attitudes are not a conceptual overlay which we may or may not place upon experience as we choose. It would be more correct to say that all experience is cultural through and through, that we experience our "world" in such a way that our culture is already present in the very experience itself.

In arguing for the significance of cultural basis for metaphors, Gibbs (1999b: 155) points out that "embodied metaphor arises not from within the body alone, and is then represented in the minds of individuals, but emerges from bodily interactions that are to a large extent defined by the cultural world". The bodily experiences that form the source domains for conceptual metaphors are themselves complex social and cultural constructions. Cultural models, "in shaping what people believe, how they act, and how they speak about the world and their own experiences", set up specific perspectives from which "aspects of embodied experience are viewed as particularly salient and meaningful in people's lives" (p. 154). That is, "social and cultural constructions of experience fundamentally shape embodied metaphor" (p. 155). In sum, according to cognitive linguistic view, conceptual metaphors emerge from the interaction between body and culture: They are grounded in bodily experience, but shaped by cultural understanding.

Empirical studies of conceptual metaphors have revealed that some of them are potentially universal, others widespread, and still others culture-specific (see Kövecses 2005 for a detailed discussion). While conceptual metaphor theory accounts for such variations in universality and culture-specificity in general terms of interaction between body and culture (e.g., Gibbs 1999b, 2003; Yu 1995, 1998, 1999, 2000, 2003a, 2008a, 2008b), which constitutes the experiential basis of conceptual metaphors, the question still remains, however, as to how such experiential basis actually works. In other words, the question is how, exactly, the interplay between body and culture gives rise to conceptual metaphors that are potentially universal, widespread, or culture-specific.

In order to answer that question, the newer version of conceptual metaphor theory puts forth a "decomposition" account based on the distinction between two kinds of conceptual metaphors: *primary metaphors* and *complex metaphors* (see Grady 1997a, 1997b; also see Kövecses 2002, 2005; Lakoff and Johnson 1999, 2003). In short, as argued, primary metaphors derive directly from our experience and very often from our common bodily experience, and therefore are more likely to be universal or widespread, whereas complex metaphors are combinations of primary metaphors and cultural beliefs and assumptions and, for that reason, tend to be culture-specific.

More specifically, the decompositional approach has an important implication for the analysis of conceptual metaphors in terms of their universality and cross-cultural variation. In their formulation of a newer version of conceptual metaphor theory, Lakoff and Johnson (1999) suggest that the decomposition account, as part of the integrated theory, has shed some new light on the question of which metaphors are universal (or at least widespread) and why. Drawing upon the distinction between primary and complex metaphors, they explain that complex metaphors are "molecular", made up of "atomic" metaphorical parts called primary metaphors (p. 46; see pp. 50–54 for a list of common primary metaphors). Primary metaphors are derived directly from experiential correlations, or "conflations in everyday experience" that "pair subjective experience and judgment with sensorimotor experience" (p. 49). In contrast, complex metaphors, "formed by conceptual blending" (p. 46), are "built out of primary metaphors plus forms of commonplace knowledge: cultural models, folk theories, or simply knowledge or beliefs that are widely accepted in a culture" (p. 60). Thus, they suggest (p. 257):

> Inevitably, many primary metaphors are universal because everybody has basically the same kinds of bodies and brains and lives in basically the same kinds of environments, so far as the features relevant to metaphor are concerned.
>
> The complex metaphors that are composed of primary metaphors and that make use of culturally based conceptual frames are another matter. Because they make use of cultural information, they may differ significantly from culture to culture.

For instance, Lakoff and Johnson (1999: 60–61) suggest that the complex metaphor A PURPOSEFUL LIFE IS A JOURNEY is composed of the following cultural belief (reformulated here as two propositions) and two primary metaphors:

PEOPLE SHOULD HAVE PURPOSES IN LIFE
PEOPLE SHOULD ACT SO AS TO ACHIEVE THEIR PURPOSES
PURPOSES ARE DESTINATIONS
ACTIONS ARE MOTIONS

Whereas the two primary metaphors (PURPOSES ARE DESTINATIONS and ACTIONS ARE MOTIONS), based on common bodily experience, are likely to be universal, the complex metaphor (A PURPOSEFUL LIFE IS A JOURNEY) is less so. This is because its validity in a particular culture depends on this culture's holding the combination of the two propositions (PEOPLE SHOULD HAVE PURPOSES IN LIFE and PEOPLE SHOULD ACT SO AS TO ACHIEVE THEIR PURPOSES) and the two primary metaphors, as listed above.

A more recent development that is related to conceptual metaphor theory is blending or conceptual integration theory (e.g., Fauconnier and Turner 1998, 2002; Turner and Fauconnier 1995, 2002). Different from conceptual metaphor theory's conceptual mapping from a source to a target domain, this theory postulates conceptual integration of two or more "input spaces" into a new "blended space" based on a "generic space" of abstract commonalities shared by the input spaces. The blended space not only inherits structure from its inputs but also contains emergent structure of its own. Here is a "trashcan basketball" example provided by Coulson (2001: 115–118). When two college students try to shoot the paper "ball" (made from a crumpled-up piece of paper) into the wastepaper basket as a competition in their own dorm room, the game of "trashcan basketball" is born. "Trashcan basketball" is a new "blended space" with emergent structure (therefore called "trashcan basketball") arising from the two "input spaces" combined or "blended" – trash disposal and conventional basketball – governed by a "generic space". The generic space represents abstract, schematic properties applying to both input spaces and, in this case, it is throwing an object (crumpled paper and leather ball) into a container (trashcan and basket consisting of the rim and net).

Such a multiple-space model can account for various metaphorical and nonmetaphorical aspects of conceptual phenomena (see also Fauconnier and Turner 1998, 2002; Grady, Oakley, and Coulson 1999; Kövecses 2002; Turner and Fauconnier 1995, 2002). A major difference between conceptual metaphor theory and blending theory is that the former is typically concerned with entrenched conceptual relationships and the ways in which they may be elaborated whereas the latter often focuses on spontaneous, real-time processes that can yield short-lived and novel conceptualizations (Coulson 2006; Grady, Oakley, and Coulson 1999). The two approaches, however, are largely complementary, with similar assumptions about the relationship between language and conceptualization (Coulson 2006). According to Grady (2005), primary metaphors, as generic metaphorical patterns or templates, also serve as inputs to the processes of conceptual blending or integration. Lakoff and Johnson (1999) refer to complex metaphors as resulting from conceptual blending.[21]

Having outlined the theoretical concern and background of this book, I now provide a sketch of its organization.

1.6. Structure of the book

This book has seven chapters. Since it aims at both a cultural and a semantic understanding of its research object, the next two chapters research its cultural background. As the concept of "heart" lies at the core of ancient Chinese thought as the cognitive agent, Chapters 2 and 3, respectively, survey the relevant remarks on the *xin* 'heart' in the texts of ancient Chinese philosophy and of traditional Chinese medicine. The latter sees the heart as both the physiological and psychological center of a person, and extensively shares the worldview of ancient Chinese philosophy.

Chapter 4, which presents a synchronic study, is the central core of the book and focuses on the usages in the present-day Chinese language. In studying the linguistic expressions involving the Chinese term *xin* 'heart', it shows that the notion of "heart" encompasses one's inner self and one's mental and emotional life, which are associated separately with the head and the heart in Western dualism. Chapter 5 applies the insights into the linguistic and cultural model gained in Chapter 4 to present-day Chinese discourse, both prosaic and poetic. The essayist discusses the loss and re-

---

21 The latest development out of conceptual metaphor theory is the "Neural Theory of Metaphor" (see Lakoff 2008), which studies various kinds of neural computations that neuronal groups in the brain must perform to characterize frames, metaphors, metonymies, mental spaces, and blends, and therefore vastly enriches the understanding of how conceptual metaphor works on the basis of neuroscience.

covery of traditional moral values in modern and contemporary China, but he discusses this in terms of *xin* 'heart'. The poet characterizes the heart as the seat of the self and the organ of moral judgment. They both demonstrate that the heart is indeed conceptualized as the central faculty of cognition that plays various mental and emotional functions.

Chapter 6 takes up a wider culture-comparative perspective. It first surveys the concepts of "heart" and "brain" in the West. It then takes a comparative look at the concept of "heart" in English and Chinese. It finally compares two different cultural traditions from a historical perspective by looking at two philosophical and/or medical theories in which the corresponding conceptualizations of the heart are rooted: the Western, i.e. Greek, four-humor theory and the Eastern, i.e., Chinese, five-element theory. Chapter 7 summarizes the findings and their significances. The study will conclude with findings of both similarities and differences between Chinese and Western cultures and insights into their respective cultural models for "heart" and "mind" and the perceived agent and subject of human cognition.

Chapter 2
The HEART in ancient Chinese philosophy

2.1. Introduction: Basic philosophical notions and constructs

In this chapter, I analyze the conceptualization of the *xin* 'heart' as the locus of the "mind" (2.2), moral sense (2.3), and governance (2.4) in ancient Chinese philosophy. I will concentrate on Confucianism, including Neo-Confucianism, and Daoism, the two most influential schools of Chinese thought, which have influenced each other in their interaction over time. I intend to show that over two thousand and five hundred years ago the heart organ was already conceptualized by both of these two schools, without variation between them in this regard, as the central organ of the human being and the locus of the cognitive agent. As will later be shown in Chapters 3–5, this conceptualization of the heart in ancient Chinese philosophy has exerted a strong influence on Chinese culture in general. Specifically, I will explore this influence on traditional Chinese medicine (Ch. 3). In effect, ancient Chinese philosophy and traditional Chinese medicine have both laid the foundation of the Chinese cultural model for the concept of *xin* 'heart'. This is richly manifested in the great number of conventionalized expressions in the present-day Chinese language (Ch. 4), and the analysis of the prosaic and poetic texts on the *xin* 'heart' from present-day Chinese discourse demonstrates that the ancient and traditional understanding of the heart has largely survived and remains a cultural conceptualization shared by the Chinese today (Ch. 5). However, let us first look into Chinese philosophy in the present chapter.

2.1.1. Confucianism and Daoism: The notion of "heart"

In *A Short History of Chinese Philosophy*, Fung Yu-lan (1966: 17–19) calls Confucianism and Daoism "the two poles of one and the same axis" because they "both express, in one way or another, the aspirations and inspirations of the farmer" or the "Value of Agriculture" in China as an agrarian country. They differ, however, in that Confucianism "emphasizes the social responsibilities of man" whereas Daoism "emphasizes what is natural and spontaneous in him" (p. 22). While Confucianism "emphasizes social order and an active life", Daoism "concentrates on individual life and tranquility" (Chan 1963: 136). In the *Zhuangzi*, it is said that the Confucians "roam within the bounds of society", while the Daoists "roam beyond it" (Fung 1996: 22). For this reason, Confucianism appears more "this-worldly" than Daoism, and Daoism more "other-worldly" than Confucianism (p. 22). Whereas Daoism "is a severe critic of Confucianism" by "opposing Confucian conformity with nonconformity and Confucian worldliness with a transcendental spirit", it is also "fully the equal of Confucianism" in "its doctrines on government, on cultivating and preserving life, and on handling things" (Chan 1963: 136). In sum, as Fung (1996: 22) puts it: "These two trends of thought rivaled one another, but also complemented each other. They exercised a sort of balance of power. This gave to the Chinese people a better sense of balance in regard to this-worldliness and other-worldliness". This balance becomes manifest in their conceptions of "heart" and "mind".

Traditionally, "the Chinese do not separate heart and mind" (Larre and Rochat de la Vallée 1996: 42; see also Godwin 2001: 61–68). In ancient Chinese philosophy, the heart is regarded as "the site of both affective and cognitive activities" (Shun 1997: 48). It is conceptualized as "the organ of thinking, reasoning and reflecting, as well as the faculty of will and the seat of the emotions" (Knoblock 1994: 297). This conception differs from that of Western philosophical tradition, at least in the last several hundred years, which upholds the "reason-emotion dichotomy", contrasting "the reasoning faculty (the mind) with the irrational, base, physical desires and passions (the heart)" (Hansen 1992: 22). To Western thinkers, beliefs and ideas come from the mind whereas the heart is the seat of desires and emotions.[22] In sharp contrast, this "distinction between 'heart' and 'mind' in the Western sense does not exist in Chinese philosophy" (Lin 2001: 202). In other words, the "heart" and the "mind", in their Western senses, are conceptualized in ancient Chinese philosophy as being one, the *xin* 'heart', which houses thoughts and feelings, ideas and emotions. The Chinese *xin* 'heart'

[22] As pointed out by an anonymous reviewer, individuals in Western society sometimes may not make a clear linguistic distinction between heart and mind; for instance, "She *knew in her heart* that it was wrong" suggests the conflation of heart and mind. I also came across this example: a driver who had stopped to rescue the victims of an auto accident said, "It wasn't anything you could drive by because *in your heart* you're going to *think* about it for the rest of your life. It was serious" [italics mine]. It seems that this kind of "conflation" may happen when emotion and/or sense of morality is involved in thinking or knowing.

is the core of affective and cognitive structure, conceived of as having the capacity for logical reasoning, rational understanding, moral will, intuitive imagination, and aesthetic feeling, unifying human will, desire, emotion, intuition, reason and thought. It is "a holistic-comprehensive structure in which all human faculties are unified and integrated" (Lin 2001: 202).

It seems that the Chinese term *xin* 'heart' conveys both cognitive and affective implications. It is, therefore, often glossed as "heart-mind" or "heart/mind", as well as either "heart" or "mind", in more recent English literature on Chinese philosophy (e.g., Chan 2002a; De Bary 1981; Hansen 1992; Liu 2003; Shun 1997; Slingerland 2003; Yearley 1990). This is done because, in translating this culture-specific concept, scholars of Chinese philosophy have taken into consideration "both the affective and cognitive concerns that the concept of *xin* encompasses" (Chan 2002c: 42). In his study of Mencius' moral psychology as related to the concept of *xin*, for instance, Cua (2002: 127) says that the "adoption by many Sinologists of 'mind-heart' as a translation of *xin* rightly presumes a Mencian rejection of an exclusive disjunction between 'reason/judgment' and the 'passions/emotions'". Hansen (1992: 20) also points out that "The common translation of *xin* as *heart-mind* reflects the blending of belief and desire (thought and feeling, ideas and emotions) into a single complex dispositional potential".

This chapter discusses three prominent aspects of the *xin* 'heart' as conceptualized in ancient Chinese philosophy, namely the *xin* 'heart' as the locus of mind, morality, and governance. Philosophy, as defined by Fung (1966: 2), is "systematic, reflective thinking on life". In this kind of thinking emerge the theories of the universe and knowledge, in addition to the theory of life itself. "The theory of the universe arises because the universe is the background of life – the stage on which the drama of life takes place. The theory of knowledge emerges because thinking is itself knowledge", and "before we start to think about life, we must first 'think our thinking'" (p. 2). What is the mental faculty with which we conduct thinking? In ancient Chinese philosophy, the locus of the "mind" is the heart.

Also according to Fung (1966: 7), many people say that Chinese philosophy is a "this-world philosophy", which "emphasizes what is in society, such as human relations and human affairs". He said that these people are to some extent right because, at least on a "superficial view", "Chinese philosophy, regardless of its different schools of thought, is directly or indirectly concerned with government and ethics", that is, "concerned chiefly with society", "with the daily functions of human relations", and "with man's present life" (p. 7). This is especially true of Confucianism, which "is the philosophy of social organization" and, for that matter, is adopted by the ruling class as "the orthodox philosophy" most of the time throughout the long history of Chinese feudalism (p. 22). Confucianism is after all a philosophy of "rectifying the heart, cultivating the self, educating the family, and governing the country (正心、修身、齐家、治国), as expounded in the *Great Learning* (《大学》).[23] Accordingly, the governance of the country depends on the education of the family, which in turn depends on the cultivation of the self; but the key to cultivating the self is rectifying or "straightening" one's heart. That is, setting one's heart right is really the key to setting right, respectively, the self, the family, and the country. So understood, the heart is the center of both an individual and a society, serving as the link between them in a holistic cosmological view.

2.1.2. Unity of nature and man: Macrocosm and microcosm

Chan (1963) characterizes the history of Chinese philosophy with one word – humanism: "If one word could characterize the entire history of Chinese philosophy, that word would be humanism – not the humanism that denies or slights a Supreme Power, but one that professes the unity of man and Heaven" (p. 3). He suggests that humanism in this sense has dominated Chinese thought from the dawn of its history.[24] Apparently, humanism in the context of Chinese philosophy is characterized by "the unity of man and Heaven". Moore (1967b: 7–8) echoes this argument when he concludes

---

[23] *The Great Learning* is one of the "Four Books" (《四书》), the most important Confucian classics, the other three being *The Analects of Confucius*, *Mencius*, and *The Doctrine of the Mean*. In Chinese, the word 正 *zheng*, as in 正心 *zhengxin*, has a primary spatial sense that means "straight", "upright", or "straighten". Therefore, 正心 *zhengxin* 'rectify the heart' literally means "to straighten the heart", which has been "crooked" or "deformed", say, by evil desires or thoughts.

[24] While pointing out that "the humanistic tendency had been in evidence long before his time", Chan credits Confucius (551–479 BC) as the one who actually turned humanism into "the strongest driving force in Chinese philosophy", giving Chinese philosophy "its humanistic foundation". He said, "Confucius exerted great influence on Chinese philosophical development in that, first of all, he determined its outstanding characteristic, namely, humanism" (Chan 1963: 15). See also Moore (1967a) for arguments for the humanistic view of ancient Chinese philosophy and culture.

that the Chinese thought-and-culture tradition may be characterized by humanism with an emphasis upon a sense of harmony with Nature and fellow human beings.

Ancient Chinese philosophy advocated the ideas that nature and man are unified (天人合一 *tian ren heyi*) and the universe and the human correspond to each other (天人对应 *tian ren duiying*).[25] The words *nature* and *universe* are both used to translate the Chinese word *tian* (天), which primarily refers to the sky or heaven, but should be interpreted to mean "the external world", including the social and cultural structures, in which people live (see, e.g., Zhang and Rose 2001: Ch. 4). Thus, for instance, the Daoists conceived of the human body as "a microcosm of the universe" (p. 86), and "always tried to understand what was happening inside the body by comparing and contrasting it with what was happening outside in nature" (Chia and Chia 1990: 14). To them, "The microcosm is a mirror image of the macrocosm", and "The universe within is the same as the universe without" (p. 15). Therefore, one can understand the entire universe by understanding one's own body and vice versa. Understanding, however, is a function of the human heart, which as the central faculty of cognition and central organ of the human body connects the human with the universe.

Before I move on to illustrate how the ancient Chinese perceived the unity and correspondence between the universe and the human, I want to mention in passing the ancient theories of metaphysics and cosmology in Chinese philosophy, namely, the theories of yin-yang and of the five elements. These theories serve as the links between the perceived parallels between the macrocosm of the universe and the microcosm of the human. The yin-yang doctrine is very simple but its influence has been extensive: "No aspect of Chinese civilization – whether metaphysics, medicine, government, or art – has escaped its imprint" (Chan 1963: 244). In simple terms, the doctrine teaches that all things and processes in nature are products of two forces: the yin, which is negative, passive and feminine, and the

---

[25] I just want to mention in passing that in the Chinese original phrases *ren* 'human; person; people' is neutral in terms of gender. In this book, I sometimes use the English word *man* in the sense of "a human being or person" or more generally "the human race or mankind", to follow the convention in the English literature on Chinese philosophy. However, I also use the word *human*, which is intrinsically neutral in gender, wherever possible or desirable. Hence, for instance, in the phrases "nature and man" and "the universe and the human" here, "man" and "human" are both used to translate the Chinese word *ren*.

yang, which is positive, active and masculine. This theory is associated with that of the five elements or phases, namely wood, fire, earth, metal, and water, which may be taken as an elaboration of the yin-yang idea but actually adds the important concept of rotation, that is, things succeed one another as the five elements take their turns.[26] These doctrines represent early Chinese attempts in the direction of addressing the questions of "the process through which things in the world have come to be and the fundamental stuff of which they are made" (p. 245). As Chan (1963) suggests, yin and yang and the five elements should be understood as forces or powers rather than material elements. The theories emphasize principles and laws of operation that combine contradiction and harmony, uphold unity in multiplicity, and realize a dynamic monism through the dialectic, giving rise to the view that things are related and reality is a process of constant transformation.

To illustrate the unity and correspondence between the universe and the human as perceived by the ancient Chinese, one example from the *Wenzi*, a classic Daoist text, should suffice:[27]

---

26 Table 1 below lists some of the correspondences between the human body as microcosm and the universe as macrocosm. Section 3.1 will present a more detailed discussion of the yin-yang and five-element doctrines, which have been serving as the guiding principles and reasoning tools of traditional Chinese medicine up to date.

27 The examples in this chapter are extracted from classic texts of ancient Chinese philosophy. The English translations are, again, my own unless otherwise acknowledged. I have referred to the following for their English translations: Le Guin (1998) and Waley, Chen, and Fu (1999) for the *Laozi* or *Daode Jing*; Bao and Lao (1992) and Legge (nd.) for the *Analects*; He and He (1992) and Legge (nd.) for the *Great Learning*; Zheng et al. (1993) and Legge (nd.) for the *Mencius*; Knoblock (1988, 1990, 1994) and Watson (2003) for the *Xunzi*; Giles (1926) and Wang, Qin, and Sun (1999) for the *Zhuangzi*; and Rickett (1985, 1998) for the *Guanzi*. Modifications of my own are made to varying degrees. In studies of ancient Chinese philosophy, translations of the original classic Chinese, from specific terms to longer texts, vary considerably. Therefore, I decided to place the English translations below their original texts in Chinese characters so that readers, if they want, can conveniently read both. To me, the English translations are provided and meant merely for readers' reference, and nothing more.

> 老子曰：人受天地变化而生，…… 头圆法天，足方象地。天有四时、五行、九曜、三百六十日，人有四支、五藏、九窍、三百六十节；大[28]有风雨寒暑，人有取与喜怒，胆为云，肺为气，脾为风，肾为雨，肝为雷。人与天地相类，而心为之主；耳目者日月也，血气者风雨也。《文子・九守》(Ji 1995, vol. 49: 82)
>
> Laozi said: Man is born in the change of Heaven and Earth, … his head is round modeled on heaven; his feet are square just like earth. Nature has four seasons, five elements, nine stars, and three hundred and sixty days; man has four limbs, five zang organs, nine apertures, and three hundred and sixty parts. Nature has winds and rains, and is affected by cold and heat; man has likes and dislikes,[29] and is affected by joy and anger. The gallbladder is the cloud, the lung the air, the spleen the wind, the kidney the rain, and the liver the thunder. Man is similar to Heaven and Earth in kind, and the heart is his master. His ears and eyes are the sun and moon, and his blood and qi are rain and wind. *Wenzi: Nine Things to Be Preserved.*

As in this passage of a quotation from Laozi (c. 581–500 BC), the founder of Daoism, various parallels, real or imaginary, are perceived between man and nature. According to the Daoist conceptions, the sky, which is yang, is round whereas the earth, which is yin, is square.[30] Therefore, man has round head and square feet (two rectangles), modeled on Heaven and Earth. The parallels then extend: nature has four seasons, and man has four limbs; nature has five elements or phases (wood, fire, earth, metal, and water), and man has five zang organs (liver, heart, spleen, lung, and kidney) that match the five elements accordingly (see Table 1); nature has nine stars (九曜 *jiuyao* refers to the Big Dipper, consisting of seven stars, plus two auxiliary ones [HYDCD 2000: 114]), and man has nine apertures or orifices (seven in the head, plus two in the lower body); nature has 360 days for a year (in

---

28 The word 大 *da,* which means "big", "large", "great", "grand", etc. in modern Chinese, once had the sense of 天 *tian* 'sky, heaven, nature, universe' in old Chinese (HYDCD 2000: 737). Similarly, the word 支 *zhi*, which occurs in the previous context, was the same as 肢 *zhi* 'limb' in ancient times (p. 1543).

29 In the original, 取与 *quyu* means "accept and give" (HYDCD 2000: 493). In general, people have things to gain or lose. I translate the word into "likes and dislikes" in the specific context.

30 The ancient Chinese conceptualized the earth as being square, under the vault of heaven that is round. For instance, the Temple of the Heaven and the Temple of the Earth in Beijing, built on these conceptions in ancient times, have almost everything in contrast between round and square shape.

the Chinese lunar calendar),[31] and man has 360 parts for his body. Man's temperament varies and emotion changes, as much as nature's climate and weather.[32] It is worth mentioning that the internal organs listed in this passage are zang organs except the gallbladder, which is a fu organ (see Table 1 below). The heart, which is one of the five zang organs, is singled out separately as the "master" of the whole body.

According to the five-element schema of Daoism that highlights the unity of microcosm and macrocosm, the heart is the organ of fire, and is classified with the Mars out in the universe, which in Chinese is known as the "Planet of Fire" (火星 *huoxing*). Given below in Table 1 is a partial list of the five-element classification, which shows the perceived correlations between the organs in the body and the planets in the universe.

---

31 The traditional Chinese lunar calendar has 360 days divided into five equal periods of 72 days each. The five periods are called "five divisions" (五运 *wuyun*), which correlate with the five phases or elements accordingly. While one year consists of four seasons of 90 days each, the last 18 days of each season belong to an extra, interim season, known as "long summer" (长夏 *changxia*), which is located in the middle of the four seasons. Thus, spring is the season of wood, summer the season of fire, long summer the season of earth, autumn the season of metal, and winter the season of water (see Zhang and Rose 2001: 27).

32 There are other "parallels" observed between the macrocosm of nature and the microcosm of man. For example, it is said that man has 12 major joints while nature has 12 months, man opens and closes his eyes and nature has days and nights, man has currents of blood and breath circulating through arteries and vessels in his body whereas nature has water flowing along rivers and streams on the earth, and so forth (see, e.g., Cai 2000: 209–210; Kuriyama 2002: 50, 157). As Dong Zhongshu (179–104 BC), the representative Confucian in the Han dynasty (206 BC–220 AD), argued, "the essence of man is rooted in Heaven, which is also his great grandfather (人之为人，本于天，天亦人之曾祖父也《春秋繁露・为人者天》)" (from Cai 2000: 209). Since "man is a replica of the universe (人副天数 *ren fu tianshu*)", they are fundamentally of the same kind (天人相类 *tian ren xianglei*), and interact with each other (天人感应 *tian ren ganying*). Heaven created the ten thousand things (万物 *wanwu*) to raise humans, whom it created to realize its own will. Heaven and human have the same physiological essence and moral nature. While Heaven's climate and weather changes affect humans, humans' behavior and mental activities evoke responses from Heaven, too (see Cai 2000: 206–212). Readers are also referred to the section "The body as representation of the Cosmos" in Lévi (1989: 105–109) for more discussions.

Table 1. Correspondences between the zang and fu organs and the planets

Elements	Zang	Fu	Planets
wood	liver	gallbladder	Planet of Wood 木星 *muxing* 'Jupiter'
fire	heart	small intestine	Planet of Fire 火星 *huoxing* 'Mars'
earth	spleen	stomach	Planet of Earth 土星 *tuxing* 'Saturn'
metal	lung	large intestine	Planet of Metal 金星 *jinxing* 'Venus'
water	kidney	bladder	Planet of Water 水星 *shuixing* 'Mercury'

Incidentally, these five planets have other names that are no longer widely known nowadays (see Table 3 in section 3.1 for a more detailed five-element categorization).

What I want to point out again at this juncture is that in ancient Chinese philosophy the *xin* 'heart' is taken as the locus of three functions: (a) as the locus of the "mind" or the faculty of knowing and understanding (心知 *xinzhi*, lit. "heart knowing and understanding") (see section 2.2), (b) as the locus of moral sense and character (see section 2.3), and (c) as the locus of governance and government (see section 2.4). In the following, I will deal with these three aspects of the conceptualization of the heart in ancient Chinese thought one by one.

2.2. The heart as the locus of the "mind"

In ancient Chinese philosophy, the heart is believed to be the organ of thinking, knowing, understanding, reasoning, and feeling and, for that matter, to be the central faculty of cognition (Yu 2007a, 2008c). As we will see below, this culturally constructed belief is expressed both literally and metaphorically.

2.2.1. The heart as the thinking and knowing organ

Ancient Chinese philosophy emphasizes the cognitive functions of the heart as the human being's thinking and knowing organ, which possesses all the mental faculties given at birth. Thus, in the *Guanzi*, the title bearing the name of Guanzi or Guan Zhong (c. 725–645 BC), a statesman and philosopher of the Spring and Autumn period (770–476 BC), a baby in the mother's womb will "take shape in five months, and be born in ten months; after the birth, the eyes will see, the ears will hear, and the heart will think" (五月而成，十月而生。生而目视，耳听，心虑《管子・水地》). It is taken for granted that humans are born with the heart to think, as much as with the eyes to see and the ears to hear, although some people make better use of these faculties than others:

> 耳司听，听必顺闻，闻审谓之聪。目司视，视必顺见，见察谓之明。心司虑，虑必顺言，言得谓之知。《管子・宙合》(Ji 1995, vol. 49: 749)
> The ear is in charge of listening. When listening, people should be prudent about what they hear. If they examine what they hear, that is acute hearing. The eye is in charge of looking. When looking, people should be prudent about what they see. If they scrutinize what they see, that is clear seeing. The heart is in charge of thinking. When thinking, people should be prudent about their views and ideas. If their views and ideas are correct and proper, that is real knowing.[33] *Guanzi: The Way of the Universe.*

As we can see from this passage, our ears, eyes, and heart are recognized as our essential faculties of cognition through which we get to know and understand the external world. While each of these faculties is in charge of an

---

33 According to HYDCD (2000: 2109), the Chinese word 顺 *shun* can be used, in one sense, as the same as 慎 *shen* or 谨慎 *jinshen*, which means "be careful, cautious, or prudent". As used in the original text, the Chinese word 聪 *cong* refers to "acute hearing" while 明 *ming* means "being sharp-eyed or clear-sighted". When these two are used together as a compound word, however, it means "intelligent, bright, smart, or clever". Thus, literally, one's intelligence depends on having "acute hearing and clear vision". In the last sentence of the original, the word 言 *yan*, according to HYDCD (2000: 360), has the meaning of 学说 *xueshuo* and 主张 *zhuzhang* in addition to its primary meanings of "speech, talk, or expression". The word 知 *zhi* has various meanings, including "know", "understand", and "knowledge", the three primary senses. It is also the ancient variant of the character 智 *zhi* 'intelligence; wisdom' (p. 1968).

important cognitive function, they are not equal, as expounded in the *Guanzi* with a special version of the CONTAINER metaphor:

> “洁其宫，阙其门”：宫者，谓心也。心也者，智之舍也，故曰“宫”。洁之者，去好过也。门者，谓耳目也。耳目者，所以闻见也。《管子・心术上》(Ji 1995, vol. 49: 784)
> “Cleanse the imperial palace and open the doors”. The “imperial palace” refers to the heart. The heart is the residence of intelligence, and therefore it is called an “imperial palace”. Those who cleanse it get rid of partiality and bias. The “doors” refer to the ears and eyes. The ears and eyes are the means for hearing and seeing. *Guanzi: Art of the Heart.*

As this quotation shows, the heart as the “imperial palace” or the center of the human body is the “residence” of intelligence or intellect, whereas the ears and eyes are the “doors” that serve as pathways or entrances for information to reach into this residence. It is important to keep these doors open to let information in, but that is still not enough for the purpose of cognition. Raw information has to be processed by the heart before it can turn into knowledge and wisdom. That is why it is necessary to “cleanse” the heart to avoid partiality and bias.

It is common sense that we should examine what we hear with our ears and what we see with our eyes. Such examination is accomplished through our heart, as is further illustrated by the conversation, recorded in the *Kongcongzi*, between Confucius (or Kongzi, c. 551–479 BC) and his grandson, Zisi:

> 子思问于夫子曰：“物有形类，事有真伪，必审之，奚由？”子曰：“由乎心，心之精神是谓圣，推数究理，不以物疑。”《孔丛子・记问》(Ji 1995, vol. 49: 390)
> Zisi asked Confucius, “Objects vary in shape and kind, and things may be true or false. Therefore, one has to examine them. But through what?” Confucius said, “Through the heart. The spirits of the heart are regarded as holy. Through inferring and reasoning, the heart studies the whys and wherefores of things, and will not be confused by them”. *Kongcongzi: Recorded Questions.*

In Confucius’ words, 精神 *jingshen*, which literally means “essence and spirit”, is the mental aspect (or the “mind”), in contrast with the physical form (or the body), of a person. The locus of that “mental half” is the heart. Through thinking the heart can gain insights into things that are otherwise confusing. Thinking results in knowing and understanding. That is why

Confucius referred to the mental function of a person as "holy". The heart, the "imperial palace", is "sacred" because it possesses mental power that is "holy".

The heart receives information through the eyes and ears, but is able to process and store it for use. Mencius (or Mengzi, c. 372–289 BC), who represented the "idealistic wing" of Confucianism (Fung 1966), distinguished the heart, the thinking organ, from the organs of ears and eyes, which do not think and which tend to be deceived by external things when in contact with them. He asserted that the function of the organ of heart is to think, and a good sense of understanding and reasoning can only be obtained through thinking.

> 耳目之官不思，而蔽于物。物交物，则引之而已矣。心之官则思，思则得之，不思则不得也。《孟子 • 告子上》(Zheng et al. 1993: 418)
> Such organs as ears and eyes do not think, so they tend to be deceived by external things. When in contact with external things, they are often led astray. The organ of heart is for thinking. If you think, you will get it; if you do not, then you will not get it.[34] *Mencius: Gaozi,* Part I.

What gives humans distinction among the creatures of Heaven and Earth is the heart. As the thinking faculty, Mencius assumed, the heart is endowed by Heaven, but is not necessarily preserved by people. Only those "great men" actually "preserve the heart" (存心 *cunxin*), make good use of it, or even "exhaust" it (尽心 *jinxin*), whereas those "petty men" or "small men" do not.

In comparison with the Confucian advocacy for active use of the *xin* 'heart' in knowing and understanding the world, Daoism appears to be more passive in this regard. Instead of "using the heart" (用心 *yongxin*) or "exhausting the heart" (尽心 *jinxin*), Daoism maintains the practice of abstaining from using the heart, namely the "fasting of the heart" (心斋 *xinzhai*).[35] For instance, Laozi maintained that it would be ideal if "the eye

---

34 Here in the English translation, "it" literally refers to the heart, but by extension it means "a good sense of understanding and reasoning" that comes with the heart. That is, we can see this as an instantiation of the conceptual metonymy CONTAINER FOR CONTAINED.

35 As pointed out by Slingerland (2003: 225), Zhuangzi's "fasting of the heart/mind" (心斋 *xinzhai*), as a CONTAINER metaphor, is designed to make the container of the heart/mind "tenuous" or "empty" (虚 *xu*) so that it will have room to "receive" or "gather" the Way.

remains sharp but does not see, the ear acute but does not hear, the mouth articulate but does not talk, and the heart unobstructed but does not think" (目明而不以视，耳聪而不以听，口当而不以言，心条通而不以思虑《文子・下德》). This is because Daoism promotes "indifference and inaction" (漠然无为 *moran wuwei*) through which to have all things accomplished (see Slingerland 2003). The key is to stay above worldly considerations and material gains. Thus, a sage, according to Laozi, as quoted in the *Wenzi*, should practice the following:

> 食足以充虚接气，衣足以盖形御寒，适情辞余，不贪得，不多积，清目不视，静耳不听，闭口不言，委心不虑。《文子・九守》(Ji 1995, vol. 49: 82)
> Eat just enough to fill the emptiness and keep qi circulating. Wear just enough to cover the body and keep it from the cold. Maintain a proper mood and reject excessive emotions. Do not have an insatiable desire for possession or accumulation. Have clear eyes but do not see; have quiet ears but do not listen. Shut the mouth and do not talk; relax the heart and do not think. *Wenzi: Nine Things to Be Preserved.*

That is, a sage, to Laozi, "should have a level heart and an easy mood and contain his spirits inside so that he would not be confused and tempted by external things" (心平志易，精神内守，物不能惑《文子・下德》). According to the Daoist doctrine, if one's spirits can be contained inside, then one will enjoy longevity. In the *Zhuangzi,* titled after Zhuangzi (c. 369–286 BC), there is a supposed sage, Guangchengzi, who taught the following to the Yellow Emperor, who wanted to learn how to access the Way and make the self last: "If the eye sees nothing, the ear hears nothing, and the heart knows nothing, your spirits will keep themselves in the body, and the body will live forever" (目无所见，耳无所闻，心无所知，女神将守形，形乃长生《庄子・在宥》). This sage believed that one should cherish that which is within oneself and shut off that which is without; for much knowledge is harmful, and if one cherishes and preserves one's own self, all the rest will prosper of itself.

Of course Daoism is not preaching the value of completely shutting down one's faculties of cognition in its literal sense. What it advocates is to rise above the worldliness and to access the Way of Heaven and Earth. Once that is accomplished, one can get beyond the self and become one with Heaven and Earth so that a sage can gain "a higher point of view" and "see things in the light of Heaven" (Fung 1966: 112). As Laozi said, quoted in the *Wenzi*, a sage can "see with the eye of all-under-Heaven, hear with the ear of all-under-Heaven, and think with the heart of all-under-Heaven" (以天下之目视，以天下之耳听，以天下之心虑《文子・上仁》).

2.2.2. The heart as the central faculty of cognition

As we have seen from the above, the *xin* 'heart' in ancient Chinese philosophy is the thinking and knowing organ. In thinking, it processes the information that it receives from other parts, especially the sense organs, of the body so that it gets to know and understand the external world. To know the universe, one needs to know and understand its essence and nature. In ancient Chinese philosophy, it is to know and understand the Way (道 *dao*) and Virtue (德 *de*), which are the beginning and the end of the knowing and understanding process. According to Laozi, *Dao,* the Way, is that by which all things come to be. In this process of coming to be, each individual thing obtains something from the universal Way, and this something is called *De* (德), the Virtue or Power, i.e., it is the power of the Way manifested in individual things. The Virtue of things is what they naturally are, or that by which they are what they are (see Fung 1966: 100). In other words, when *Dao* is possessed by individual things, it becomes their Character or Virtue, *De* (see Chan 1963: 136). That is, *De* is *Dao* individualized in the nature of things, or particularized when inherent in a thing (Chan 1963). This is the ancient version of what is known as human cognition in contemporary terms. As the thinking and knowing organ, the heart is conceptualized in ancient Chinese thought as the central faculty of cognition, by which one connects with the Way and Virtue and understands the external world.

According to Xunzi (c. 313–238 BC), the representative of the "realistic wing" of Confucian philosophy (Fung 1966), what is crucial in human understanding is the connection between the heart of an individual and the Way of the universe. The Way keeps the world in balance.

> 何谓衡？曰：道。故心不可以不知道。心不知道，则不可道而可非道。《荀子・解蔽篇》(Ji 1995, vol. 49: 362)
> What is the balance? I say that it is the Way. This is why it is inadmissible for the heart not to know the Way. If the heart does not know the Way, then it may reject what is accordant with the Way and accept what is contrary to the Way. *Xunzi: Dispelling Blindness.*

It is interesting to note that in modern Chinese "to know" literally is "to know the way" (知道 *zhidao*), so that if you know something, you actually "know the way or principle" of that thing. In ancient times, however, knowing the Way means thorough and deep understanding that results in not only knowledge, but also wisdom, the great Virtue, as suggested in the *Zhuangzi*:

> 目彻为明，耳彻为聪，鼻彻为颤，口彻为甘，心彻为知，知彻为德。《庄子・外物》(Ji 1995, vol. 49: 61)
> The eye that sees everything is sharp; the ear that hears everything is keen; the nose that smells everything is sensitive; the mouth that tastes everything is exquisite; the heart that knows everything is wise; the intellect that reaches everything is virtuous. *Zhuangzi: Contingencies.*

It is certainly virtuous for the heart to know the Virtue of things, and hence the Way of the universe. Through various sense organs the heart gets to know and understand the world. It has some special qualities that make it the central faculty of cognition, as argued by Xunzi:

> 人何以知道？曰：心。心何以知？曰：虚壹而静。心未尝不臧也，然而有所谓虚；心未偿不满也，然而有所谓一；心未偿不动也，然而有所谓静。《荀子・解蔽篇》(Ji 1995, vol. 49: 362)
> How does a man get to know the Way? I say it is through the heart. How does the heart know? I say by its emptiness, unity, and stillness. The heart never stops storing; nonetheless it possesses what is called emptiness. The heart never lacks diversity; nonetheless it possesses what is called unity. The heart never stops moving; nonetheless it possesses what is called stillness. *Xunzi: Dispelling Blindness.*

Here, Xunzi discusses how one can know the world through the heart knowing the Way. He characterized the heart as having three important qualities. First, it should be "empty", "void", or "vacuous" (虚 *xu*) as a receptacle. That is, the heart-container should always be open and receptive to new things even though it may have already stored up many old things. One should not let the old things preoccupy the heart-container and keep it from accepting new things. Second, the heart should remain as a "unified one" and maintain its "oneness" (壹 *yi*). That is, it should be unified with one focus. In its learning process, the heart accepts different kinds of things. One should not let this diversity interfere with the unity or singleness of the heart, or let one thing interfere with the other. Thus, Xunzi argued, "The world does not have two Ways, and the sage does not have two hearts" (天下无二道，圣人无两心《荀子·解蔽篇》). That is, the unity of the heart is as important as the unity of the Way. In a similar vein, as we can see here, the heart to the sage is the same as the Way to the universe. The sage gets to know the world through his heart knowing the Way. The heart should follow the Way, and should not go astray. This is because "if the heart branches off, it will lack understanding; if it tilts, it will lack acuity; and if it is divided, it will be filled with doubts and delusions" (心枝则无知，倾则不精，贰则疑惑《荀子·解蔽篇》). That is why it is said, "A single heart can serve a hundred gentlemen, but a hundred hearts cannot serve a single gentleman" (一心可以事百君，百心不可以事一君《孔丛子·诘墨》). Third and last, Xunzi believed that the heart should be "still" or "quiescent" (静 *jing*). "In general", he argued, "when examining things about which there are doubts, if the heart is not inwardly settled, then external things will not be clear" (凡观物有疑，中心不定，则外物不清《荀子·解蔽篇》). In other words, one should keep one's mental state calm and free from emotional disturbances. This is especially important since the heart, which hosts such mental functions as reason and judgment, houses emotions and desires too (see 2.2.4 below).

What should be noted is the fact that Xunzi already suggested the embodied nature of human cognition over 2,000 years ago. He believed that the human mind and cognition depend on the human body and perception. In his own words, "the spirits are born when the body takes shape" (形具而神生《荀子·天论篇》). That is, the "mind" arises from the body and mental force is based on physical form. Through the functioning of their sense organs, namely the eye, ear, nose, mouth, and body, which represent the five perceptual senses, namely sight, hearing, smell, taste, and touch, humans gather information about the external world. The contact between the body and the world initiates cognition and constitutes its first step through perception. What follows next is the processing of the information, which the five sense organs have gathered, by the thinking organ of heart, the central faculty of cognition. Xunzi called this second step of cognition "levy and understand" (征知 *zhengzhi*), that is, "through its thinking processes and activities, 'the heart' classifies, differentiates, and accepts or rejects the knowledge obtained by such sense organs as ears, eyes, nose, and mouth, so as to further understand external reality" (HYDCD 2000: 918). In his words, "The heart is capable of levying and understanding" (心有征知《荀子·正名篇》). It is through this "levying and understanding", or information gathering and processing, that lower perceptual knowledge rises into mental rational knowledge (see also Cai 2000: 84–85).

According to Mencius, the "heart is an integral part of a total cosmic system" (Hansen 1992: 173). Understanding Heaven means that one's own heart is connected with the Way of Heaven so that it penetrates Heaven and Earth and the ten thousand things (万物 *wanwu*) in between. The heart is not only the center of a person, but also the passage to Heaven. Through their heart, people can understand their common human nature endowed by Heaven. In so doing they can also understand Heaven itself:

> 尽其心者，知其性也。知其性，则知天矣。存其心，养其性，所以事天也。《孟子・尽心上》(Zheng et al. 1993: 466)
> One who exhausts the heart understands human nature. To understand human nature is to understand Heaven. To preserve the heart and to cultivate human nature is thus to serve Heaven. *Mencius: Exhausting the Heart,* Part I.

That is, through exhausting one's own heart and knowing one's own nature, which is endowed by Heaven, man "can not only know Heaven, but can also become one with Heaven" (Fung 1966: 77). He has become a "citizen of Heaven" (天民 *tianmin*). As such, he feels no distinction between himself and others or between the individual and the universe, and "becomes identified with the universe as a whole" (p. 77). Mencius put the content of Heaven into the heart. In understanding Heaven one does not have to explore the external world, but to probe into the inner world of the self. Understanding Heaven means understanding one's own heart. He said, "The ten thousand things are all within me. There is no greater delight than to realize this in self-examination" (万物皆备于我。反身而诚，乐莫大焉《孟子・尽心上》).

Mencius' notion of "exhausting the heart" is echoed by a representative Neo-Confucian of the Song dynasty (960–1279), Cheng Hao (1032–1083), who is known as one of the major exponents of the "Learning of the Principle" (理学 *lixue*). He believed that the human heart is not separable from external things, thus getting rid of the distinction between the subject and the object of knowing. He argued: "The individual heart is Heaven. If you exhaust it, then you know human nature; if you know human nature, then you know Heaven" (只心便是天，尽之便知性，知性便知天《遗书・卷二》). Now that the human heart is the source of knowledge and truth, human cognition is the process of "exhausting the heart" in search of the Principle of Heaven. He declared:

> 己之心，无异圣人之心，广大无垠，万善皆备，欲传圣人之道，扩充此心焉耳。《宋元学案・明道学案》(from Cai 2000: 291)
> Our heart is not different from the sage's heart. It is vast and boundless, possessing all the goodness. If we want to disseminate the Way of the sage, we just need to expand and strengthen this heart. *Study Cases of Song and Yuan: Mingdao*.

To Cheng Hao, a scholar's task is to "recognize benevolence" (识仁 *shiren*), which is rooted in the heart, as Mencius had argued, since a benevolent person is integrated and united with Heaven and Earth and the ten thousand things (see Cai 2000: 290–291).

According to Zhu Xi (1130–1200), the leading Neo-Confucian of the "Learning of the Principle" of the Song dynasty, the Principle (理 *li*) is the highest and most fundamental concept of all, abstracted from physical phenomena but existing independently of all physical existence. It is prior to Heaven and Earth, the ten thousand things, and human beings, and is regarded as the root and origin of the universe. Although humans are born with principles for everything in their heart, they cannot directly know them from within, but have to "investigate things" (格物 *gewu*) in the external world in order to recognize their principles contained in their heart. This is just like an ancient bronze mirror covered by dust: Only after the dust is removed can you see yourself in the mirror. In short, to Zhu Xi, the Principle is the foundation of the universe while the heart is posterior to it (see Cai 2000: 298–312).

On the contrary, Lu Jiuyuan (1139–1193), the leading Neo-Confucian of the "Learning of the Heart" in the Song dynasty, believed that the principles for things exist only inside the human heart. While he did not deny Zhu Xi's idea of universality of the Principle, he argued that its existence is verified only by and in the human heart. The Principle inside the heart is not only in connection with, but also the best manifestation of, the Principle of the universe (see Cai 2000: 307–312). To him, the heart is the origin of all things: "The behavior of the heart is like that of the things that are capable of reproduction" (心之所为，犹之能生之物《陆九渊集・敬斋记》). Thus, he said:

> 万物森然于方寸之间，满心而发，充塞宇宙，无非此理。《陆九渊集・语录上》(Ji 1995, vol. 50: 2383)

> The ten thousand things are dense in the square-inch. They cram the heart and go beyond it to pervade the universe. This is nothing but the Principle. *Collected Writings of Lu Jiuyuan: Quotations,* Part I.

That is, according to Lu Jiuyuan, all things originate in the "square inch" of the heart, and then disperse into the universe. To get hold of the Principle of Heaven and Earth and the ten thousand things people just need to probe deep into their own hearts. Therefore, it is a similar but much stronger version of Mencius' claim for getting to know human nature and Heaven through "exhausting the heart". Lu Jiuyuan's view can be summarized by his thesis that "What all people have is the heart, what all hearts possess is the Principle, and the heart is the Principle" (人皆有是心，心皆具是理，心即理也《陆九渊集・与李宰》).

As the leading figure of Neo-Confucianism and the master exponent of the "Learning of the Heart" in the Ming dynasty (1368–1644), Wang Yangming (1472–1529) further developed Lu Jiuyuan's "Learning of the Heart". He posited that the heart and the Principle are inseparable, the latter being the substance of the former, and there is no Principle of things independent of the heart. In short, he argued, "There exist no things, no affairs, no principles, no righteousness, and no goodness outside the heart" (心外无物，心外无事，心外无理，心外无义，心外无善《王阳明集・与王纯甫》). In his view, the principles (or the Principle) are all rooted in the heart, which is their administrator or manager, and from which they extend to the ten thousand things:

> 心虽主乎一身，而实管乎天下之理，理虽散在万事，而实不外乎一人之心。《王阳明集・传习录中》(Ji 1995, vol. 54: 17)
> Although the heart governs one body, it actually takes charge of all the principles under Heaven. Although the principles scatter in the ten thousand things, they actually exist inside the heart of a single person. *Collected Writings of Wang Yangming: Record of Instructions*, Part II.

Again, apparently, the heart is the very core of the universe. This view accords with Wang Yangming's definition of the relationship between the human and the universe: "Man is the heart of Heaven and Earth" (夫人者，天地之心《王阳明集・传习录中》). That is, in the macrocosm of the universe, the human is the "heart" of Heaven and Earth, whereas Heaven and Earth are but the "body" of the human. This relationship is parallel to the microcosm of man, where the heart is the source of the "divine light".

盖天地万物与人原是一体，其发窍之最精处，是人心一点灵明。《王阳明集・传习录下》(Ji 1995, vol. 54: 43)
Thus, Heaven and Earth and the ten thousand things are harmoniously integrated with man into one body, its finest place of aperture being that one dot of divine light of human heart.[36] *Collected Writings of Wang Yangming: Record of Instructions*, Part III.

Here, the heart is the "one dot of divine light" in the whole universe of which man is an integral part. As the light source of the universe, the heart shines and radiates the light beams of principles to Heaven and Earth and the ten thousand things. Since the heart is the origin of the universe, its state affects the state of the universe. Thus, "the changes of Heaven and Earth and the ten thousand things are all changes of my heart (天地万物之变化皆吾心之变化)" (from Cai 2000: 329). This claim makes good sense within the HEART AS LIGHT SOURCE metaphor: The changes of the light source will change the visual perception of the things in the light of this light source.

2.2.3. The heart as the "ruler" and "master"

As suggested before, the idea that the heart is the thinking and knowing organ and the central faculty of cognition is a basic proposition in ancient Chinese thought, which, needless to say, constitutes a cultural belief. While the heart is literally believed to possess and perform abstract mental functions, it is also seen in some metaphorical uses, for instance, as a "receptacle" for storing information and knowledge or the "residence" of intelligence or wisdom. In this section I will discuss another and more fundamen-

---

36 Two things are worth mentioning here. First, the Chinese word 窍 *qiao* means "hole" or "aperture, orifice" of the body. The ancient Chinese believed that the organ of heart has an aperture or orifice, called 心窍 *xinqiao* 'heart aperture', through which thinking is conducted (see HYDCD 2000: 1129). This compound word also means, metonymically, "capacity for clear thinking" (p. 1128). Since man is conceptualized as the "heart" of the universe, his heart then becomes the "heart aperture" of the universe. Therefore, as in the above sentence, the word 窍 *qiao* 'aperture; orifice' actually refers to man's heart, not the "aperture" of the heart. The second point worth noting is that the compound word 灵明 *lingming* 'divine light' is actually synonymous to 神明 *shenming*, which is translated as "spiritual light" as in the previous context.

tal metaphorical understanding of the heart, namely its roles as the "ruler" and the "master".

In ancient Chinese philosophy the heart is conceptualized literally as "the most valuable part of the self" and, metaphorically, as "the ruler of the other parts" (Slingerland 2003: 229). For example, Xunzi employed the HEART AS RULER or MASTER metaphor when he argued that the heart is the "ruler of the body" and the "master of the spiritual light":

> 心者，形之君也，而神明之主也，出令而无所受令。…… 故口可劫而使墨云，形可劫而使诎申，心不可劫而使易意。是之则受，非之则辞。《荀子·解蔽篇》(Ji 1995, vol. 49: 362)
> The heart is the ruler of the body and master of the spiritual light, who issues commands but does not receive commands. … Thus, the mouth can be forced to be silent or to speak; the body can be forced to crouch down or stretch out, but the heart cannot be forced to change its ideas. It will accept what it thinks is right, and reject what it thinks is wrong. *Xunzi: Dispelling Blindness.*

In this passage, the "spiritual light" (神明 *shenming*), which is also translated as "spirit light" (Wiseman and Feng 1998), "spiritual brightness" (Slingerland 2003), "spiritlike clarity" (Shun 2002), "spiritual intelligence" (Knoblock 1988), "godlike intelligence" (Watson 2003), and "godlike insights" (Cua 2002), refers to the totality of spiritual and mental aspects of a person. It is also a general term for all the supernatural, divine forces in nature (HYDCD 2000: 1835). The fact that it refers to the "invisible half", which operates and manipulates the "visible half", of both nature and man, manifests the claims for the unity and correspondence between nature and man. The image of the heart as a light source certainly fits into the five-element categorization of the heart as the organ of fire and the metaphorical conceptualization of the heart as the sun (see Ch. 3). The heart is the organ that enlightens and warms the whole body. A synonym of 神明 *shenming* is its shortened form 神 *shen*, which means "gods", "deities" or "divinities" in nature, and "spirits" of the human. The human "spirits", manifested in various mental states, processes, and activities, are governed by the heart, the "ruler" of the body. For instance, it is said in the *Wenzi* that "the heart is the master of the body, and the spirits are treasures of the heart" (心者形之主也，神者心之宝也《文子·九守》). That is, the heart, the "master" of the body, controls all "spirits-treasures". According to traditional Chinese medicine, there are five kinds of "spirits" (五神 *wushen*) in a person. They are conceptualized as being controlled and commanded by the heart, but stored separately in the five zang organs (see Ch. 3). The first of the five kinds, which is called "spirit" (神 *shen*), the same name as the general term for all five kinds, is stored in the heart (心藏神 *xin cang shen*). According to Wiseman and Feng (1998: 550), the "Chinese concept of spirit is what normally makes us conscious and alert during the day, what becomes inactive during sleep, and thus corresponds to the concept of the English word 'mind' in the sense of the mental capacity to think, feel, and respond". This "mind" as conceptualized in Chinese, however, lodges in the heart. The heart commands the other parts of the body by controlling all mental states, processes, and activities of a person.

As the "ruler" or "master", the heart has authority over other parts of the body. This authority is illustrated in Xunzi's passage above: Whereas both mouth and heart are parts of the body, the former is commanded by the latter. The mouth acts according to the orders from the heart, but the heart acts of its own will. This kind of sovereign-subject relationship is further brought out by the HEART AS RULER metaphor in the following passage from the *Xunzi*:

> 耳目鼻口形能，各有接而不相能也，夫是之谓天官。心居中虚以治五官，夫是之谓天君。《荀子・天论篇》(Ji 1995, vol. 49: 352)
> Ears, eyes, nose, mouth, and body each have the capacity to provide sense contact, but their capacities are not interchangeable; they are therefore called the heavenly officials/faculties. The heart dwells in the central cavity and governs the five officials/faculties, and hence it is called the heavenly ruler. *Xunzi: On Heaven.*

The heart takes the central position of the body both in the physical and metaphorical senses. It is the supreme leader, the "heavenly ruler", of the "government", regulating and coordinating the functions of other parts or "officials" of the body. The loss of the command from the heart leads to the disfunctionality of other parts: "When the heart is not employed, the eyes will not see black and white right in their front, or the ears will not hear thunders or drums sounding at their side" (心不使焉，则白黑在前而目不见，雷鼓在侧而耳不闻《荀子・解蔽篇》). It is worth mentioning here that the Chinese word 官 *guan* has both bodily and societal meanings that reflect the fundamental view on body and society as microcosm and macrocosm of each other: i.e. "organ" or "faculty", such as sense organs or faculties of eyes and ears, and "official", "officer", or "office" that officials or officers hold. Therefore, 天官 *tianguan* 'heavenly organs or faculties' and 五官 *wuguan* ‘five organs or faculties’ in the above passage can be translated respectively as “heavenly officials” and “five officials”, which instantiate the HEART AS RULER and the BODY AS SOCIETY metaphors.

As the master exponent of the “Learning of the Heart” in the Ming dynasty (1368–1644), Wang Yangming also deployed the HEART AS RULER metaphor and argued that “The heart is the dictator of the body” (心者身之主宰《王阳明集・传习录下》). In his teaching to his disciples, he defined the heart, shown in the following passage, as the locus of the mind that “dictates” the other parts of the body:

> 这视听言动皆是汝心。汝心之视，发窍于目；汝心之听，发窍于耳；汝心之言，发窍于口；汝心之动；发窍于四肢。若无汝心，便无耳目口鼻。所谓汝心，亦不专是那一团血肉。若是那一团血肉，如今已死的人，那一团血肉还在，缘何不能视听言动？所谓汝心，却是那能视听言动的，这个便是性，便是天理。有这个性才能生，这性之生理便谓之仁。这性之生理，发在目便会视，发在耳便会听，发在口便会言，发在四肢便会动，都只是那天理发生，以其主宰一身，故谓之心。这心之本体，原只是个天理，原无非礼，这个便是汝之真已，是躯壳的主宰。若无真已，便无躯壳。真是有之即生，无之即死。《王阳明集・传习录上》(Ji 1995, vol. 54: 15)
> The actions of seeing, hearing, speaking, and moving are all conducted by your heart. Your heart sees through its apertures of eyes, hears through its apertures of ears, speaks through its aperture of mouth, and moves through its command of the four limbs. Without your heart, there would not be ears, eyes, mouth, or nose. The so-called heart does not exclusively refer to that lump of blood and flesh. If it were that lump of blood and flesh, why can’t those people who are dead now, but in whom that lump of blood and flesh is still there, see, hear, speak, or move? The so-called heart is that which can see, hear, speak, and move. It is human nature; it is the Principle of Heaven. Only with this nature can one live. The principle of life of this nature is called benevolence. This principle of life of human nature can see when it reaches the eyes, can hear when it reaches the ears, can speak when it reaches the mouth, can move when it reaches the four limbs. It is all because the Principle of Heaven takes effect. What dictates the whole body with the Principle of Heaven is the heart. The essence of the heart is just the Principle of Heaven, and has nothing indecorous about it. That is your true self, and the dictator of your outer form. Without the true self, there will be no outer form either. The presence of that trueness means life; its absence means death. *Collected Writings of Wang Yangming: Record of Instructions*, Part I.

Two important things distinguish Wang Yangming from his predecessors. First, he assigned a more active role to the heart. Instead of making other parts of the body act, the heart acts itself, with the help of other body parts, which have more of an instrumental role under the absolute control of the heart. In accordance with this view, Wang Yangming used a stronger version of the HEART AS RULER metaphor, namely THE HEART IS THE DICTATOR. A "dictator" (主宰 *zhuzai*) leaves little or no room for initiative on the part of those who are under his ruling. Secondly, Wang Yangming explicitly pointed out that the so-called "heart" is not just that physical organ, the "lump of blood and flesh", which is but the locus of what is called the "mind" in English. The physical organ of heart is nothing but an "outer form" of the mind, as much as the body is merely the "outer form" of the heart. Then what is the "mind"? To Wang Yangming, it is "human nature", that which distinguishes humans from other things or animals. Its "principle of life" is benevolence, the first of the classical virtues put forward by Mencius (see section 2.3). More importantly, this "human nature" is itself the "Principle of Heaven".

2.2.4. The heart as "water" and "mirror"

As seen above, the Chinese *xin* 'heart' is conceptualized metaphorically as the "ruler of the body" and the "master of the spiritual light". Also, the "spirits", the spiritual and mental aspects of the person, are conceptualized metaphorically as "treasures" stored in the heart as a container. Although in these cases metaphor plays an important role, the conception that the heart is the locus of the "mind", however, is a literal belief.

This section discusses the other two metaphors of the heart as the central faculty of cognition, i.e., the HEART AS WATER and the HEART AS MIRROR metaphors. Xunzi used the HEART AS WATER metaphor or analogy to make his point:

> 故人心譬如盘水，正错而勿动，则浑浊在下而清明在上，则足以见须眉而察理矣。微风过之，湛浊动乎下，清明乱于上，则不可以得大形之正也。心亦如是矣。《荀子・解蔽篇》(Ji 1995, vol. 49: 362)
> Hence, the human heart can be compared to a pan of water. If you place the pan on a level and do not stir the water up, the heavy sediment will settle to the bottom, and the water on top will be clear so that you can see your beard and eyebrows and examine the lines on your face. However, if a faint wind passes over the top of the water, the heavy sediment will be stirred up from

the bottom and the clear water will become mingled with it, so that you can no longer get a clear reflection of even a large object. The heart is just the same. *Xunzi: Dispelling Blindness.*

The heart, like water, can reflect things only when it is still and clear. It distorts reality when disturbed and unsettled. The word *qingming* 清明 literally means "clear and bright". As Knoblock (1994: 93) points out, metaphorically, "clear" can mean both "understanding" and "enlightened" whereas "bright" has the extended meanings of "brilliant" and "intelligent". When the heart is still, like still water, it is "clear and bright" and can get a truthful reflection of the external world.

Stillness and emptiness, associated with the heart, are also central concepts in Daoism. Thus Laozi is quoted as saying that "stillness and indifference are the residence of the spiritual light; emptiness and nothingness are the house of the Way" (静漠者神明之宅，虚无者道之所居《文子・九守》). That is, in the stillness of the heart, the spiritual light, namely the mental power, functions at its best; with its emptiness, the heart-container is able to accept the Way with full capacity. In the *Classic of the Yin Signs,* supposedly written by the Yellow Emperor, one line reads:

心欲安静，虑欲深远，心安静则神明荣，虑深远则计谋成。《阴符经・实意》(Ji 1995, vol. 49: 1077)
The heart wants to be tranquil and still, and thinking wants to go deep and far. When the heart is tranquil and still, then the spiritual light will be prosperous; when thinking goes deep and far, then the scheme will be constructed. *Classic of the Yin Signs: Real Intention.*

As can be seen, if the heart is still, the spiritual light will become prosperous, and that is when thinking can go deep and far. The stillness of the heart gives rise to knowing and understanding. This brings us back to the HEART AS WATER metaphor found in the *Xunzi*. It is found in the *Zhuangzi* too:

圣人之静也，非曰静也善，故静也。万物无足以铙心者，故静也。水静则明烛须眉，平中准，大匠取法焉。水静犹明，而况精神！圣人之心静乎，天地之鉴也，万物之镜也。《庄子・天道》(Ji 1995, vol. 49: 37)
The stillness of the sage is such that it is not because it is said that being still is good, he therefore wants to be still. He is still because none of the ten thousand things can ever disturb his heart. When water is still, it clearly re-

> flects the beard and the eyebrows. It gives the accuracy with a level surface, and from it the great master acquires his model. If water thus derives lucidity from stillness, how much more so do the spirits! The heart of the sage is still and, therefore, it is the reflector of Heaven and Earth, and the mirror of the ten thousand things. *Zhuangzi: The Way of Heaven.*

The quality of water is such that when it is still, it has a level surface that can give an accurate reflection of things outside it, like a mirror. The mirror, however, is a man-made object meant to reflect things, with its level and bright surface. Levelness and brightness are necessary conditions and intrinsic characteristics of a mirror. In the *Zhuangzi*, therefore, the HEART AS MIRROR metaphor is also employed to describe the heart of a sage as in the above passage, and of a "perfect man" as in the line below:

> 至人之用心若镜，不将不逆，应而不藏，故能胜物而不伤。《庄子・应帝王》(Ji 1995, vol. 49: 30)
> The heart of the perfect man is used like a mirror. It does not move with things, nor does it move against them. It responds to things, but does not retain them. Therefore, the perfect man can deal successfully with things without being harmed by them. *Zhuangzi: Competent Emperors and Kings.*

While a mirror always remains passive and inactive, it can catch an accurate reflection of the external world. With his heart like a mirror, the sage or perfect man is able to gain insights into things and will not be led astray by them. In so doing, he can manipulate things without being affected by them in any negative way.

When the heart is "still" (心静 *xinjing*), it is "level" (心平 *xinping*). As Laozi said, quoted above, a heart that is "level" will not be confused or tempted by the external things. Similarly, if the heart is "settled" (心定 *xinding*) into stillness (cf. Xunzi's words quoted above), it can extend to Heaven and Earth and connect with the ten thousand things. As is said, "One heart settled into stillness is to rule all under Heaven" and "One heart settled into stillness has sovereignty over the ten thousand things" (一心定而王天下；一心定而万物服《庄子・天道》). Once the heart is "settled", the person can have all under Heaven and the ten thousand things on Earth "housed" in it. Small as it is, the heart connects with the great Way. For that reason, the person who "transcends the distinction between the self and the world" and becomes one with the universe is a sage (Fung 1966: 110). The sage's heart does not worry over anything. With such a state of "mind", or rather "heart", the sage enters a harmonious integration into the processes of Heaven and Earth, and the forces of yin and yang. It may sound esoteric and mysterious, as Daoism itself is perceived to be, but it demonstrates the Daoist belief in a supreme mental state of "settledness", "stillness", and "levelness", which are qualities unified under the HEART AS WATER metaphor, a twin version of the HEART AS MIRROR metaphor. Such a mental state transcends the worldly, encompasses great wisdom, and is the key to true knowing and understanding.

In the Song dynasty, Wang Yangming also used the HEART AS MIRROR metaphor in his exposition of critical function of the heart in cognition. He said:

> 圣人之心如明镜，只是一个明，则随感而应，无物不照，……。只怕镜不明，不怕物来不能照。《王阳明集・传习录上》(Ji 1995, vol. 54: 5)
> The sage's heart is like a clear mirror. It is all about clarity. When it is clear, it will respond and reflect all the things when in interaction with them, … You merely have to worry about the fact that the mirror is not clear, and when it is clear you do not have to worry that it will not reflect things that have come into its sight. *Collected Writings of Wang Yangming: Record of Instructions*, Part I.

Through his teaching, his students came to realize the importance of the clarity of the mirror. As one of his students suggested, the heart is like a mirror: Whereas a sage's heart is a clear mirror, an ordinary man's is a dim one. If the mirror is dim, any effort to reflect things with it is useless. Therefore, an effort should be made to shine the mirror instead. Once the mirror is clear, it will produce sharp and accurate images of everything it reflects. The metaphor used highlights the importance of "rectification of the heart" in knowing and understanding the external world. As Chan (1963: 655) points out, Wang Yangming's approach is "moral" rather than "intellectual" like that of Zhu Xi. His whole emphasis was on moral values. He was convinced that if the heart-mind "is divided or devoted to external things, it will be concerned only with fragmentary details and will lack the essentials" (Chan 1963: 655–656). This moral function of the heart is further explored in the next section.

2.3. The heart as the locus of moral sense

In ancient Chinese philosophy, the heart is also conceived of as the locus of one's moral sense and moral character. It is worth noting that this aspect of the "heart" conceptualization is closely related to the cultural belief that the heart is the "residence" and "governor" of the "spiritual light" or, in more general terms, the locus of the "mind", as discussed in the previous section. Since the heart is the thinking and reasoning organ, it is equipped with the mental power necessary to make a rational evaluation of one's behavior in accordance with one's moral norms and values. It is therefore believed that the heart is the locus of one's moral sense and character. In metaphorical terms, the heart as a "mirror" is capable of reflecting and self-reflecting when making a moral judgment on what is right or wrong. As the "ruler" the heart has the authority to determine the moral direction for the person to follow.

In the Chinese language, the word for "morality" and "ethics" is 道德 *daode*, which literally means the "Way and Virtue". That is, people are moral and ethical if they follow the Way and uphold the Virtue. The title of the famous Daoist text, Laozi's *Daode Jing* (《道德经》), literally means the "Classic of the Way and the Virtue". It is also the classic of morality or ethics. Laozi accounted for the difference between the moral and the immoral in terms of "qi" and "heart". As quoted in the *Wenzi*, he related one's moral sense to the Way and the Virtue, as physically manifested in the qi, the gaseous vital force inside the body, which originates in the heart:

> 老子曰：人有顺逆之气生于心，心治则气顺，心乱则气逆。心之治乱在于道德，得道则心治，失道则心乱。心治即交让，心乱即交争，让则有德，争则生贼。有德即气顺，贼生即气逆，气顺则自损以奉人，气逆则损人以自奉。《文子・符言》(Ji 1995, vol. 49: 87)
>
> Laozi said: People have both "downstream" qi and "upstream" qi, which originate from the heart. If the heart is in order, qi will go with the current; if the heart is in disorder, qi will go against the current. The order and disorder in the heart depend on the Way and the Virtue. Those who obtain the Way will have their heart in order; those who lose the Way will have their heart in disorder. Those whose hearts are in order yield to each other; those whose hearts are in disorder contend against each other. Those who yield have the Virtue, and those who contend become evil. Having the Virtue makes qi move with the current, and becoming evil makes qi go against the current. If qi moves downstream, one will attend to others at the expense of oneself; if qi moves upstream, one will harm others to benefit oneself. *Wenzi: Magic Words.*

Thus, the regulation of qi, whose behavior manifests virtue or evil, depends on the regulation of the heart, which in turn depends on the connection between the heart and the Way.

As the "ruler" of the body, the heart is the organ that makes moral judgments. It dominates the sense organs of the body, and oversees their functions and behaviors from the height of moral diagnosis. It has the authority to deny what it sees as improper assessments of the individual sense organs, and stop them from acting inappropriately. The heart's moral authority is illustrated in the following statement by Shizi (c. 390–330 BC), a well-known Eclectic philosopher of the Warring States period (475–221 BC) who borrowed extensively from both Daoism and Confucianism:

> 目之所美，心以为不义，弗敢视也；口之所甘，心以为不义，弗敢食也；耳之所乐，心以为不义，弗敢听也；身之所安，心以为不义，弗敢服也。《尸子・贵言》(Ji 1995, vol. 49: 1085)
> If the heart believes that it is not righteous to do so, the eyes should not dare to see what looks beautiful, the mouth should not dare to eat what tastes delicious, the ears should not dare to hear what sounds delightful, and the body should not dare to do what seems pleasurable. *Shizi: Valuable Words.*

The heart, as the ruler of the body, bears great moral responsibility as it makes moral judgments and issues authoritative commands.

> 然则令于天下而行，禁焉而止者，心也。故曰：心者，身之君也。天子以天下受令于心，心不当则天下祸；诸侯以国受令于心，心不当则国亡；匹夫以身受令于心，心不当则身为戮矣。《尸子・贵言》(Ji 1995, vol. 49: 1085)
> Therefore, the heart is what issues, under Heaven, orders to be implemented or bans to be imposed. That is, as is said, the heart is the ruler of the body. The Son of Heaven receives commands from the heart on behalf of all under Heaven. If the heart is not right, then all under Heaven will suffer from disasters. Princes or dukes receive commands from the heart on behalf of their state. If the heart is not right, then their state will perish. Ordinary people receive commands from the heart on behalf of themselves. If the heart is not right, then they themselves will be punished.[37] *Shizi: Valuable Words.*

---

[37] The Chinese word 身 *shen* can mean both "body" and "self". The latter is adopted in the English translation, but the former seems to make good sense in the context too. That is, "Ordinary people receive commands from the heart on behalf of their body. If their heart is not right, then their body will be punished".

As can be seen, all the people, up from the monarch down to commoners, rely on the heart, the command-issuing organ, for moral direction. There will be dire consequences if their hearts make wrong judgments.

Ancient Chinese philosophy seems to have attributed immorality mainly to desires and emotions, both located in the heart. This is because, apparently, both desires and emotions interfere with rational thinking, reasoning, and for that matter one's moral sense, which are all localized in the heart too. In the following two subsections (2.3.1 and 2.3.2), I will discuss remarks on desires and emotions by ancient philosophers. It will be shown that Daoism and Confucianism are differentiated by their views on emotions: Daoism believes that all emotions lead to interference with one's moral sense; Confucianism, instead, only regards negative emotions as interfering with one's moral judgment. In 2.3.3, I will focus on two opposing views on human nature as related to morality, held by Mencius and Xunzi, the two leading Confucian philosophers during the Warring States period (475–221 BC). I will then turn to the views of Neo-Confucians in the Song (960–1279) and Ming (1368–1644) dynasties. It will become apparent that Mencius' view on human nature and morality exerted greater influence on Neo-Confucianism, and this influence has extended to the present day.

2.3.1. Desires in the heart and immorality

According to ancient Chinese thought, evil arises from desires, which will deprive people of their senses, and of the function of the heart that controls the senses. Laozi, for instance, advocated restraining desires aroused by external temptations stimulating one's sense organs, because, as he put it in the *Laozi* or *Daode Jing*: "The five colors blind the eyes; the five notes deafen the ears; the five flavors dull the taste;[38] and racing, chasing, and hunting drive people's hearts crazy" (五色令人目盲，五音令人耳聋，五味令人口爽，驰骋田猎令人心发狂《老子・检欲第十二》). While bodily desires impair all the sense organs, the key is that they make the heart lose its thinking power: "Many desires make the heart loose; the heart be-

[38] In this example of Laozi, the "five colors", "five (sound) notes", and "five flavors" are again instantiations of the five-element schema with which the universe is classified. Other examples include five sense organs, five grains, five atmospheric conditions, five metals, five virtues, five feelings, five social relations, etc.

ing loose makes the will weak; and the will being weak makes thinking obstructed" (多欲则心散，心散则志衰，志衰则思不达也《阴符经・养志》). That is, the heart distracted by too many desires will lose its focus and will, and one's thinking will also lose its power and will "reach nowhere" (不达 *buda*). Apparently, the moral aspect of the heart will affect its mental aspect. That is why Laozi said that desires will "drive the heart crazy". They interfere with the workings of the heart and drag it away from functioning properly.

As the ruler of the body, the heart that is affected by desires will lose its command of, and control over, other parts of the body. Thus, "when the heart has desires, things passing across the eyes will not be seen, and sounds coming to the ears will not be heard" (夫心有欲者，物过而目不见，声至而耳不闻也《管子・心术上》). The use of the HEART AS RULER metaphor in the *Guanzi* makes the point clearer:

> 心之在体，君之位也；九窍之有职，官之分也。心处其道，九窍循理；嗜欲充益，目不见色，耳不闻声。故曰：上离其道，下失其事。《管子・心术上》(Ji 1995, vol. 49: 783)
> The heart holds the position of the monarch in the body. The functions of the nine apertures are the separate responsibilities of officials. If the heart follows the Way, the nine apertures will perform their functions properly. Should sensual desires occupy it to the full, the eyes will not see colors, nor will the ears hear sounds. Therefore, it is said, if the supreme one above departs from the Way, those below will lose their functions accordingly. *Guanzi: Art of the Heart*, Part I.

When the monarch above, i.e. the heart, is filled with desires, the officials below, i.e. the organs such as eyes and ears, will not be able to perform their functions properly. As a matter of fact, the same is also true if the metaphor is taken literally, that is, as if the passage were addressing the government of a country. Remember that the Daoist view is that a body is a microcosm of a state. In fact, Laozi, in his *Daode Jing*, advised that restraining desires is the key to the governance of a country, as much as it is the key to the maintenance of morality and ethics on the individual basis. He proposed to do it by all means, even though it may appear to be quite negative:

> 不尚贤，使民不争。不贵难得之货，使民不为盗。不见可欲，使心不乱。是以圣人治，虚其心，实其腹，弱其志，强其骨，常使民无知无

> 欲；使夫知者不敢为也。为无为，则无不治。《老子·安民第三》(Ji 1995, vol. 49: 3)
> Not praising the meritorious keeps people from competing. Not prizing rare treasures keeps people from stealing. Not seeing the desirable keeps the heart in order. Therefore, the sage who governs people would empty their hearts, fill their stomachs, weaken their will, and strengthen their bones, which often keeps them from knowing or desiring, and keeps those who do know from daring to do anything. Do not-doing, and nothing will be out of order. *Laozi: Chapter 3 Pacifying the People.*

Thus, Laozi's way of pacifying the people is to keep them from seeing the desirable and from desiring to attain them. That is, to pacify the people one needs first to pacify their hearts. The order is achieved in making the people do nothing. Two things are worth noting here. First, as Le Guin (1998: 6) points out, Laozi's concept of "doing not-doing" or "action by inaction", though seemingly not susceptible to logical interpretation, is "a concept that transforms thought radically", of which the whole book of *Daode Jing* is an explanation and demonstration. Second, as Fung (1966) points out, there is a fundamental difference between Confucianism and Daoism in terms of what the sage-ruler should do to govern the country. According to the Confucians, a sage-ruler should try to do many things for the people, whereas according to the Daoists, the duty of the sage-ruler is not to do things, but rather to undo or not to do at all. The reason for this, according to Laozi, is that "the troubles of the world come, not because there are many things not yet done, but because too many things are done" (p. 102). That is to say, in effect, Laozi's philosophy "is not for the hermit, but for the sage-ruler, who does not desert the world but rules it with noninterference". Daoism "is therefore not a philosophy of withdrawal. Man is to follow Nature but in doing so he is not eliminated; instead, his nature is fulfilled" (Chan 1963: 137).

In Confucianism, desires are also seen as sources of evil. In the *Analects*, for instance, Confucius said that it was only after he turned seventy years old that he could follow what his heart desired without transgressing what was right (七十而从心所欲，不逾矩《论语》). To uphold morality and virtue, according to his teaching, one should practice the cultivation of the self, which should proceed from the rectification of the heart: "One who wishes to cultivate the self must first rectify the heart" (欲修其身者，先正其心《大学》). Why should this be so? The reason is that the heart is the seat of desires, as well as of emotions, which are regarded as negative, especially when they are excessive. In cultivating themselves, according to

Xunzi, people should do whatever will enhance peace in the heart and add to the virtue of righteousness, even though it means much labor for their body and little profit for themselves (身劳而心安，为之；利少而义多，为之《荀子・修身篇》). "Those who put righteousness before profit are honorable; those who put profit before righteousness are disgraceful" (先义而后利者荣，先利而后义者辱《荀子・荣辱篇》).

2.3.2. Emotions in the heart and immorality

In Daoism, it seems, all emotions, negative or positive, are perceived as being evil or astray from the Way and the Virtue. For instance, it is said in the *Zhuangzi*:

> 悲乐者，德之邪。喜怒者，道之过。好恶者，德之失。故心不忧乐，德之至也。《庄子・刻意》(Ji 1995, vol. 49: 41)
> Sorrow and joy are deviations from the Virtue; happiness and anger are violations of the Way; and likes and dislikes lead to the loss of the Virtue. Thus, if the heart is unconscious of sadness or happiness, that is the perfection of the Virtue. *Zhuangzi: Self-Conceit.*

The Daoists wanted "to disperse emotion with reason" (Fung 1966: 108). They maintained that the sage has no emotions because he has a complete understanding of the nature of things. This, however, does not mean that he lacks sensibility; rather it means that he is not disturbed by the emotions, and enjoys what may be called "the peace of the soul" (p. 109). The Daoist doctrine seems to seek absolute "settledness", "stillness", and "levelness" of the heart. Anything that may disturb the heart is evil.

In contrast, Confucianism seems to be mainly on guard against negative or excessive emotions. After all, to Confucians, only negative and excessive emotions disturb the heart in a real sense. Thus, according to Confucius' teaching, negative emotions and desires, if unsuppressed, will make rectification of the heart impossible, as is explained in the *Great Learning*:

> 所谓修身在正其心者，身有所忿懥，则不得其正；有所恐惧，则不得其正；有所好乐，则不得其正；有所忧患，则不得其正。心不在焉，视而不见，听而不闻，食而不知其味。此谓修身在正其心。《大学》(He and He 1992: 12)
> That self-cultivation depends on rectification of the heart means that rectification of the heart is impossible if one is burning with anger, or trembling

> with fear, or given to addiction and pleasure, or laden with sorrow and distress. When the heart is not present, one looks but does not see, listens but does not hear, and eats but does not know the taste. This is what is meant by saying that self-cultivation depends on rectification of the heart. *The Great Learning*.

One has to rectify the heart, which means to rid the heart of its negative emotions and desires, before one can cultivate the self. This is because when the heart-ruler above is "crooked" or "deformed", all the organs-officials below will lose their functions as a result. If the heart is not "upright" or "straight", it cannot rule the self properly; instead, it will only lead the self astray. That is to say, no self-cultivation is ever possible under the wrong leadership of the heart.

Xunzi also argued that the heart, as the seat of emotions, is subject to the impact of both positive and negative emotions. When this happens, the heart will pass the emotional impact to other parts of the body accordingly and, as a result, affect the function of the body and its interaction with the external world:

> 心忧恐则口衔刍豢而不知其味，耳听钟鼓而不知其声，目视黼黻而不知其状，轻暖平簟而体不知其安。…… 心平愉，则色不及庸而可以养目，声不及庸而可以养耳，蔬食菜羹而可以养口，粗布之衣、粗紃之履而可以养体，屋室、庐庾、葭槁蓐、尚机筵而可以养形。《荀子・正名篇》(Ji 1995, vol. 49: 365)
> If the heart is anxious or fearful, then although the mouth is filled with fine meats, it will not be aware of their taste. Although the ear hears bells and drums, it will not be aware of their sound. Although the eye beholds fine embroidered patterns, it will not be aware of their appearance. And although the body is clothed in warm, light garments and rests on a fine bamboo mat, it will not be aware of their comfort. … If the heart is serene (lit. level) and happy, then colors that are less than mediocre can nurture the eye. Sounds that are less than average can nurture the ear. A diet of vegetables and a broth of greens can nurture the mouth. Robes of coarse cloth and shoes of rough hemp can nurture the body. And a cramped room, reed blinds, a bed of dried straw, plus a stool and mat can nurture the bodily form. *Xunzi: Rectifying Names.*

That is why Xunzi attached great importance to "the art of controlling the qi and nourishing the heart" (治气养心之术), which he saw as an essential aspect of the cultivation of the self. This is because, in traditional Chinese culture, emotions are conceived of as various behaviors of qi, and as being centrally regulated by the heart (see Ch. 3). In nurturing the heart, gentlemen should be sincere (君子养心莫善于诚《荀子・不苟篇》). If they have a "sincere heart" (诚心 *chengxin*), they will try to maintain benevolence and serve righteousness. With good practice and right principle, they will gain in their heart spirituality (神 *shen*) and clarity (明 *ming*), the qualities of "spiritual light" (神明 *shenming*), which will make all the difference.

2.3.3. Human nature in the heart: Innately good or bad?

Mencius, who lived in "a period of political struggle, moral chaos, and intellectual conflicts" (Chan 1963: 49), proposed his own theory of morality, which has been seen as a great contribution to Confucianism. He argued that human nature is innately good. Specifically, he posited that the heart is an organ of moral direction, serving as the behavior-guiding mechanism, which distinguishes between right and wrong, between good and bad, and thus guides action, conduct, and behavior. He believed that moral character is rooted in the heart and consists of "four seeds", which under appropriate cultivation will grow and blossom into the four classical virtues. These four virtues will together make up a mature moral character (Hansen 1992: 20, 162–164). In his words:

> 恻隐之心，仁之端也；羞耻之心，义之端也；辞让之心，礼之端也；是非之心，智之端也。人之有是四端也，犹其有四体也。《孟子・公孙丑上》(Zheng et al. 1993: 114)
> The heart of compassion is the seed of benevolence; the heart of shame is the seed of righteousness; the heart of modesty is the seed of propriety; the heart of right and wrong is the seed of wisdom. Humans possess these four seeds just as they possess four limbs.[39] *Mencius: Gongsun Chou,* Part I.

[39] In the English translation, "heart", as in the "heart of compassion", etc., is the more literal translation of the Chinese *xin* 'heart', which could have been translated as "sense" or "feeling" as well. Note that the heart is conceptualized as a container or an object, while the "four seeds" and the "four virtues" are conceptualized as the contents inside the container or elements that compose the object. Here, therefore, the use of "heart" is metonymic, namely, CONTAINER FOR CONTAINED or WHOLE FOR PART.

In Mencius' view, therefore, the "four seeds" are innate, as much as human beings are born with their four limbs. Furthermore, he argued that the four classical virtues, which grow out of the four seeds, are also innate in the sense that their "seeds" are intrinsic:

> 仁义礼智，非由外铄我也，我固有之也，弗思耳矣，故曰："求则得之，舍则失之"。《孟子·告子上》(Zheng et al. 1993: 400)
> Benevolence, righteousness, propriety, and wisdom are not infused into us from outside; they are in our essence. Only we are not aware of them in us. Hence the saying: "Seek and you will find them; neglect and you will lose them". *Mencius: Gaozi,* Part I.

The heart, as the locus of moral character, is the center of the body. However, it still shares with other parts of the body some characteristics that define human beings. Mencius explored this relationship in his reasoning and teaching about the heart:

> 口之于味也，有同嗜焉；耳之于声也，有同听焉；目之于色有同美焉。至于心，独无所同然乎？心之所同然者何也？谓理也，义也。《孟子·告子上》(Zheng et al. 1993: 404)
> All mouths have the same preference in taste; all ears have the same preference in sound; all eyes have the same preference in beauty. Are hearts an exception to this general rule? What is common to all hearts are principle and righteousness. *Mencius: Gaozi,* Part I.

As argued in this passage, all humans have similar preferences in taste, and have similar likings in appreciation of sound and beauty. In a similar fashion, all humans have something in common in their hearts: principle and righteousness. To Mencius, this commonality among all human hearts defines human nature. Because humans have principle and righteousness deeply rooted in their heart, it is possible for them to restrain the growth of desires that lead to immorality. Although humans also have "lower instincts", the elements that humans share in common with other living creatures, these elements "represent the 'animal' aspect" of human life, "and therefore, strictly speaking, should not be considered as part of the 'human' nature" (Fung 1966: 69).

As Hansen (1992: 164) points out, the novelty of Mencius' view lies in the claim of innateness of the moral dispositions in the heart. That is, the heart comes with all the internal dispositions to moral behavior innate in its own structure. The innate dispositions grow and flower like a seed. Socialization will either reinforce or interfere with what is already there. Thus, the heart has predispositions toward goodness, and being ethical is a matter of preserving the predispositions of the heart (Shun 1997). The essential practice is to cleanse the heart and reduce the number of desires, and to preserve the heart and cultivate human nature (清心寡欲，存心养性). To resist attractions of selfish desires one should have an "unmoved heart" (不动心 *budong xin*) and a "constant heart" (恒心 *hengxin*), which both represent mental control and maturity (see also Shun 1997; Chan 2002b, 2002c; Cua 2002). While Mencius knew that many selfish desires would lead to immoral behavior, he also understood that humans could not completely do without material possessions and, for that matter, desires. Therefore, he taught people to reduce rather than eliminate desires. He advised, "For the nurturing of the heart there is nothing better than to reduce the number of desires" (养心莫善于寡欲《孟子·尽心下》). Apparently, this view is different from Xunzi's view that the best way for a gentleman to nurture the heart is to be sincere.

Mencius argued that "great people" know how important it is to "preserve the heart" (存心 *cunxin*). By preserving one's own heart, one promotes mutual love and respect in society:

> 君子所以异于人者，以其存心也。君子以仁存心，以礼存心。仁者爱人，有礼者敬人。爱人者，人恒爱之；敬人者，人恒敬之。《孟子·离娄下》(Zheng et al. 1993: 300)
> A gentleman differs from ordinary people in that he preserves his heart. He preserves his heart with benevolence, and with propriety. A man of benevolence loves others; a man of propriety respects others. One who loves others is always loved by others; one who respects others is always respected by others. *Mencius: Li Lou,* Part II.

That is, a gentleman is distinguished from ordinary people in that he has classical virtues of benevolence and propriety stored in his heart, which he tries to preserve. Virtuous people love and respect others and, in return, they are loved and respected by others. This is how an ideal society can be established, but it originates in a gentleman's heart, in which the four classical virtues are rooted, and from which energy and vitality are radiated to the whole body:

> 君子所性，仁义礼智根于心，其生色也睟然，见于面，盎于背，施于四体，四体不言而喻。《孟子·尽心上》(Zheng et al. 1993: 480)
> The nature of a gentleman lies in the fact that benevolence, righteousness, propriety and wisdom are deeply rooted in his heart, manifested in his mild,

> gentle looks and manners, shown on his face, presented by his back, and expressed by his four limbs, which can convey the message without the use of language. *Mencius: Exhausting the Heart,* Part I.

As we can see, the heart is truly a central organ of the body, which it commands. A different heart is manifested in a different body, its looks and manners, with messages conveyed without the use of language. Mencius attached prime importance to the cultivation of his "floodlike qi" (浩然之气 *haoran zhi qi*), the vast and indomitable vital energy that fills the body and interacts with the heart (see also Chan 2002c; Fung 1966; Heng 2002; Slingerland 2003). If nourished with steady accumulation of righteousness, this energy can be omnipresent, pervading all between Heaven and Earth and integrated with the Way.

Although the heart has a predisposition toward goodness, it does not mean that it can remain morally healthy regardless of circumstances. It may also catch diseases that are not of a physical nature, as explained by Mencius, who would proceed from bodily experiences in his account:

> 饥者甘食，渴者甘饮，是未得饮食之正也，饥渴害之也。岂惟口腹有饥渴之害？人心亦皆有害，人能无以饥渴之害为心害，则不及人不为忧矣。《孟子・尽心上》(Zheng et al. 1993: 488)
> Any food tastes delicious when one is hungry, and any drink tastes sweet when one is thirsty. One's mouth fails to taste the real flavor of food and drink because it has been harmed by hunger and thirst. Are mouth and belly the only parts subject to harm by hunger and thirst? So is the heart. If a man can keep his heart from being harmed by hunger and thirst, then he does not have to worry about failing to keep pace with others. *Mencius: Exhausting the Heart,* Part I.

Just as the mouth cannot get the right taste of food and drink due to hunger and thirst, the heart cannot think and reason right if it lacks proper nutrition from education. This claim fits well into the PLANT metaphor. Seeds have the potential of growing into plants, but they will not sprout without, say, air, water and sunlight. The heart will not be able to serve as the organ of moral direction if it is "crooked" for not being "preserved" in its right form and constitution. Since, to Mencius, the heart guides behavior and conduct, and is the center and root of a society, he set for himself the task of "rectifying (or straightening) people's hearts" (正人心 *zheng renxin*).

As Hansen (1992: 174–179) has discussed, Mencius used a PLANT metaphor for the cultivation of the heart-mind. Selfish desires, which are motivations of the other organs of the body, are weeds that grow together with the virtues rooted in the heart. If we ignore desires-weeds, they will weaken, shrivel, and die while the heart grows. Conversely, if we cater to the bodily desires for food, sex, and leisure, they get the nourishment and the sprouts of the heart withers. Every time we follow a moral intuition rather than a bodily desire, we strengthen our heart against the weeds and vice versa. Unfortunately, many people do not really cultivate their hearts, by choice or not, and they are instead interested only in material possessions, out of their selfish desires. In Mencius' words, these people have lost their hearts of benevolence:

> 仁，人心也；义，人路也。舍其路而弗由，放其心而不知求，哀哉！人有鸡犬放，则知求之；有放心而不知求。学问之道无他，求其放心而已矣。《孟子·告子上》(Zheng et al. 1993: 414)
> Benevolence is the human heart; righteousness is the human road. It is sad if people do not go on the road of righteousness or seek to recover the lost heart of benevolence! When their chickens or dogs are missing, people will look for them; but when their heart is missing, they will not try to seek it back. The pursuit of learning is nothing but to recover this lost heart. *Mencius: Gaozi,* Part I.

In this passage, benevolence, the first of the four classical virtues and the core concept of Confucian and Mencian thought, is seen as the heart itself while righteousness, the second virtue, is conceived of as the road of one's life journey. Thus, those who do not uphold the virtue of righteousness are those who have departed from their road of life and are going nowhere in their life. It is similarly sad that those who have lost their heart of benevolence do not want to seek it back whereas they want to recover their material possessions. To Mencius, the purpose of learning and education is nothing but to seek the lost heart back. Only after people regain their possession of the heart can they preserve it and make use of it.

To illustrate his point that "petty people" value the body over the heart, Mencius used an example of a person whose ring finger was crooked and could not stretch straight. Though it caused no pain, nor any inconvenience in his work, he would not hesitate to travel all the way from the state of Qin to the state of Chu to seek its treatment, simply because he could not bear to have his finger inferior to other people's. "When his finger is inferior to other people's, he is displeased; yet when his heart is inferior to other people's, he is not displeased at all. This is what is called making no distinction between the minor and the major" (指不若人，则知恶之；心不若人，则不知恶，此之谓不知类也《孟子・告子上》).

Although Mencius and Xunzi were both representative thinkers of Confucianism, they had a fundamental difference. Xunzi attacked Mencius' view of the innateness of good human nature. Instead, he argued that man's nature is evil, although "he can be reformed by education and the effects of acculturation" (Knoblock 1994: 139). His thesis is that "the nature of man is evil" and his goodness is acquired by training (Fung 1966: 145). According to him, nature is the unwrought material, only to be refined by culture. "Without nature there would be nothing upon which to add the acquired. Without the acquired, nature could not become beautiful of itself" (p. 145). Thus, training is especially important to Xunzi. "If a man lacks a teacher and the model, then his heart will be just like his mouth and stomach" (人无师无法，则其心正其口腹也《荀子・荣辱篇》). A gentleman, he asserted, "should explain his ideas to others with a benevolent heart, listen to others with a learning heart, and make his judgments with a fair heart" (以仁心说，以学心听，以公心辨《荀子・正名篇》). He should train himself against the evil and toward the good, as related in the following passage:

> 使目非是无欲见也，使耳非是无欲闻也，使口非是无欲言也，使心非是无欲虑也。及至其致好之也，目好之五色，耳好之五声，口好之五味，心利之有天下。《荀子・劝学篇》(Ji 1995, vol. 49: 320)
> He trains his eyes so that they desire only to see what is right, his ears so that they desire to hear only what is right, his mouth so that it desires to speak only what is right, and his heart so that it thinks only what is right. When he has reached the limit of such perfection, he finds delight in it. His eyes then find greater enjoyment in the five colors, his ears in the five sounds, his mouth in the five tastes, and his heart benefits from possessing all that is under Heaven. *Xunzi: Encouraging Learning.*

From this passage we can see that, while all other organs of the body carry out very specific functions in their division of labor, the heart, the central mechanism of cognition, reflects and understands the whole world.

Regarding human nature, Xunzi argued that "everything that is good and valuable is the product of human effort" (Fung 1966: 144). "Value comes from culture and culture is the achievement of man" (p. 144). With and without training, a gentleman and a petty man differ in their heart, the locus of moral character. Although both of them may have a heart of the same size, a "big heart" (大心 *daxin*) or a "small heart" (小心 *xiaoxin*), the content inside distinguishes between them:

> 君子，小人之反也。君子大心则敬天而道，小心则畏义而节。…… 小人则不然，大心则慢而暴，小心则淫而倾。《荀子·不苟篇》(Ji 1995, vol. 49: 322)
> The gentleman is the opposite of the petty man. When the gentleman is bold of heart (lit. big-hearted), he reveres Heaven and follows its Way. When faint of heart (lit. small-hearted), he is awe-inspired by his sense of moral duty and regulates his conduct to accord with it. … The petty man does not behave in this way. When he is bold of heart (lit. big-hearted), he is haughty and irritable. When faint of heart (lit. small-hearted), he is wicked and crooked. *Xunzi: Nothing Indecorous.*

In classic Chinese, "being big-hearted" (大心 *daxin*) has two very different meanings, one complimentary and the other derogatory. In its positive sense, it means "having lofty aspirations" or "cherishing high ambitions"; in its negative sense, however, it means "being arrogant, haughty, and self-important" (HYDCD 2000: 739). This is also true of "being small-hearted" (小心 *xiaoxin*). It can mean both "being careful, cautious" and "being petty, narrow-minded" (p. 774). The differences in meaning characterize well the differences in moral character between a gentleman and a petty man. Basically, it is not the size or capacity of the heart-container, but the content inside, that makes the difference.

What is distinctive of Xunzi is his view that desires come from human nature received at birth. He tried to prove that "man is born with an inherent desire for profit and sensual pleasure" (Fung 1966: 145). "It is human nature", he argued, "that people want to eat their fill when hungry, keep warm when cold, and take a rest when tired" (饥而欲饱，寒而欲暖，劳而欲休，此人之情性也《荀子·性恶篇》). This also comes to the fore in his words:

> 若夫目好色，耳好声，口好味，心好利，骨体肤理好愉佚，是皆生于人之性情者也，感到自然，不待事而后生之者也。《荀子·性恶篇》(Ji 1995, vol. 49: 366)
> Phenomena such as the eye's fondness of colors, the ear's fondness of sounds, the mouth's fondness of tastes, the heart's fondness of profits, and the body's fondness of pleasure and ease – all these are products of man's essential and inborn nature. They are instinctive and spontaneous. People do not have to do anything to produce them. *Xunzi: Man's Nature Is Evil.*

In his view, desires are common to all people: sage-kings or tyrant-emperors, gentlemen or petty men. However, they can be controlled and moderated by the heart, the behavior-guiding mechanism, as explained in the following passage:

> 故欲过之而动不及，心止之也。心之所可中理，则欲虽多，奚伤于治！欲不及而动过之，心使之也。心之所可失理，则欲虽寡，奚止于乱！故治乱在于心之所可，亡于情之所欲。《荀子·正名篇》(Ji 1995, vol. 49: 365)
>
> Therefore, when desires run to excess, actions do not follow to that point because the heart stops them short. If what the heart permits coincides with the principle, then although the desires are manifold, how could they do harm to order! Conversely, even though desires are not running far, actions may exceed the desires because the heart orders them to do so. If what the heart permits conflicts with the principle, then although the desires are few, how could they stop disorder! Therefore, order or disorder depends on what the heart permits, and not on the desires of the emotional nature. *Xunzi: Rectifying Names.*

As Xunzi argued in this passage, actions are not directed by desires, but by the heart. What really matters is whether or not the heart holds to the principle. People do not have to try to reduce the number of desires because, to him, having desires means life whereas lack of desires means death, and their contrast has nothing to do with order or disorder (有欲无欲，异类也，生死也，非治乱也《荀子·正名篇》). What really is important is nurturing or nourishing the heart with good education so that it gets to know and understand the Way. That is what he meant when he asserted that "Man's nature is evil; his goodness is acquired through conscious effort" (人之性恶，其善者伪也《荀子·性恶篇》).

This view sets Xunzi apart from Mencius, who asserted the innate goodness of human nature and the reduction of the number of desires in the first place. In the final analysis, however, Mencius and Xunzi's positions are not far apart from each other, as noted by many scholars (see, e.g., Cai 2000: 85; Knoblock 1994: 139–150). For Mencius, man's nature is good, but can be smothered by desires, which should be reduced via good education so as to keep the heart good. For Xunzi, conversely, man's nature is evil, but desires can be regulated by a heart of goodness acquired via good education. That is, they started from the opposite ends but ended up meeting in the middle. As Wang Yangming of the Ming dynasty suggested, "Goodness and evil are just one thing" (善恶只是一物《王阳明集·传习

录中》). While believing that goodness is the essence of the heart, he argued that it could change into evil when fluctuating out of the appropriate degree of being good. It is just a matter of degree in quantity.

2.3.4. Morality and the "Learning of the Heart"

From a historical point of view, Xunzi "exerted far greater influence up through the Han period (206 BC–AD 220) than did Mencius" because "both psychology and logic advanced greatly in him, but not in Mencius" (Chan 1963: 115). After the Han period, however, Mencius was regarded as being in the direct line of transmission from Confucius, probably because Xunzi was too "tough-minded" for the Chinese, who preferred "tender-minded" Mencius (Chan 1963: 115). For our specific interest here, it seems that Mencius' view on morality and human nature has been more influential than Xunzi's. It was accepted and adopted as the orthodox Confucian doctrines by most Confucian scholars later in time. One such example is Lu Jiuyuan, a representative exponent of the "Learning of the Heart" of the Song dynasty, who explicated Mencius' view that the best way to nurture one's heart is to reduce the number of one's desires. He started by saying:

> 将以保吾心之良，必有以去吾心之害。何者？吾心之良，吾所固有也。吾所固有，而不能以自保者，以其有以害之也。有以害之，而不知所以去其害，则良心何自而存哉？
> To protect the goodness of our heart we must remove the harm from our heart. What does that mean? The goodness of our heart is what we possess intrinsically. Although we intrinsically have goodness, we cannot protect it because there is something that harms it. When something is harming the goodness yet we do not know how to get rid of it, then how is it possible for the good heart to preserve itself?

As we can see, following Mencius, Lu Jiuyuan claimed that the heart possesses goodness intrinsically although the "good heart" (i.e. conscience) may not be necessarily preserved simply because people do not know how to protect it from being harmed. He continued:

> 故欲良心之存者，莫若去吾心之害。吾心之害既去，则心有不期存而自存者矣。夫所以害吾心者何也？欲也。
> Therefore, to preserve the good heart there is nothing better than to remove the harm from our heart. Once the harm in our heart is removed, our heart

> will preserve itself without being expected to do so. Then what is the thing that harms our heart? It is desire.

Here, Lu Jiuyuan made it clear that desires are the thing that harms the goodness of the heart. Thus, the best way to preserve the "good heart" is to rid it of the harm – the desires. This is because of the following:

> 欲之多，则心之存者必寡，欲之寡，则心之存者必多。故君子不患夫心之不存，而患夫欲之不寡，欲去则心自存矣。然则所以保吾心之良者，岂不在于去吾心之害乎？《陆九渊集・拾遗》(Ji 1995, vol. 50: 2365)
>
> If there are many desires, then what the heart preserves must be few. If there are few desires, then what the heart preserves must be many. Therefore, the gentleman is not afraid that the heart is not preserved, but that the desires are not few. Once the desires are gone, the heart will preserve itself. Thus, is it not the case that the protection of the goodness of our heart lies in the removal of the harm from our heart? *Collected Writings of Lu Jiuyuan: Supplementary Amplifications.*

Lu Jiuyuan's reasoning is simple and clear. The heart as a container has a fixed capacity. If the storage for one thing goes up, the room for the other has to go down. Besides, if something rotten is stored in the same place as the good thing, it will change the quality of the good thing and make it go bad. Furthermore, since the heart can preserve itself if the harm of desires is removed, reducing the number of desires is thus the best way to nourish the heart and preserve its goodness. This view, of course, does not accord with Xunzi's. According to Xunzi, the heart stores desires in the first place, and a strong heart "contains" them with proper control and moderation.

Wang Yangming, the master exponent of the "Learning of the Heart" of the Ming dynasty, also held a view similar to that of Lu Jiuyuan in this regard. He said, "The heart governs the body, human nature resides in the heart, goodness originates in human nature, and Mencius was right when he said that human nature was good" (夫心主于身，性具于心，善原于性，孟子之言性善是也《王阳明集・与王纯甫》). He believed in the "intuitive knowledge" or, literally, "good knowledge" (良知 *liangzhi*) that can distinguish between the right and the wrong. This knowledge is "the inner light" of our heart (Fung 1966: 315). He said:

> 是非之心，不虑而知，不学而能，所谓良知也。良知之在人心，无间于圣愚，天下古今之所同也。《王阳明集·传习录中》(Ji 1995, vol. 54: 32)
> The heart of right and wrong is what one knows without thinking, and what one is capable of without learning. That the intuitive knowledge exists in the human heart is true to both sages and fools, and is the same all under Heaven from ancient time to the present. *Collected Writings of Wang Yangming: Record of Instructions*, Part II.

That is, this "intuitive knowledge" is universal and eternal to all humans, regardless of their status of being sages or fools. The "extension of the intuitive knowledge" (致良知 *zhi liangzhi*), as advocated in the *Great Learning*, is nothing but the "manifestation of the illustrious virtue" (明明德 *ming mingde*). The problem, however, is that this knowledge can be smothered by selfish desires, as he explained below:

> 人心是天渊。心之本体无所不该，原是一个天。只为私欲障碍，则天之本体失了。心之理无穷尽，原是一个渊。只为私欲窒塞，则渊之本体失了。如今念念致良知，将此障碍窒塞一齐去尽，则本体已复，便是天渊了。《王阳明集·传习录下》(Ji 1995, vol. 54: 38)
> The human heart is heaven and abyss. The essence of the heart possesses all, and is originally a heaven. Only due to the blockage by selfish desires is this essence of heaven lost. The Principle of the heart has no limit, and is originally an abyss. Only due to the stuffing of selfish desires is this essence of abyss lost. Now, with devoted effort to extend the intuitive knowledge, we can get rid of the blockage and stuffing all together so that the essence of our heart will be restored, and our heart will become heaven and abyss again. *Collected Writings of Wang Yangming: Record of Instructions*, Part III.

Here, we see a similar scenario as that of Mencius. Man is born with goodness in his heart, but this goodness is edged out by selfish desires, so his task is to recover it. Wang Yangming also maintains the Confucian doctrine that cultivation of the self depends on rectification of the heart because, to him, "The heart is the dictator of the body" (心者身之主宰《王阳明集·传习录下》). The other body parts, such as eyes, ears, mouth, and four limbs, all act according to the dictates of the heart. Thus:

> 主宰一正，则发窍于目，自无非礼之视；发窍于耳，自无非礼之听；发窍于口与四肢，自无非礼之言动。此便是修身在正其心。《王阳明集·传习录下》(Ji 1995, vol. 54: 48)

> Once the dictator is straightened (i.e. rectified), its straightness will get through to its apertures of eyes, ears, mouth and four limbs, so that the eyes will not see anything against propriety, the ears will not hear anything against propriety, the mouth and four limbs will not say or do anything against propriety. This is why cultivation of the self depends on rectification of the heart. *Works of Wang Yangming: Record of Instructions*, Part III.

He also used the PLANT metaphor to illustrate the importance of nurturing the heart in promoting virtues: "Those who plant trees must cultivate their roots; those who plant virtues must nurture their hearts" (种树者必培其根，种德者必养其心《王阳明集・传习录上》). Apparently, virtues are plants that grow out of the heart.

Like Mencius, Wang Yangming attached prime importance to knowing Heaven through knowing one's own heart. He said, "The heart is the Way, and the Way is Heaven; knowing the heart you also know the Way and Heaven" (心即道，道即天，知心则知道、知天《王阳明集・传习录上》). That is, it is possible for the heart to be connected with the Way and Heaven through human nature, which is akin to what Mencius argued for. However, there is a fundamental difference between Mencius and Wang Yangming. That is, for Mencius, the heart is linked to Heaven as its appendix, but to Wang Yangming, the heart is linked with Heaven as its origin. He unified Heaven and Earth and the ten thousand things into the human heart, whose nature is good and benevolent. Thus, it is possible to attain the ideal state: the "benevolence of the Oneness of Heaven and Earth and the ten thousand things" (天地万物一体之仁《王阳明集・传习录中》). Since the heart possesses the innate "intuitive knowledge" about morality, people can access it as long as they "exhaust the heart".

2.4. The heart as the locus of societal governance

In ancient Chinese philosophy, the heart is also conceptualized as the locus of governance and government. There are two sides to this thesis. First, the ruler's governance is grounded in his heart. Second, the government of the country is grounded in the hearts of its people.

2.4.1. The ruler as the "heart" of the state

It is worth noting at this point that, while the heart of a person is understood as the ruler of a nation, as shown previously in section 2.2.3, the reverse is also true. That is, the ruler of a state is also understood as the heart of a person. The bidirectional and reciprocal mappings attest to the philosophical view that there is a correspondence between nature and man, the former including the political and social structures in the form of a country. In the *Wenzi*, for instance, a passage quotes Laozi as saying: “The sovereign is the heart of the state. When the heart is under control, all parts of the body are in order; when the heart is disturbed, all parts will be in disorder” (主者，国之心也。心治则百节皆安，心扰则百节皆乱《文子・上德》). It is very important that the ruler be self-disciplined and under self-control. If not, the whole nation will be in trouble and disorder. The maintenance of the “upper virtue” should lead to the desirable governing situation in which “one starts singing and ten thousand will follow suit, like the body following the heart” (一人唱而万人和，如体之从心《鹖冠子・天则》). In keeping with its doctrine of “inaction” or “nonaction”, however, Daoism believed that “the best way of governing is through nongovernment”, because the result will be opposite to what is expected “when uniform codes of laws and morals are enforced by government and society upon the individual” (Fung 1966: 106). Thus, both Laozi and Zhuangzi advocated “government through nongovernment”, although for somewhat different reasons. Laozi emphasized his general principle that reversing is the movement of the Way. The more one governs, the less one achieves the desired result. Zhuangzi, however, emphasized the distinction between what is of nature and what is human. The more the former is overcome by the latter, the more there will be misery and unhappiness (see Fung 1966: 106–107).

The quotation below presents another example of the RULER AS HEART metaphor from the *Guanzi* in the form of a simile:

> 君之在国都也，若心之在身体也。道德定于上，则百姓化于下。戒心形于内，则容貌动于外矣。《管子・君臣下》(Ji 1995, vol. 49: 777)
> The monarch in the capital of the country is like the heart in the body. The ethics (lit. the Way and Virtue) are established above, and the masses will follow below. The heart of vigilance takes shape inside, and the looks will change outside. *Guanzi: Monarch and Subjects,* Part II.

It is crucial for the ruler to provide good moral leadership, for the masses will follow wherever their leader is going. If the ruler is on guard against immorality, the nation as a whole will display an ethical difference. A good ruler should govern on the basis of morality. He should respect and trust his officials, who are to carry out his governance. Mencius had this advice to the ruler: "If a ruler sees the officials as his hands and feet, then the officials will see the ruler as their belly and heart" (君之视臣如手足，则臣视君如腹心《孟子·离娄下》).[40] If the ruler follows the Way of a monarch in his governance, then this is what will happen:

> 故天子不视而见，不听而聪，不虑而知，不动而功，块然独坐而天下从之如一体、如四肢之从心。《荀子·君道篇》(Ji 1995, vol. 49: 344)
> Thus, the Son of Heaven does not look yet sees, does not listen yet hears, does not think yet knows, and does not move yet accomplishes. Like a clod of earth he sits alone on his mat, and the world follows him as though it were of a single body of his, just as the four limbs follow the dictates of the heart. *Xunzi: On the Way of a Monarch.*

That is, by following the Way, the monarch, also known as the "Son of Heaven" in ancient China, can accomplish everything while doing nothing himself. His ruling of the country is as easy as the heart commands the four limbs and the whole body. In a similar fashion, it is argued in the *Guanzi* that the monarch who upholds the Virtue can "be quick without movement, know without being told, accomplish without action, and reach the goal without being guided" (Ji 1995, vol. 49: 772).

> 故天不动，四时云，下而万物化。君不动，政令陈，下而万功成；心不动，使四肢耳目，而万物情。《管子·戒》(Ji 1995, vol. 49: 772)
> Thus, while Heaven does not move, with four seasons evolving, the ten thousand things beneath it will grow and transform. While the monarch does not move, with administrative orders distributed, the ten thousand tasks beneath him will be accomplished; while the heart does not move, deploying four limbs, and ears and eyes, it can appreciate the ten thousand things. *Guanzi: Admonitions.*

Here, three-way parallels are observed, and the line in the middle is the monarch. Upholding the Virtue, the monarch, the Son of Heaven and the

---

[40] In the Chinese original of Mencius' advice to the ruler, the word 腹心 *fuxin* means "belly/stomach and heart". They are more important than hands and feet because they take the "central position" of the body, as the ruler does of the country. In a different collocation, however, 腹 *fu* 'belly/stomach' may be derogatory. For example, 口腹之欲 *koufu zhi yu* means "the desires of mouth and stomach", i.e., the bodily desires for good food and drinks, or for material gains in general.

heart of the state, can behave in similar ways as Heaven or heart. The passage again highlights the Daoist belief in the harmonious integration of nature and man and the unified correspondence between body and world.

2.4.2. The heart as the center of governance

In the *Guanzi*, it is also argued that the heart is the center of governance. The ruler's heart has to be well regulated and at peace before he can govern his country peacefully.

> 圣人裁物，不为物使。心安是国安也，心治是国治也。治也者心也，安也者心也。治心在于中，治言出于口，治事加于民，故功作而民从，则百姓治矣。《管子·心术下》(Ji 1995, vol. 49: 785)
> The sage manipulates things, and is not to be utilized by them. His heart being at peace, his country is also at peace. His heart being well regulated, his country is also well regulated. Being regulated is a matter of the heart; being at peace is also a matter of the heart. A well-regulated heart lies inside him, well-regulated words issue from his mouth, and well-regulated policies are applied to his people. Thus, if meritorious services are performed and the people are responsive, then all the commoners will become well regulated as well. *Guanzi: Art of the Heart,* Part II.

To govern a country is to govern its people, and to govern the people is to govern their hearts. As Confucius suggested in the *Analects*, a successful ruler is the one who has "all the people under Heaven turn their hearts toward him" (天下之民归心焉 《论语》). Laozi also said, "The sage has no heart of his own; he uses the heart of the people as his heart" (圣人无常心，以百姓心为心《老子·任德第四十九》). As quoted in the *Wenzi*, he asserted that the foundation of successful ruling is winning people's hearts:

> 能成霸王者，必德胜者也。能胜敌者，必强者也。能强者，必用人力者也。能用人力者，必得人心者也。《文子·符言》(Ji 1995, vol. 49: 87)
> Those who can become overlords must win with virtue. Those who can defeat their enemy must be strong people. Those who can be strong must make good use of personnel. Those who make good use of personnel must win people's hearts. *Wenzi: Magic Words.*

Guanzi saw people's hearts, or their will, as a great trend that is unstoppable. The government will prosper if it goes with it, and will collapse if it goes against it. "Success in government lies in following the hearts of the people. Failure in government lies in opposing them" (政之所兴，在顺民心；政之所废，在逆民心。《管子・牧民》)

Mencius's conception of the heart also has a strong social component. For instance, he believed that people fall into two classes: those who work with their hearts, and those who work with their hands. Although they depend on each other in different ways, those who work with their hearts are apparently superior as rulers:

> 故曰，或劳心，或劳力；劳心者治人，劳力者治于人；治于人者食人，治人者食于人，天下之通义也。《孟子・滕文公上》(Zheng et al. 1993: 184)
> As the saying goes, people work either with their hearts (i.e. mind) or with their strength. Those who work with their hearts rule others; those who work with their strength are ruled by others. Those who are ruled feed others; those who rule are fed by others. This is a principle universally accepted. *Mencius: Duke Wen of Teng,* Part I.

Given that the heart is conceptualized metaphorically as the ruler that dictates the body, it follows that those who work with their heart should rule those who work with their strength associated with the body. Mencius' division of labor is simply an entailment of the HEART AS RULER metaphor.

Mencius advocated the "practice of benevolent government" (施仁政 *shi renzheng*), which above all is grounded *in* and *on* people's hearts. People's hearts represent people's will, and people's will, to him, is Heaven's will. The people are the most important element in a state whereas the sovereign is the least: "If a ruler lacks the ethical qualities that make a good leader, the people have the moral right of revolution" (Fung 1966: 74). He argued as follows: "The root of all under Heaven is the state, the root of the state is the family, and the root of the family is the individual" (天下之本在国，国之本在家，家之本在身《孟子・离娄上》). As shown above in the previous sections, Mencius believed that the root of an individual person is the heart. It follows that a benevolent government depends on winning the hearts of its people:

> 得天下有道：得其民，斯得天下矣。得其民有道：得其心，斯得民矣；得其心有道：所欲与之聚之，所恶勿施，尔也。《孟子・离娄上》(Zheng et al. 1993: 254)

> There is a way to win the world: Win the people and you will win the world. There is a way to win the people: Win their hearts and you will win the people. There is a way to win the people's hearts: Collect for them what they desire and do not force on them what they hate. That is all. *Mencius: Li Lou,* Part I.

The key is to govern with the Virtue: "People submit to force not because they do so at heart, but because they are not strong enough to resist it; people who submit to the virtuous rule do so after their own heart" (以力服人者，非心服也，力不赡也；以德服人者，中心悦而诚服也《孟子·公孙丑上》). According to Mencius, there are two ways of governing: the "kingly way" (王道 *wangdao*) and the "tyrannical way" (霸道 *badao*). The former carries out the government through moral instruction and education, and the latter through force and compulsion. He advocated good education, rather than "good government", to win people's hearts. Only when everyone has received some education and has come to an understanding of human relationships, does the kingly way become complete (see Fung 1966: 73–77). He said, "Good government is feared by the people while good education is loved by them. Good government gains people's wealth while good education gains their heart" (善政，民畏之；善教，民爱之。善政得民财，善教得民心《孟子·尽心上》). Adhering to the principle that the people are more important than the ruler, he aimed to advise the ruler to attach great importance to the people's will and pay close attention to their sufferings. He said:

> 人皆有不忍人之心。先王有不忍人之心，斯有不忍人之政矣。以不忍人之心，行不忍人之政，治天下可运之掌上。《孟子·公孙丑上》 (Zheng et al. 1993: 114)
>
> All people have the heart that cannot bear to see the sufferings of others. As the early kings had this unbearing heart, they likewise had an unbearing government. Running such a government with an unbearing heart, a king should find it as easy to rule all under Heaven as to roll something on the palm of his hand. *Mencius: Gongsun Chou*, Part I.

The practice of benevolent government in the kingly way is nothing but the nurturing of the "unbearing heart" (i.e. a heart sensitive to the sufferings of others) common to all humans (see Fung 1966: 75–77). Mencius actually developed Confucius' idea of self-cultivation and extended its application to government and politics, so that it became a principle not only for "sageliness within", but also for "kingliness without" (Fung 1966: 76).

The idea of the heart as the locus of governance figured prominently in later periods of Chinese history. For instance, in the Han dynasty (206 BC–AD 220), Dong Zhongshu (179–104 BC), the leading Confucian of the time, argued that the ruler needs to rectify his heart in order to rectify, successively, the court, the officials, the people, and the country. It was believed that the court is the basis of the country, the ruler the basis of the court, and the heart the basis of the ruler. That is, the governance of the country is ultimately rooted in the heart of the ruler. To rectify the ruler's heart is to connect and align it with the Way, the ultimate principle. If the ruler's heart is rectified, and the Way followed, then the country will be in order. Otherwise, it will be in disorder. Therefore, it was said, order depends on the Way and lies in the heart (see De Bary 1981: 115–116). To Dong Zhongshu, the emperor, the Son of Heaven, governs the people according to the will of, and with power endowed by, Heaven. The rectification of the emperor's heart is the key to the communication and interaction between Heaven and humans.

According to Neo-Confucianism, cultivation of the self and rectification of the heart are the keys to the "Learning of the Emperors" (De Bary 1981: 116). Zhu Xi of the Song dynasty believed that self-cultivation through heart rectification is the root of ruling. The emperor's "rectified heart with sincere will" (正心诚意 *zhengxin chengyi*) lays down the foundation for a peaceful world. If his heart is nourished with the principle, it is bright and clear; if it is obscured by the desires for personal gains, then it is deluded. Rulers' hearts must be at peace before they can govern peacefully. Following Confucianism, the Neo-Confucian doctrines "asserted self-cultivation as the basis of rulership and then rectification of the heart as the basis of self-cultivation" (p. 116). It was believed that universal self-cultivation through rectification of the heart is the principal means of governance and the best way to govern the people or the country. This belief was based on the realization that "the world can be won by military might, but it cannot be governed by military might" (p. 148). The governance is based on the Way whereas the Way is rooted in the heart. If the heart, the ruler of the self, is clear, laws and systems will operate unhindered, public discipline will be maintained, and the world will be at peace.

2.5. Summary and discussion

In this chapter I have attempted to trace the conceptualization of the *xin* 'heart' in ancient Chinese philosophy based on a survey of linguistic data extracted from classic texts of Confucianism and Daoism. I concentrated on three aspects: (a) the heart as the locus of the mind, (b) the heart as the locus of moral sense and character, and (c) the heart as the locus of governance and government. The second and third aspects stem directly from the first one. That is, because the heart is conceptualized as playing the functions of thinking, knowing and feeling, it is regarded as the locus of moral sense and character, and of governance and government as well. In this final section I intend to put my survey of the data in this chapter into perspective. To me, the significant finding is that the Chinese *xin* 'heart' conceived of as the central faculty of cognition is largely understood in metaphorical terms.

First, in order to make this claim clearer, I want to point out the nonmetaphorical aspect of this understanding. The conceptualization of the heart as the locus of the "mind" is indeed nonmetaphorical; it arises from a cultural belief that is propositional in nature, expressed linguistically in the subject-verb collocations. For instance, as listed below, the first two are recurrent collocations that show up in many examples.

> The heart *thinks* and *contemplates* (思 *si* and 虑 *lü*).
> The heart *knows* and *understands* (知 *zhi*).
> The heart *examines*, *infers* and *reasons* (审 *shen*, 推数究理 *tuishu jiuli*).
> The heart *feels uncertain* or *confused* (疑 *yi* and 惑 *huo*).

That is, the heart is the organ that hosts various mental activities, processes, and states. In terms of division of labor, the heart thinks, knows, and understands, just as the eyes see, the ears hear, the nose smells, the mouth tastes and speaks, and the four limbs move and act. Since the heart carries out the mental functions of a person, it is the part that commands all the other parts of the body. This conceptualization leads to its metaphorical understanding.

The conceived authoritative mental role assigned to the heart prompted a very popular conceptual metaphor of the heart in terms of social structure and hierarchy:

> THE HEART IS THE RULER OF THE BODY

This metaphor emphasizes the perceived correspondences between the physiological system of the body and the social system of the country: The heart to a person is what the emperor, monarch, or sovereign is to a country. It needs to be pointed out that this conceptual metaphor is a complex one that presumes the combination or blending (in the sense of Lakoff and

Johnson 1999) of the following more fundamental cultural understandings, both propositional and metaphorical:

> THE HEART IS THE LOCUS OF THE MIND (a proposition)
> A PERSON IS A SOCIETY (a metaphor)

Here the first is a proposition reflecting a cultural belief or assumption whereas the second is a metaphor, which in turn is combined from the following more generic metaphorical mappings or entailments:

> PHYSIOLOGICAL SYSTEM IS SOCIAL SYSTEM
> PHYSIOLOGICAL STRUCTURE IS SOCIAL STRUCTURE
> PHYSIOLOGICAL FUNCTION/OPERATION IS SOCIAL FUNCTION/OPERATION

These metaphorical mappings are governed by the fundamental worldview that equates microcosm and macrocosm: Thus, PHYSIOLOGICAL IS SOCIAL, and vice versa.

As we can see, the propositional component THE HEART IS THE LOCUS OF THE MIND, which reflects a cultural belief or assumption, makes the complex metaphor THE HEART IS THE RULER OF THE BODY quite culture-specific. Thus, this conceptual metaphor reflects the culturally constructed and culturally bound view of the mind-body relationship in ancient Chinese philosophy: While the mind controls the body, it is also located in a part of the body rather than being split from it. Therefore, it is indeed a holistic and "embodied" view of mind, in sharp contrast to, say, the Cartesian dualism in Western philosophical tradition, where the mind is "disembodied," seen as being severed from the body, with mental substance utterly different from physical substance (Damasio 1994; Lakoff and Johnson 1999). It is interesting to note that recent cognitive science advocates the slogans "to put the body back into the mind" (Johnson 1987) and "to look for the mind inside the body" (Sharifian et al. 2008b).

In accordance with the predominant beliefs in the unity and correspondence between the universe and the human, the metaphor emphasizes the perceived parallels between the macrocosm of the universe and the microcosm of the human. Its mappings and entailments include, but are not limited to, the following:

THE HEART IS THE RULER OF THE BODY		
Country	→	Body
Ruler (monarch, sovereign, emperor)	→	Heart
Central government/court	→	Central physiological system

Political power	→	Mental power
Governmental activities, processes, states	→	Mental activities, processes, states
Governmental officials	→	Bodily organs
Governmental functions, operations	→	Physiological functions, operations
Political situations of the country	→	Physiological conditions of the body

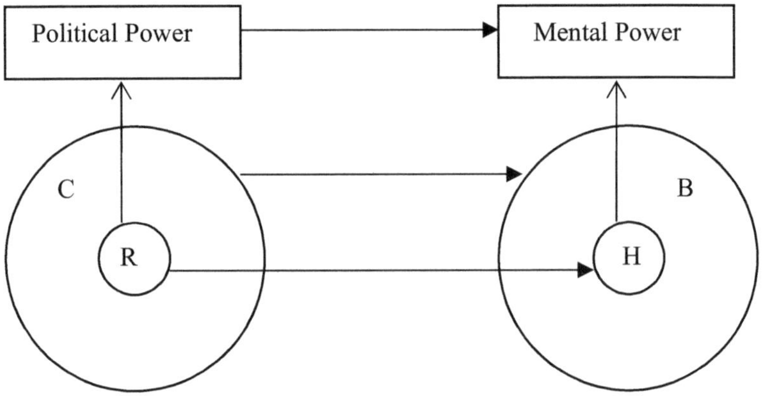

Figure 1. Schematic illustration of the metaphorical mappings from Ruler to Heart

The key aspect of the metaphor THE HEART IS THE RULER OF THE BODY is the mental power that distinguishes humans from lower animals. Humans are superior to other species of animals in that the former are uniquely equipped with mental power, i.e., the "mind", which enables them to think, know, understand, and reason. In ancient Chinese philosophy, this "mind" is seen to be located in the heart.

Figure 1 is a schematic illustration of the metaphorical mappings from the ruler to the heart. In this figure, the horizontal lines with solid arrows indicate the direction of the metaphorical mappings: The ruler is mapped onto the heart, the country onto the body, and political power onto mental power. The vertical lines with open-headed arrows represent the relationship of "possession", that is, the ruler possesses political power and the heart possesses mental power. As shown in the illustration, it is apparent that the conceptual metaphor is based on the center-peripheral image-schema. The heart is the center of the body just as the ruler is the center of the country. In addition, the political power of the ruler grounds his status as being the center of the country whereas the mental power of the heart grounds its status as being the center of the body. Thus, the key is the mapping from the political power of the ruler to the mental power of the heart. It is this metaphorical projection that triggers off the mappings and entailments from the country to the body, from the ruler to the heart, and so forth.

It is interesting to note that the mental power of the heart itself is also understood metaphorically: MENTAL POWER IS SPIRITUAL LIGHT. This mental power is "spiritual" in that, although formless and intangible, it operates behind and above what is physical and obvious, as much as how supernatural spirits, deities, divinities, and gods operate mysteriously in nature. This power is "light" in that it "enlightens" in a metaphorical sense derived from physical and bodily experience. Whereas light enables seeing, mental power enables thinking, knowing, understanding, and reasoning. The heart, however, is both the source of mental power, which enables one to think, know and understand, and the source of "spiritual light", which enables one to "see". While mental power is "spiritual light", thinking, knowing or understanding is "seeing". In other words, the metaphor MENTAL POWER IS SPIRITUAL LIGHT actually entails the common primary metaphor THINKING, KNOWING, or UNDERSTANDING IS SEEING, based on the following conceptual associates in contrast between "darkness" and "light": obscurity, blockage, restriction, ignorance, and stupidity versus enlightenment, penetration, expansion, knowledge, and wisdom.

The reason why the heart is said to be the "ruler of the body" is that it is conceptualized as possessing the "supreme power" or the "spiritual light", with which it commands and governs other parts of the body. This conceptualization is expressed via the metaphor THE HEART IS THE MASTER OF THE SPIRITUAL LIGHT, which simultaneously maps two pairs of source concepts onto one pair of target concepts, as shown below:

THE HEART IS THE MASTER OF THE SPIRITUAL LIGHT

Master	→	Heart	←	Light Source
Social Power	→	Mental Power	←	Spiritual Light

Being the "master" with social power and the "source" of the spiritual light at the same time, the heart "possesses" the mental power at its disposal in the same way as the ruler possesses the political power as the foundation of his ruling. A different version of this metaphor is one in which the mental power and its functions are understood as valuable possessions, as expressed in the couple of metaphors: (a) THE HEART IS THE MASTER OF THE SPIRITS, and (b) THE SPIRITS ARE TREASURES OF THE HEART. Again, that the heart can be in its unique position of being the "ruler of the body" is because it is "the master of the spirits", or "the commander of the mental functions". The "spirits", which are functions of mental power, are further extended metaphorically as "treasures", namely, "valuable possessions" of the heart. Note that treasures are not only valuable, but also shining, so "light" is an entailment of this metaphor too. The ownership of such "treasures-spirits" is a privilege that puts the heart in the supreme position of a ruler.

Another metaphor for the heart that is related to the "light" is THE HEART IS THE SUN (see Ch. 3). The sun is a light source. The heart radiates its "light" to various parts of the body as it exerts its mental power in the direction and operation of those body parts. Light from the sun comes with heat, and they both are essential factors that give rise to life. In the body, the heart is believed to be "the generator of light and heat" that gives rise to the mental and physical dimensions of human life. That is why the heart is also said to be "the root of life". Note that both "light" and "heat" associated with the heart as the "sun" are also culturally consistent with the fact that in Chinese the heart is regarded as an organ of "fire". Another possible parallel between the sun in the universe and the heart in a person is that the sun is the center of a constellational system whereas the heart is the center of a physiological system. This perceived parallelism between cosmology and biology manifests the beliefs in the unity and correspondence between the universe and the human.

As we have seen, with the "Learning of the Heart" in Neo-Confucianism, the social structure metaphor THE HEART IS THE RULER OF THE BODY has a stronger version or variant that reflects the doctrines of its philosophical thought:

THE HEART IS THE DICTATOR OF THE BODY

Here, the "dictator" (主宰 *zhuzai*) suggests a more active and authoritative use of power than the ordinary "ruler" (君 *jun*) does in the governance of the country. A dictatorial ruler wants absolute control over his subjects and direct involvement in governmental affairs. The heart in the body was assigned a similar role by Neo-Confucians like Wang Yangming. Thus, the heart does not *cause* the other parts of the body to act; it *acts* with the help of other parts of the body. That is, the heart no longer sits there passively giving orders to, and receiving briefings from, the major organs of the body. Instead, it works actively, deploying the major organs to act according to its commands. Besides, Wang Yangming went further to make even stronger metaphorical claims such as in the following couple:

MAN IS THE HEART OF THE UNIVERSE
THE HEART IS THE MASTER OF THE UNIVERSE

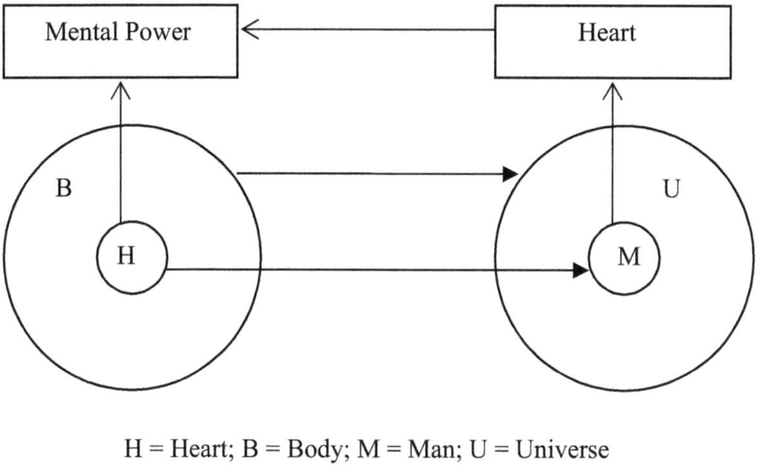

Figure 2. Schematic illustration of MAN IS THE HEART OF THE UNIVERSE

While man is the center of the universe, his heart governs not just his body, but also the whole universe. A stronger claim in philosophical doctrine is expressed by a stronger version of metaphor. The first metaphor of the above couple is schematically illustrated in Figure 2. In this figure, again, the lines with solid arrows indicate the direction of metaphorical mappings whereas the lines with open-headed arrows represent the relationship of possession. In this case, the heart is mapped onto man, and the body is mapped onto the universe. The reason why man can be the center of the universe is that he has the heart, which in turn possesses mental power. In the source domain, it is possible for the heart (H), as the center of the body, to be mapped onto man in the target domain, again, because it possesses mental power. Therefore, the fact that the heart is conceptualized as possessing that mental power is the root of the metaphor under consideration.

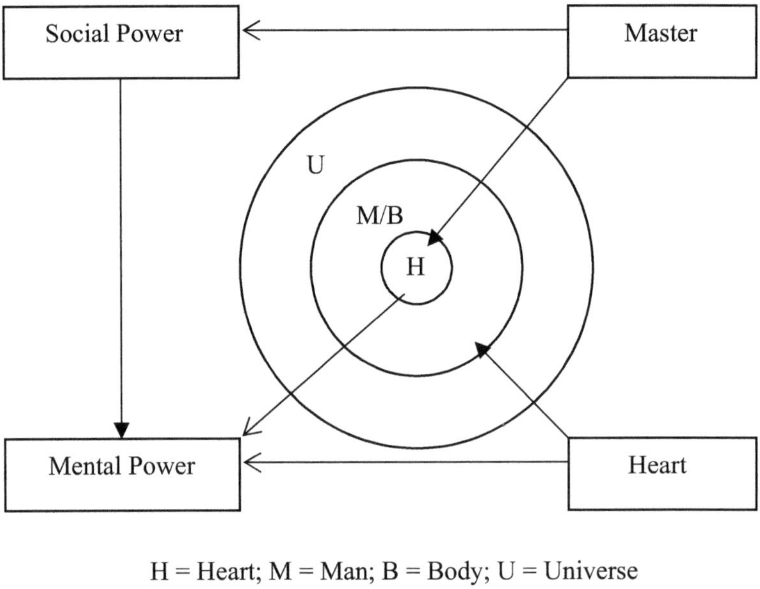

Figure 3. Schematic illustration of HEART IS THE MASTER OF THE UNIVERSE

The second metaphor of the previous couple can be illustrated schematically in Figure 3. In this figure, the heart, as the center of man or body, is the master of the universe. The master is mapped onto the heart because a master has social power, which is mapped onto mental power possessed by the heart. Moreover, the heart that has mental power is also mapped onto man, represented by the middle circle, to result in the first metaphor of the couple: MAN IS THE HEART OF THE UNIVERSE. As we can see from Figures 2 and 3, the two metaphors are both based on the cultural conception or assumption that the heart possesses mental power. To the Neo-Confucians of the "Learning of the Heart", like Wang Yangming, the mental power of the heart, called the "divine light" (灵明 *lingming*), is lifted to a supreme height, even higher than Heaven and Earth, and supernatural beings. Little wonder the heart, with its "divine light", is regarded as the center of the universe. These metaphorical conceptualizations represent the strongest expression of humanism characteristic of ancient Chinese philosophy, as discussed earlier.

In section 2.4, I discussed the view that the heart is the key to governance and the foundation of government. That is, the ruler's governance, effective or ineffective, moral or immoral, is attributed to his heart. If his heart is "straight and upright", his governance will be so as well. The ruler, in order to govern his country successfully, has to win his people's support. In order to win his people's support, he must win their hearts. That is, "winning the people's hearts" (得民心 *de minxin*) is the key to the ruler's successful governance, which however depends on his own heart being "straight and upright". In other words, if the ruler's own heart is "straight and upright", he will be able to "obtain the people's hearts". The people's hearts are the foundation of the ruler's government for ruling the country. That is the so-called "benevolent government", promoted by Mencius, again as an expression of the ideal of humanism.

I have shown, in this chapter, that there exist in ancient Chinese philosophy two-way mappings between the heart and the ruler. That is, THE HEART IS THE RULER OF THE BODY, and THE RULER IS THE HEART OF THE COUNTRY. According to the theory of conceptual metaphor (e.g., Lakoff 1993, 1994; Kövecses 2002), however, metaphors mapping across conceptual domains are asymmetric, that is, such mappings are usually unidirectional, from one source domain to another target domain, but not vice versa. The case under consideration is a culture-specific exception to that general principle.[41] Let us see how and why. The bidirectional mappings, namely THE HEART IS THE RULER OF THE BODY and THE RULER IS THE HEART OF THE COUNTRY, can be seen as instances of more general metaphors: A BODY/PERSON IS A SOCIETY/COUNTRY and A SOCIETY/COUNTRY IS A BODY/PERSON. Empirical studies of conceptual metaphors have shown that the human body, with its bodily experience, is a potentially universal source domain, whereas society is a common target domain (see, e.g., Kövecses 2002: 16–25). This means that A SOCIETY/COUNTRY IS A BODY/PERSON should be more widespread across cultures than A BODY/PERSON IS A SOCIETY/COUNTRY. But why is the latter such an important metaphor in ancient Chinese philosophy (e.g., the heart as the monarch, and sense organs as officials)? This question brings us back to my earlier argument that this metaphor is the key to understanding the mind-body relationship in ancient Chinese philosophy: The heart as the locus of the "mind" is the "ruler" of the body. The embodied nature of this metaphor also lies in the biological fact that our heart organ, which pumps blood

---

41 Other instances may include THE COMPUTER IS A BRAIN and THE BRAIN IS A COMPUTER, and ANGER IS A STORM and A STORM IS ANGER. See Kövecses (2002: 24–25) for the discussion and the conclusion that conceptual metaphors are mostly unidirectional.

throughout our body to maintain its functioning, is the center of our physiological system.

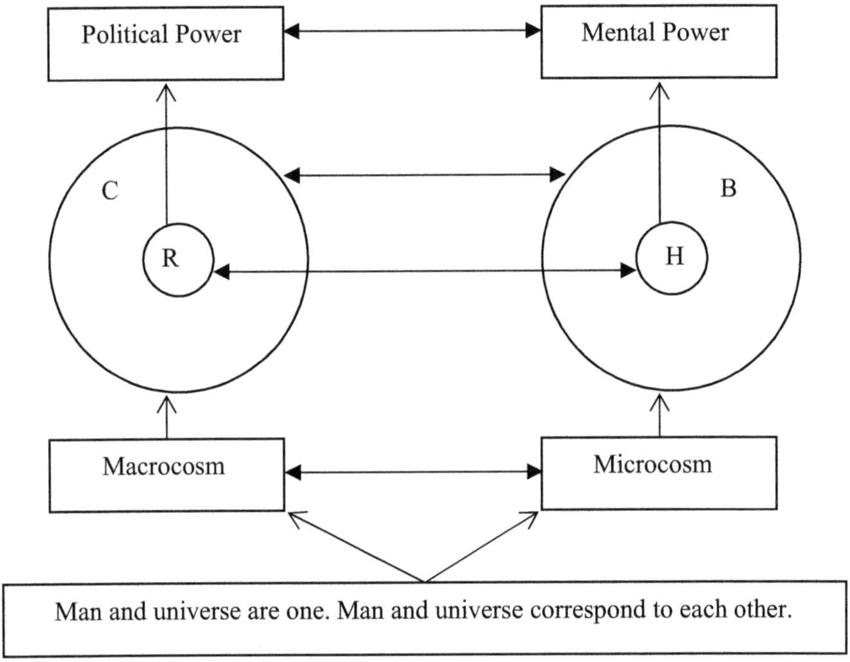

R = Ruler; C = Country; H = Heart; B = Body

Figure 4. Illustration of the bidirectional mappings between Ruler and Heart

As I have tried to explain above, the existence of the bidirectional mappings between HEART and RULER, and BODY and SOCIETY results from and at the same time constitutes the culture-specific understanding of the "mind", and its relationship with the body, of ancient Chinese philosophy in its historical context. In fact, these bidirectional mappings, as twin metaphors, converge on and constitute a more fundamental cultural model in Chinese cosmology, as is illustrated schematically in Figure 4. In this figure, there are two-way mappings between the ruler and the heart, the country and the body, and political power and mental power. These bidirectional mappings are possible and natural in the context of ancient Chinese philosophy and politics because the two sides, or domains, of the mappings are conceived of as parallel correspondences labeled as macrocosm and microcosm of each other. Thus, it is believed that one can try to understand the microcosm by comparing it with the macrocosm and vice versa. This belief is built on the foundation of the claim for the unity and correspondence between the universe and the human (天人合一 *tian ren he yi*; 天人相类 *tian ren xiang lei*), as an expression of the major tendency of humanism in ancient Chinese philosophy.

As an internal organ inside the body, the heart is also understood via other metaphors that may not be consistent with each other. These metaphors include the following:

THE HEART IS A CONTAINER.
THE HEART IS AN OBJECT.
THE HEART IS WATER.
THE HEART IS A MIRROR.
THE HEART IS SOIL.
THE HEART IS A PLANT.

In order to get full transparency, I will, in what follows, discuss these metaphors one by one. The first is the one in which the heart is conceptualized as a container.

THE HEART IS A CONTAINER

Heart	→	Container
Eyes and ears	→	Entrances of the container
Mental capacity	→	Physical capacity of the container
Things mental and emotional	→	Contents in the container
Things to learn mentally	→	Things to be put into the container
Things to lose mentally	→	Things to be removed from the container

An important characteristic of a container is that it has a physical capacity. That is, its storage is limited and it can only contain a certain number of things or a certain amount of substance. If there is little room left but more needs to be put into it, then what is already in there has to be taken out to make room. If many different kinds of things or substances are put into it, then the space for each of them is limited accordingly. What is bad has to be removed from the container so that good things or substances in its contact or vicinity will not turn bad.

It is interesting to note that the eyes and ears, as important organs of cognition, serve only as entrances, but not as exits, of the container. Thus, in the *Guanzi*, the heart is said to be the "residence" of intelligence or wisdom, and the ears and eyes as the "doors" of the residence. We can imagine things "entering" through these doors, but hardly things "exiting" them. Anyway, HEART AS IMPERIAL PALACE is but a special instantiation of the more general HEART AS CONTAINER metaphor.

With the CONTAINER metaphor, the heart is conceptualized as a container for affective and cognitive constituents of a person: emotions, thoughts, intellect, knowledge, moral values and judgments, etc. For instance, Xunzi argued that it is possible for people to learn and understand things because their heart is "empty" inside so that it can receive things for storage and use. Although it has already stored up many things, as long as the person is, or tries to be, "empty-hearted" (虚心 *xuxin*), the heart-container should never be too full to accept new things. Besides, Xunzi also seemed to suggest that the heart, although characterized by diversity of things stored in it, should maintain its "unity" (壹 *yi*) when receiving things, concentrating on one thing at a time. The focus will be lost when reception of many things at the same time divides the attention-capacity of the heart-container.

In Mencius' metaphor system, the heart also seems to be a container. As a container, it stores, as its content, innate good human nature, including the four "seeds" that will turn into four classic virtues under the circumstances that the content of the heart-container is "preserved". Unfortunately, many people lose the content of the container and do not seek to recover it. Comprehended as such, "preserving the heart" (存心 *cunxin*) and "exhausting the heart" (尽心 *jinxin*) are instances of metonymy CONTAINER FOR CONTAINED. That is, it is the content inside the container that is preserved or exhausted. At the same time, to preserve or exhaust the content of the heart is also metaphorical, for no such content of the heart can be preserved or exhausted literally. Mencius' reasoning about desires is metaphorical, too. Given a fixed capacity of the container, the more desires it contains, the less room there is for good human nature that is originally in there. While it is impossible to eliminate human desires completely from the heart, one should always try to "reduce the number of desires" (寡欲 *guayu*) so as to preserve the good nature and to make room for the growth of classic virtues in the heart.

When Laozi talked about pacifying the people by "emptying their heart" (虚其心 *xu qi xin*), the CONTAINER metaphor is also involved. There is at least one difference between Laozi and Mencius: Instead of reducing the number of desires as suggested by Mencius, Laozi seemed to suggest that desires be eliminated from the heart-container altogether, which may be characteristic of Daoist doctrine. Thus, Zhuangzi resorted to the CON-

TAINER metaphor in a similar way when he talked about the "fasting of the heart" (心斋 *xinzhai*). He wanted to "empty the heart" so that it would not be disturbed by any emotions, desires, etc., in its state of stillness. It is worth noting that Xunzi and Laozi differed widely when they talked about "emptying the heart". For Xunzi, to empty the heart is to make room for new things to learn and understand; for Laozi, it is to eliminate desires in his effort to become "empty" within and "indifferent" without.

In the metaphor THE HEART IS AN OBJECT, "object" is actually the superordinate of "container", since a container is necessarily an object whereas the reverse may not be true. In Mencius' metaphor system, for instance, the heart can sometimes be interpreted as a valuable object when its internal structure is not under consideration. Since human nature, as the substance of the heart, is innately and inherently good, people should maintain this good nature of the heart-object and make sure that it will not change in quality. That explains the necessity of keeping a "constant heart" (恒心 *hengxin*). Furthermore, the heart-object is the most valuable and precious thing to a human being. Unfortunately, many people do not recognize its real value and desire material possessions instead. In a different and very popular conception, the heart as a valuable object has its own shape, but its outer form can be, and very often is, twisted and crooked by negative forces such as desires. The deformed heart will not function properly unless it is restored to its original normal shape. The process of restoring the heart from its deformed shape to its original shape is called "straightening (i.e., rectifying) the heart" (正心 *zhengxin*). Rectification of the heart is taken as the base of self-cultivation. Thus, the HEART AS OBJECT metaphor has the following mappings or entailments:

THE HEART IS AN OBJECT		
Valuable object	→	Heart
Substance of the object	→	Good human nature with moral character
Original shape of the object	→	Proper function of the heart
Deformed shape of the object	→	Malfunction of the heart
Restoration to its original shape	→	Restoration to its proper function
Loss of the object	→	Loss of human nature and morality
Recovery of the object	→	Recovery of human nature and morality

As shown by this list of mappings and entailments, the HEART AS OBJECT metaphor emphasizes two parameters: the deformed and straightened heart, and the loss and recovery of the heart.

The metaphor THE HEART IS WATER is basically used to conceptualize and describe the heart as the central faculty of cognition and judgment, and the organ of knowing, understanding, and reasoning. It also highlights the fact that the function of this faculty is constrained by various factors. The following is a list of its mappings and entailments:

THE HEART IS WATER		
Water	→	Heart
Stillness of the water	→	Peace of the heart
Level surface of, settlement of sediments in, the water	→	Optimal working conditions of the heart
Clarity of the water in reflection	→	Correctness of the heart in cognition
Disturbance of the water	→	Loss of the heart's cognitive ability
Forces that disturb the water	→	Desires and emotions, etc. that disturb the peaceful state of the heart

That is, the heart should maintain a quiescent state, free from the disturbance of desires and emotions. Only when it is quiescent can the heart obtain truthful understanding and right judgment. That is why Mencius believed that it is meritorious to maintain an "unmoved heart" (不动心 *budong xin*). Such a heart is not to be stirred up by any worldly attractions. It is a supreme state of mind acquired after constant self-cultivation. Besides, the WATER metaphor is also responsible for such compound words as "level heart" (平心 *pingxin*), "quiet (or quiescent) heart" (静心 *jingxin*), and "settled heart" (定心 *dingxin*), often used by Daoists and Confucians to describe a calm mental state.[42]

The HEART AS MIRROR metaphor is the combination of both the HEART AS OBJECT and the HEART AS WATER metaphors. An artificial product for the purpose of reflecting, the mirror is superior to the still water in this regard in that it is "constant" and "unmoved", with far more clarity, brightness and accuracy. Little wonder that both Zhuangzi and Wang Yangming

---

42 In Buddhism, according to Godwin (2001: 15–16), the "heart level" represents the advanced achievement of consciousness in an individual where "a light is lit in the heart" for the first time, and from this point on, one is no longer dependent on "reflected light", but can at last "see directly for oneself". This conception of the heart is in fact very similar to the Confucian and Daoist conceptions of the heart as "master" or "governor" of the "spiritual light" (神明), discussed in 2.2.3 (see also Ch. 3). For a cognitive linguistic study of metaphors and paradoxes in Buddhism's *Heart Sutra*, a primary representative text of Buddhist literature, see Lu and Chiang (2007).

reserved this metaphor for the heart of a "sage" (圣人 *shengren*) or a "perfect man" (至人 *zhiren*). Of course, even a mirror needs care to keep it from being covered by dust. Dust on it, when too thick, will interfere or even block its images or reflections of reality.

Both THE HEART IS SOIL and THE HEART IS A PLANT are agricultural metaphors.[43] Mencius employed them in line with his view of human nature being "domesticated" (Slingerland 2003), as part of his ethical value system. The former involves the following mappings and entailments:

THE HEART IS SOIL

Soil	→	Heart
Seeds	→	Human senses and feelings in human nature
Sprouts	→	Virtues
Weeds	→	Desires
Cultivating sprouts	→	Cultivating virtues
Reducing the number of weeds	→	Reducing the number of desires
Fertilizing the soil	→	Nurturing the heart

The heart as soil contains good seeds of human nature endowed by Heaven. The seeds, with appropriate cultivation, can sprout into classic virtues. The process of cultivation includes reducing the number of desires-weeds and fertilizing the heart-soil. Without such cultivating measures, the weeds will smother the sprouts, and the soil will turn from fertile to barren. THE HEART IS A PLANT is a related metaphor in which the heart is conceived of as a plant that needs to be "nurtured" or "nourished" (养心 *yangxin*) to maintain human nature endowed by Heaven, and to blossom into flowers, and bear fruits, of classic virtues.

In sum, the Chinese *xin* 'heart' holds a supreme position in ancient Chinese philosophy. This is because it is conceptualized as fulfilling both physiological and mental functions of a person. As the center of a person's physiological system, the heart transports blood and qi to all parts of the body. More importantly, as seen in the folk theory, the heart is the central faculty of cognition, which hosts all mental activities or processes, includ-

43 According to the five-element classification in Chinese medicine, however, the spleen and stomach, which form a pair of zang and fu, are the organs of "earth". It is said that earth or soil is "the mother of the ten thousand things", from which "the ten thousand things grow", and that as long as the spleen and stomach are in normal condition, they will be able to absorb all the nutrition from the food, as needed for the health of the body (Chen 1989a: 995).

ing thinking, knowing, understanding, judging, inferring, reasoning, as well as feeling. With its mental power, known as the "spiritual light" or "divine light", the heart commands other parts of the body. In ancient Chinese philosophy, the human body is seen as the microcosm of the universe, nature, or society, which is seen as the macrocosm. The ancients try to understand the microcosm in comparison with the macrocosm, and vice versa. Relationships are perceived parallel between the heart to the body and the ruler to the country. Thus, the heart is conceptualized metaphorically as the "ruler" of the body, and the ruler as the "heart" of the country. It is argued that the two-directional metaphorical mappings between the heart and the ruler, culture-specific as they are, represent manifestations of the predominant beliefs in the unity and correspondence between the universe and the human, or between the macrocosm and the microcosm, in ancient Chinese thought.

As will be seen in the next chapter, the conceptions of the heart in ancient Chinese philosophy are echoed in traditional Chinese medicine, which has borrowed extensively from the former.

Chapter 3
The HEART in traditional Chinese medicine

3.1. Introduction: Basic theories of traditional Chinese medicine

The primary goal of this book is to delineate and characterize the Chinese cultural conceptualization of the heart. In the preceding chapter, I showed that the notion of *xin* 'heart' is a central construct in ancient Chinese philosophy because the heart organ is understood in this philosophy as the central faculty of cognition or the locus of the cognitive agent. In this chapter, I turn to traditional Chinese medicine, which is an important part of the Chinese cultural heritage, for its understanding of the heart.[44] After a brief introduction to some of its basic theories, I focus on how this medical tradition understands the heart and its physiological functions in the theory of internal organs. As will become clear, traditional Chinese medicine and ancient Chinese philosophy share some basic conceptions in their understanding of how the heart is related to the rest of the body and how the body is related to nature. Throughout history, apparently, ancient Chinese philosophy has exerted a very strong influence on traditional Chinese medicine, with the major doctrines of the former serving as the guiding principles and reasoning tools in the development of the latter. In return, ancient Chinese philosophy must have as well absorbed nutrients from the development of traditional Chinese medicine.

Traditional Chinese medicine is a mixture of folk and scientific medicine, with a recorded history of several thousand years (Chen 1989a). It is composed of various theories, such as theories of yin-yang and the five elements (or five phases), the theory of the qi, the theory of the internal

---

44 My primary source for this chapter is Wang et al. (1997), *Theory of Internal Organs in Chinese Medicine* (*Zhongyi Zangxiang Xue* 《中医藏象学》), an over-1000-page, comprehensive book that defines the field and its basic concepts, surveys its formation and development from both theoretical and clinical perspectives, and addresses physiological functions and pathological changes of the internal organs. My main references also include Larre and Rochat de la Vallée (1991, 1992, 1995, 1996), Wiseman and Feng (1998), Yin and Shuai (1992), and Zhang (2001). Of these the latter three at the same time serve as my major references for English translation. Other sources are used wherever relevant.

organs, the theory of channels (or meridians) and network vessels (or collaterals), and so on. All these theories, philosophical or medical, converge on and revolve around the fundamental conception that the heart is the central organ of the human body. This conception unfolds in the following view of the human body in the theory of the internal organs from a contemporary perspective (Wang et al. 1997: 5):

> Under the guidance of ancient Chinese naïve dialectic theories of yin-yang and the five elements, the visceral manifestation doctrine sees the human body as an organic whole. That is, the body is centered on the five zang organs and dominated by the heart; it is composed of parts, connected through channels and network vessels, that each carry out their functions in cooperation with other parts; and it is interrelated with natural environment.

As can be seen from this view, the medical theory of internal organs shares some doctrines and views of ancient Chinese philosophy. These include, in addition to the yin-yang and five-element doctrines, the view that the human body is an organic whole and in unity and correspondence with nature. Most importantly for my purpose of the present chapter, this medical statement shares with ancient Chinese philosophy the view that the heart is the "dominant" or "leading" (主导 *zhudao*) part of the body and defines it as the very core of the body's central physiological system composed of the five zang organs. It does not seem to be accidental that in Chinese today, the words for "center" and "core" literally mean "central heart" (中心 *zhongxin*) and "core heart" (核心 *hexin*) respectively.

Before I focus on the notion of "heart" in traditional Chinese medicine, I will first briefly introduce its theories of yin-yang and the five elements, of the qi, and of the internal organs, which are all crucial in the holistic understanding of the heart and the body within the framework of traditional Chinese medicine.

3.1.1. Theories of yin-yang and the five elements

In traditional Chinese medicine, theories of yin-yang and the five elements and the theory of the qi are borrowed from ancient Chinese philosophy. "Indeed, one of the chief differences between traditional Chinese medicine and modern medicine is the comprehensive system of philosophical constructs which served as the basis of medical theory in ancient China and have survived until the present as the functioning rationale for medical interventions" (Zhang and Rose 2001: 85).

As pointed out in Chapter 2, the ancient Chinese held the overarching philosophical view that nature and man are a unified one and the universe and the human correspond to each other. While the human heart as the central faculty of cognition is conceived of as the center of the body and the core of the universe, the unity and correspondence between nature as macrocosm and man as microcosm are defined and characterized in terms of the yin-yang and five-element doctrines. Applied in Chinese medicine, these two philosophical theories constitute the theoretical framework of Chinese medicine and, as such, serve as the tools of reasoning and exposition (Wang et al. 1997).

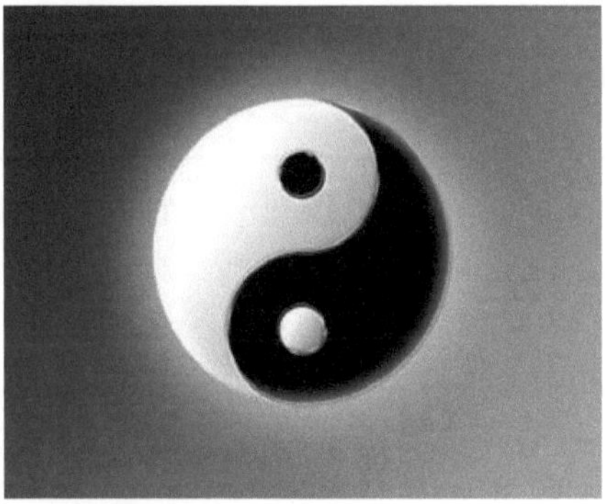

Figure 5. The yin-yang symbol of Daoism

According to the yin-yang doctrine, all phenomena and things in the universe, the human body included, are governed by the law of unity between opposites represented by two Chinese words: 阴 *yin* 'feminine; negative' and 阳 *yang* 'masculine; positive'. This ultimate law states that yin and yang are both opposed to and dependent on each other, and can even turn into each other. The dynamic relationship of the unity between the two opposites is perfectly expressed by the yin-yang symbol of Daoism, which has existed for about 2,500 years. As shown in Figure 5, this symbol has the shape of a circle, which symbolizes the "Great Harmony" (大同 *datong*) of the universe, its "oneness". Within this circle of unity, however, there exist two opposite forces symbolized respectively by the colors of black and white. These two opposites evenly divide the total size of the circle, which symbolizes two even forces in their ideal formation. Also, each of the opposing forces actually conceives its opposite within itself, as symbolized by the two small circles of either black or white located in the area of the opposite color. Finally, instead of a straight line dividing the circle into two even semicircles, the curve line, which resembles a reversed letter *S*, gives rise to a dynamic sense of both balance (between the two opposing forces) and change (of one into the opposite force).

Table 2. Some opposites of yin and yang

Yin	Moon	Earth	Night	Cold	Water	Winter
Yang	Sun	Heaven	Day	Heat	Fire	Summer

Table 3. Some binary properties of yin and yang

Yin	Static	Controlled	Dim	Cold	Soft	Weak
Yang	Dynamic	Excited	Bright	Hot	Hard	Strong
Yin	Passive	Covert	Internal	Lower	Downward	Fluidic
Yang	Active	Overt	External	Upper	Upward	Gaseous

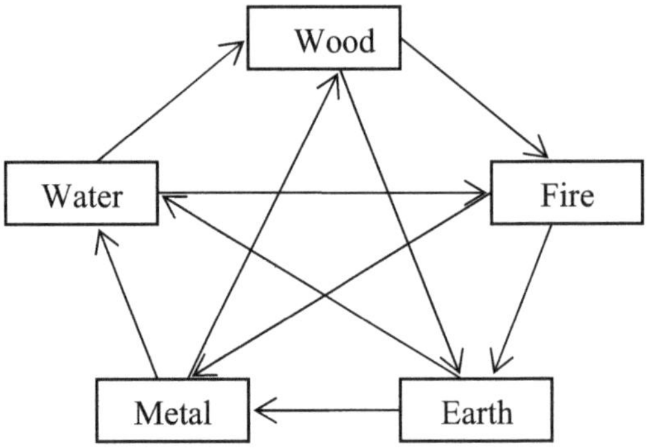

Figure 6. Relation of mutual promotion and restraint between the five elements

Table 4. A system of five-element categorization

Elements	Wood	Fire	Earth	Metal	Water
Nature					
Location	east	south	center	west	north
Season	spring	summer	long summer	autumn	winter
Climate	windy	hot	humid	dry	cold
Planet	Wood Pl. (Jupiter)	Fire Pl. (Mars)	Earth Pl. (Saturn)	Metal Pl. (Venus)	Water Pl. (Mercury)
Animal	chicken	sheep	ox	horse	pig
Crop	wheat	millet	foxtail millet	rice	bean
Life Cycle	birth	growth	ripeness	harvest	storage
Odor	rancid	scorched	fragrant	fishy	putrid
Flavor	sour	bitter	sweet	spicy	salty
Color	blue/green	red	yellow	white	black
Human					
Zang Org.	liver	heart	spleen	lung	kidney
Fu Org.	gallbladder	small intestine	stomach	large intestine	bladder
Sense Org.	eyes	tongue	mouth	nose	ears
Tissue	tendons	vessels	flesh	skin/body hair	bones
Emotion	anger	joy	overthinking	grief	fright
Indicator	nails	complex-ion	lips	body hair	hair
Expression	shouting	laughing	singing	wailing	moaning
Spirit	ethereal soul	spirit	purpose	corporeal soul	will

As two mutually complementary and opposing principles in Chinese thought, yin and yang categorize phenomena of like quality and relationship. They are rooted in, and interdependent on, each other, divisible but inseparable (Wiseman and Feng 1998: 705–708; see also Chen 1989b; Wang et al. 1997: 11–13). Some examples of yin and yang opposites in nature are listed in Table 2, and some of their binary properties are given in

Table 3 (Chen 1989b: 997). The human body, though an organic whole, can be classified in various ways according to the yin-yang schema. For example, its upper body is yang, and its lower body is yin. Its exterior is yang, and its interior is yin. With its exterior, the back is yang, and the front is yin. The outer side is yang, and the inner side is yin. The six fu organs are yang, and the five zang organs, the heart included, are yin. The network vessels are yang, and the channels are yin.

According to the five-element theory, the universe is composed of five basic elements – wood, fire, earth, metal, and water – which are in a relation of mutual promotion and restraint, as shown in Figure 6 (from Chen 1989b: 1000). In this figure, the lines forming the outer pentagon indicate the relation of promotion, and the lines forming the inner five-pointed star indicate the relation of restraint, with arrowheads indicating directions of promotion or restraint (see also Yu 1995, 1998). In traditional Chinese medicine, the theory of the five elements is applied to define nature and the human body as well as the perceived relations between them. Natural phenomena, human organs, related senses, emotions, and spirits are classified by their properties into five categories headed by the five elements. Some examples are given in Table 4 (from Wang et al. 1997: 14).

The five elements or phrases, like yin and yang, are categories of quality and relationship. The ancient Chinese saw phenomena within the universe as the products of the movement and mutation of the five elements representing qualities that relate to each other in specific ways (Wiseman and Feng 1998: 205–207; see also Chen 1989b; Wang et al. 1997: 13–16; section 6.4).

3.1.2. Theory of the qi

The theory of the qi also originates in ancient Chinese philosophy (Wang et al. 1997). As a philosophical concept, the qi in general, or the "essential qi" (精气 *jingqi*) in particular, "refers to the most essential substance from which life begins and on which life depends for its sustenance" (Zhang and Rose 2001: 6). It is "the original substance composing the ten thousand things" (Wang et al. 1997: 18). Since the universe and the human are "one" and the human is a "copy" of the universe, the qi is also "the basic substance that composes human beings" (p. 18). Just as it is "seen to drive the winds through the atmosphere, accumulate in mountains and forests, and flow through rivers to the sea", it "must certainly circulate throughout the body itself" (Zhang and Rose 2001: 86). For instance, the *Guanzi* says,

"The qi is the substance of the body" (气者，身之充也《管子・心术下》). In traditional Chinese medicine, the function of qi as the basic corporeal substance and its relationship with the body are summarized in the two statements below:

> 气聚则形成，气散则形亡。(Wang et al. 1997: 32)
> When the qi gathers, the body takes shape; when the qi disperses, the body is dead.
> 形可化气，气可生形。(Wang et al. 1997: 19)
> The body can generate the qi, and the qi can produce the body.

Here, the Chinese word 形 *xing* originally means "form" in general in the material world. Since the human is a "replica" of the universe, the human body is but a kind of "form" in this material world. In the second statement, *xing* 'form; body' specifically refers to the five zang organs that produces and stores the essential qi. That is, the five zang organs transform the extract from food into the essential qi whereas the essential qi strengthens the five zang organs and the body as a whole. As such, the qi is conceptualized as the material basis of human life with both physical and mental activities.

The qi has a very close relationship with the blood, which is the unity of the opposites of yin (blood) and yang (qi), and which is expressed by a metaphorical statement: "The blood is the official residence of the qi, and the qi is the commander in chief of the blood" (血为气之府，气为血之帅 Wang et al. 1997: 38). The qi is generated in the blood, and is responsible for the circulation of the blood when pumped by the heart organ. Therefore, as is said, "The exploiter of the qi is the blood, whereas the transporter of the blood is the qi" (采气者既是血，运血者既是气 p. 38). Since they coexist and depend on each other, they affect each other pathologically.

3.1.3. Theory of internal organs

It is said that the theory of the internal organs is the "core" and "axis" of Chinese medicine (Wang et al. 1997: i–ii). It deals with the physiological functions and pathological changes of the internal organs, which include *zang* 'viscera' and *fu* 'bowels' (see Table 4) and extraordinary fu organs.[45]

---

[45] The "extraordinary fu organs" is a "collective term for brain, marrow, bones, vessels, gallbladder and uterus" (Zhang 2001: 622). They are distinguished from the fu organs because they do not decompose food or convey waste, and

It holds a "holistic view" of the human body (as an organic unity centered on the five zang organs) and its unity and correspondence with nature. This view reveals itself in two aspects: "the five zang organs form one system (五脏一体 *wuzang yiti*)" and "nature and man form one system (天人一体 *tianren yiti*)" (p. 53). Here, the Chinese word 体 *ti* can mean both "system" and "body". After all, a system is a "body", and a body is a "system".

Specifically, the internal organs of the body are divided into two major classes (see Table 4). The five organs of primary importance are called zang: liver, heart, spleen, lung, and kidney. Each of them is matched with and related to an organ of secondary importance called fu: respectively, gallbladder, small intestine, stomach, large intestine, and bladder. An extra fu organ is called *sanjiao* 'triple heater/burner'. According to the yin-yang theory, all the zang organs belong to the yin, whereas all the fu organs belong to the yang.[46] In the five-element theory, liver and gallbladder belong to wood, heart and small intestine to fire, spleen and stomach to earth, lung and large intestine to metal, and kidney and bladder to water. With the relationship of mutual promotion, for instance, the essence of the kidneys (water) can nurture the liver (wood), and the liver (wood) can supply the heart (fire) with blood that it produces and stores. With the relationship of mutual restraint, for example, the earth of the spleen can stop the flooding of the kidney water, while the moisture of the kidneys (water) can prevent the heart fire from blazing.

Having laid out the relevant background information, I now show how traditional Chinese medicine conceptualizes the heart as the central organ of the body. As will be seen, its conceptualization of this bodily organ is

---

from the zang organs because they do not produce and store essence (Wiseman and Feng 1998). The gallbladder poses a special case because it is classed both as a fu and as an extraordinary fu organ. It is considered a fu organ because it plays a role in the processing and conveyance of food, and stands in an interior-exterior relationship with its paired zang, the liver. However, the bile that it produces is regarded as a "clear fluid" rather than as waste; hence it is also classed among the extraordinary fu organs.

46 It is worth noting that the yin-yang classification is dynamic, not static. Thus, the zang organs are yin as a group, but each of them can be yin or yang within that group. Furthermore, each zang or fu organ itself can be divided into two opposite sides. For instance, the heart as a member of the zang group is yin, but it is also yang within the zang group, and it has two opposite sides: the heart yin and the heart yang (see Wang et al. 1997:11–13). That is to say, yin and yang are relative to the levels of a hierarchical system, and this relativity in distinguishing between yin and yang reflects a dialectical viewpoint.

fundamentally metaphorical in nature, framed by two socially-based metaphors: (1) THE HEART IS THE RULER OF THE BODY, the same metaphor utilized by ancient Chinese philosophers, as discussed in Chapter 2; and (2) THE HEART IS THE GRAND MASTER OF THE INTERNAL ORGANS, which is specific to the medical context. In the next two sections (3.2 and 3.3) respectively, I will discuss the manifestation of these two metaphors in the medical literature.

3.2. The heart as the ruler of the body

As mentioned earlier, traditional Chinese medicine holds the view that the five zang organs form one system. That is, the internal organs inside the human body form a unified system, with each of them carrying out its own function but at the same time depending on the functions of other organs. In this organic system the five zang organs, while each representing a functional subsystem, compose its central operating system, of which the supreme commander is the heart. Hence, the heart is conceptualized as the "ruler" of the body, which in turn is conceived of as the microcosm of a state.

3.2.1. The heart as the "ruler"

Traditional Chinese medicine bears much similarity with ancient Chinese philosophy in its conceptions of the heart. The *Yellow Emperor's Internal Classic* (《黄帝内经》*Huangdi Neijing*), the earliest existent medical text in China first written during the Warring States period (475–221 BC), consists of two parts, the *Elementary Questions* (《素问》*Suwen*) and the *Magic Pivot* (《灵枢》*Lingshu*). The former includes the following definition of the heart based on the metaphor THE HEART IS THE RULER OF THE BODY, which is part of the metaphor characterizing the body, THE BODY IS A STATE.

> 心者，君主之官也，神明出焉。《素问》(Ji 1995, vol. 65: 10)
> The heart holds the office of monarch, whence the spiritual light emanates. *The Elementary Questions.* (Translation adopted from Wiseman and Feng 1998: 264)

The heart is to the body as the monarch is to the country. The *Internal Classic* describes the functions of the internal organs by the GOVERNMENT metaphor. Just as the monarch leads the nation and embodies its consciousness, so is the heart considered to be the seat of consciousness in the body (Wiseman and Feng 1998). It is therefore regarded as the source of the "spiritual light" or mental power. In his exposition of this definition, Zhang Jingyue, a theorist of Chinese medicine in the Ming dynasty (1368–1644), says:

> 心为一身之君主，禀虚灵而含造化，具一理而应万机，脏腑百骸，唯所是命，聪明智慧，莫不由之，故曰神明出焉。(Wang et al. 1998: 53)
> The heart is the monarch of the whole body. Empty and intelligent in character, it contains nature all in itself. Upholding one principle, it handles a myriad of state affairs. All the zang and fu organs and bones and parts follow its orders. Intelligence and wisdom arise solely from it. Therefore, it is said that the spiritual light emanates from the heart.

Note that when the heart is said to be "empty", "void", or "vacuous", it refers to its quality of being a "container" willing and ready to receive and incorporate. This is also a central image of the heart in ancient Chinese philosophy, as seen in Chapter 2. Indeed, this characterization shows that the heart, with its "spiritual light", takes the "ruling" position in the body. It really mirrors the conceptions of the heart in ancient Chinese philosophy, exemplifying its overall influence on traditional Chinese medicine.

Given below is a medical definition of the heart by the famous ancient doctor of the Han dynasty (206 BC–AD 220), Hua Tuo.

> 心者，脏之尊号，帝王之称也。与小肠为表里，神之所舍。又主血，属于火，旺于夏，手少阴是其经。《中藏经》(Wang et al. 1997: 193)
> The "heart" is the honorary title for the zang organ that bears the name of "emperor". It stands in an exterior-interior relationship with the small intestine, and is the home of the spirits. It also governs the blood, belongs to fire, and prospers during the summer. The hand lesser yin is its channel. *The Central Organ Classic*.

The first sentence is an instantiation of the HEART AS RULER metaphor, but also suggests its reverse metaphor THE RULER IS THE HEART OF THE STATE discussed in Chapter 2. These two metaphors are really the two sides of one coin, given that nature (including the social structure it contains) and man are one. In this definition, the heart mentally houses the spirits, and physiologically governs the blood. As a zang organ, which is yin, it pairs with the small intestine, a fu organ that is yang, to form the exterior-interior relation. It belongs to fire and is most vigorous during the summer (see Table 4). Finally, of the twelve channels in the body, the one that homes to the heart and nets the small intestine is called the "hand lesser yin heart channel".[47] While the "hand lesser yin" (手少阴 *shou shaoyin*) is the channel of the heart, all twelve channels in the body are commanded by the heart as the "ruler".

> 十二经皆听命于心，故为君，位南方，配夏令，属火，故为君火。十二经之气皆感而应心，十二经之精皆贡而养心，故为生之本，神之居，血之祖，脉之宗。盖神以气存，气以精宅，其理洵不诬也。《心病源流》(Wang et al. 1997: 194)
> The twelve channels all receive commands from the heart, which is the ruler. The heart is located in the south and matched with the summer season. It belongs to fire, and is thus the monarch fire. The qi of all twelve channels reacts and responds to the heart, and the essence of all twelve channels pays tribute to and nurtures the heart. Therefore, the heart is the root of life, the residence of the spirits, the ancestor of the blood, and the forefather of the vessels. Thus, the spirits live on the qi, and the qi resides in the essence. This is indeed a right observation. *The Sources of Heart Diseases.*

As the ruler, the heart commands the twelve channels and receives tribute or nutrients from them. Besides, it is also understood as the "ancestor of the blood" and the "forefather of the vessels" by the genealogical metaphor, as the "root of life" by the PLANT metaphor, and as the "residence of the spirits" by the CONTAINER metaphor. Another example of the HEART AS RULER metaphor is from a medical text of the Tang dynasty (618–907).

> 心主神，神者，五脏专精之本也。为帝王，监领四方。夏王七十二日，位在南方，离宫火也。《心脏脉论第一》(Wang et al. 1997: 193)
> The heart governs the spirits, which are rooted in the essences of the five zang organs. It is the emperor, supervising and leading all in the four directions. It is the king of the summer of 72 days, when it stays in the south, its temporary imperial palace being the fire. *On the Heart and Vessels: Chapter One.*

---

47 According to Chinese medicine, the human body has "twelve channels" that form the basic structure of the channel system comprising six of the hand and six of the foot. The "hand lesser yin heart channel" is the channel that homes to the heart and nets the small intestine (Wiseman and Feng 1998).

The spirits governed by the heart derive from the essences produced by all the five zang organs. As the emperor, the heart dominates the whole body, which is metaphorically understood as the country with a center and a vast expanse of land stretching out in four directions. As one of the five zang organs, the heart has its own specific properties in contrast with the other four. Its natural season is the summer that lasts 72 days; its location or direction is the south; and its element, metaphorically understood as the "temporary imperial palace", is the fire.

What is noteworthy is the distinction between the physical and mental aspects of the heart. A medical text of the Ming dynasty defines the heart and describes its physical or "formal" aspect and mental or "spiritual" aspect in the following passage.

> 心者，一身之主，君主之官。有血肉之心，形如未开莲花，居肺下肝上是也。有神明之心。神者，气血所化，生之本也，万物由之盛长，不著色象，谓有何有，谓无复存，主宰万事万物，虚灵不昧者是也。然形神亦恒相因，凡心之病皆因忧愁思虑，而后邪得以入之。《医学入门》 (Wang et al. 1997: 194)
>
> The heart is the master of the whole body, and the organ of monarch. There is a heart of blood and flesh, whose shape is like a lotus flower not yet in blossom, and which is located beneath the lungs and above the liver. There is a heart of spiritual light. The spirits are those into which the qi and blood have transformed. They are the roots of life, from which the ten thousand things grow prosperously. They do not have a form or appearance. They are there but invisible, formless yet existent. They dictate the ten thousand affairs and the ten thousand things. They are empty yet divine, and never become dim or dark.[48] However, the form and the spirit are always interrelated. All the diseases of the heart start with worry, anxiety, sorrow, and overthinking, and thereafter the pathogenic evils are able to intrude into it. *Gateway to Medicine.*

---

48 In the Chinese original, 灵 *ling* means both "divine" and "intelligent" (HYDCD 2000: 1779). The word 昧 *mei* means both "dim; dark" and "foolish; confused" (p. 1608). In the English translation, I use the first of these two possible choices in conformity with the metaphor of the "spirits" as "spiritual light". Note that this metaphor is an instantiation of such conceptual metaphors as INTELLIGENCE IS LIGHT and KNOWING/UNDERSTANDING IS SEEING (Sweetser 1990; Lakoff and Johnson 1999; see also Jäkel 1995; Radden 1996; Turner 1991; Yu 2003d, 2004).

This passage really reminds us of Wang Yangming, the famous Neo-Confucian of the Ming dynasty, who argued that the heart is not only a "lump of blood and flesh", but also a mental "half", which he called "nature", the "origin of the universe", the "Principle of Heaven", the "true self", or the "divine light" on various occasions (see 2.2). As defined metaphorically in this passage, the heart is the "master", "monarch", "dictator" of the body, which echoes the metaphorical conceptions of the heart in ancient Chinese philosophy. What makes the passage medical is its description of the heart from apparently anatomical and pathological viewpoints. Here, the distinction between the "heart of blood and flesh" and the "heart of spiritual light" gives rise to the two aspects of the heart: the form and the spirit (形神 *xingshen*). The "form" refers to the physical organ of the heart, whereas the "spirit" refers to the mental power of the heart, which derives from the qi and blood and is stored in the heart. Though "empty" and "formless", the spirits of the heart "dictate the ten thousand affairs and the ten thousand things". As is argued in the passage, the two aspects of the heart, its form and spirit, are closely interrelated. Thus, for instance, the heart diseases are often caused by psychological or emotional factors that belong to the mental aspect of the organ.

As discussed earlier, though one of the zang organs that belong to the yin as a class, the heart is conceptualized in traditional Chinese medicine as "the sun of the human body" (人身之日 *renshen zhi ri*). This conceptualization reflects the dominant ancient cosmological vision that the universe and the human are one and correspond to each other, as is exemplified in the following quotation from an ancient medical text:

> 盖人与天地相合，天有日，人亦有日，君父之阳，日也。《医学实在易》(Wang et al. 1997: 84)
> Therefore, the human being corresponds to Heaven and Earth. Heaven has the sun, so does the human being. The yang of monarch and father is the sun. *Essentials of Medicine.*

Here, the "yang of monarch and father" refers to the heart. Note that the heart is the "master" of the body and both in Confucianism and in traditional Chinese culture in general, the "father" is the "master" of the family and household as much as the monarch is the "master" of the country. Note that there is something common to the sun, the monarch, and the father. That is, they are all centers in a certain sense: The sun is the center of a constellational system, the monarch the center of a country, and the father the center of a family. Of these, the monarch as the center of the country and the father as the center of the family are views that, while originally promoted by Confucianism, are deeply entrenched in the ethical value system of traditional Chinese culture.

As shown in the previous examples, the heart is the organ of fire according to the five-element categorization. One medical text of the Qing dynasty (1616–1911) says this:

> 心者，君主之官，神明出焉。盖心为火脏，烛照事物，故思神明。神有名而无物，即心中之火气也。然此气非虚悬无着，切而指之，乃心中一点血液，湛然朗润，以含此气。故气时有精光发见，即为神明。心之能事，又主生血，而心窍中数点血液，则又血中之最精微者，乃生血之原泉，亦出神之渊海。……包络者，心之外卫，心为君主之官，包络即为臣，故心称君火，包络称相火……。《血证论》(Wang et al. 1997: 194)
>
> The heart holds the office of monarch, whence the spiritual light emanates. Thus, the heart is the organ of fire, illuminating all affairs and things, so it takes charge of the spiritual light.[49] The spirits have a name, but no shape. They are just the fire qi in the heart. However, this qi is not something grounded in nothing; to be exact, it is the drop of blood in the heart that, bright and shiny, contains this qi. This qi sometimes sheds bright light, and that is the spiritual light. The heart is capable of coping with things, and is also in charge of producing the blood. The several drops of blood in the heart aperture are the best and finest of all blood. Therefore, the heart is the original spring that produces the blood, and it is also the deep and vast sea from which the spirits emerge. … The pericardiac network is the external defense of the heart. The heart is the organ of monarch, while the pericardium is the subject. Thus, the heart is called the monarch fire, and the pericardium is called the prime minister fire… *On Symptoms of Blood Diseases.*

By virtue of its spiritual light, the heart commands the body as the "organ of monarch", and "enlightens" it as the "organ of fire". The passage actually grounds the heart's mental power, or spirits, on a material basis of substances of qi and blood. It claims that the spirits stored in the heart are its "fire qi" residing in the blood inside its "aperture". It is the "fire qi" that sheds the "spiritual light". The explanation that the heart's mental power arises from the qi and blood is consistent with the earlier statement, a metaphorical one, about the relationship between the qi and blood that the

---

49 The Chinese word 思 *si* can, in one of its senses, be used as the same sense as 司 *si* 'take charge of; manage' (HYDCD 2000: 1139).

blood is the official residence of the qi whereas the qi is the commander in chief of the blood. Because the heart produces the blood and possesses the "best and finest" drops of blood in its "hole" or "aperture" that hosts and nurtures the "fire qi" or the "spirits", it is described metaphorically as the "original spring" from which the blood flows and the "deep and vast sea" from which the mental power arises. In keeping with the HEART AS RULER metaphor, the passage describes the enveloping pericardiac network of the heart as its "defense", its "subject", and its "prime minister". That is, the HEART AS RULER metaphor is only part of a more general metaphor THE BODY IS A SOCIETY. These metaphors manifest the predominant philosophical view that the human body is a microcosm of the external world including the social and political structure of a state.

3.2.2. Other organs as "officials" ruled by the heart

Indeed, the GOVERNMENT metaphor is an extensive metaphor system in both ancient Chinese philosophy and traditional Chinese medicine, "because there is no difference in the Chinese mind between the well-organized political body and the human body" (Larre and Rochat de la Vallée 1996: 2). In ancient Chinese philosophy, as seen in Chapter 2, the sense organs are often metaphorized as "officials" or "subjects" in support of the "ruler", the heart. In traditional Chinese medicine, however, the GOVERNMENT metaphor is applied more to define the functions and relations of the internal organs, highlighting their interrelationships as a unified system. For instance, the five zang organs, which represent five functional subsystems in physiology and compose the central operating system of the body, are each assigned a "governmental office" under the heart as the supreme ruler. Their positions are similar to those of the officials of the central court directly under the emperor. The fu organs are assigned an office, too.

For instance, the liver, the zang of wood, is said to be the "organ of general" with an "unyielding" character (肝为刚脏 *gan wei gang zang*):

> 肝者，将军之官，谋虑出焉。《素问》(Ji 1995, vol. 65: 10)
> The liver holds the office of general, whence strategies emanate. *The Elementary Questions.* (Translation from Wiseman and Feng 1998: 358)

In the original, the word 谋虑 *moulü* means "contemplation and deliberation". Thus, just as "the heart governs the spiritual light" (心主神明 *xin zhu shenming*), "the liver governs the making of strategies" (肝主谋虑 *gan zhu moulü*). According to the theory of the internal organs, the ability to make plans is dependent upon a healthy liver because liver qi depression can give rise to rashness, impatience, and anger and liver qi insufficiency manifests itself in a tendency toward fright. These emotional tendencies can prevent the individual from "keeping a cool head" in matters of planning (Wiseman and Feng 1998: 358). Chinese medicine attributes or relates people's mental capacity to their physiological condition. Only when the liver is physiologically healthy can it make the right strategic plans. After all, Chinese medicine regards the qi and blood as the physiological basis of mental ability.

The gallbladder, a fu organ, pairs with the liver, a zang organ, in an exterior-interior relationship, with both belonging to wood. Seen as a righteous, unbiased, and selfless official, the gallbladder is perceived as possessing the mental capability and function of making judgments and decisions (Chen 1989c; Wang et al. 1997).[50]

> 胆者，中正之官，决断出焉。《素问》(Ji 1995, vol. 65: 10)
> The gallbladder holds the office of justice, from which decision emanates. *The Elementary Questions.* (Translation from Wiseman and Feng 1998: 235)

That is, "the gallbladder governs decision" (胆主决断 *dan zhu jueduan*). In the theory of the internal organs, this means that "the ability to maintain balanced judgment in the face of adversity is attributed to the gallbladder" (Wiseman and Feng 1998: 234). When gallbladder qi is weak and timid, people would show signs of lacking courage and decision, and timidity, doubt and suspicion. In modern terms, "the gallbladder governs decision" can be interpreted to mean that "certain aspects of the nervous system are traditionally ascribed in Chinese medicine to the gallbladder" (p. 234).

Also, the gallbladder is closely related to the liver, as a pair of zang and fu organs, in two senses. Physiologically, the gallbladder is attached to the liver, storing and excreting bile produced by the liver. The disease in one organ often affects the other. Psychologically, the gallbladder and the liver are also closely connected. Thus, "the liver is the organ of general, in

---

50 Readers are referred to Yu (2003a) for a study of the conceptualization of the gallbladder in Chinese culture and language. It is argued there that the culture-specific understanding of the gallbladder as the organ that makes judgments and decisions and determines one's degree of courage forms the base of the cultural model for the abstract concept of courage.

charge of contemplation and deliberation, but it relies on the gallbladder for judgment and decision" (Wang et al. 1997: 750): "The liver is the general in the center, but it relies on the gallbladder for decision" (夫肝者，中之将也，取决于胆《素问》). So defined, the liver is the "strategy-planning general" while the gallbladder is the "decision-making top advisor". The mutually dependent and complementary relationship between the two is also summarized by the statement below:

> 胆附于肝，相为表里，肝气虽强，非胆不断，肝胆相济，勇敢乃成。(Wang et al. 1997: 758)
> The gallbladder is attached to the liver, and they stand in exterior-interior relationship. Although the liver is strong with its qi, it always depends upon the gallbladder to make decisions. When the liver and the gallbladder complement each other, bravery is established.

In fact, the gallbladder is the only fu organ that is involved in mental processes and activities. It has a dual identity, both as a fu and as an extraordinary fu organ. As an extraordinary fu organ, it is categorized with the brain, which also plays a role in mental activity (see section 3.4 below).

In the theory of the internal organs, the heart and the gallbladder entertain a special relation too. The heart is the organ of emperor, dictating all psychological and mental activities (Wang et al. 1997). However, it is the gallbladder as the organ of justice that makes judgments and decisions, guided by the heart. The disease of the gallbladder will affect the functions of the heart. For instance, if the gallbladder qi rises to trouble the heart, the patient will display unusual states of emotion. If the qi in the heart and the gallbladder is "weak" or "vacuous" (虚 *xu*), the patient may feel scared for any or no reason. If the emperor (heart) and the minister (gallbladder) help each other, they will together promote vitality and preserve life (君相相辅，推动生机).

The spleen and the stomach form another pair of zang and fu organs that stand in an interior-exterior relationship and that belong to earth, from which plants, including crops, grow. According to the *Elementary Questions*,

> 脾胃者，仓廪之官，五味出焉。《素问》(Ji 1995, vol. 65: 10)
> The spleen and stomach hold the office of the granaries, whence the five flavors emanate. *The Elementary Questions*. (Translation from Wiseman and Feng 1998: 554)

The spleen and the stomach are like officials responsible for the national grain stores, providing nourishment for the whole body. Since traditionally the effect of food was understood in terms of qi and flavor, the term "five flavors" denotes the five different nutritive properties of food (Wiseman and Feng 1998: 554). That is, both organs function in close cooperation in performing the main part of digestion and assimilation. The stomach governs intake and decomposition of food, preparing it for further digestion and assimilation by the spleen. The spleen governs movement, the transformation of food, and the distribution of its essence.

The zang organ, the lungs, also has an official position in the system of "government" headed by the heart. The *Elementary Questions* says:

> 肺者，相傅之官，治节出焉。《素问》(Ji 1995, vol. 65: 10)
> The lung holds the office of assistant, whence management and regulation emanate. *The Elementary Questions*. (Translation from Wiseman and Feng 1998: 376)

While the heart holds the office of monarch, the lung serves as its assistant in promoting and regulating the circulation of the blood. The heart governs the blood, whereas the lung governs the qi. The lung therefore helps the heart to carry blood to all parts of the body so that they are all nourished (Wiseman and Feng 1998).

Finally, the kidney is the zang organ of water that stores the seminal essence and governs the fluid and reproduction. In the *Elementary Questions*, it also has an official function:

> 肾者，作强之官，伎巧出焉。《素问》(Ji 1995, vol. 65: 10)
> The kidney holds the office of labor, whence agility emanates. (Translation from Wiseman and Feng 1998: 328)

Here, "labor" actually refers to the healthy state of being mentally energetic and physically vigorous, whereas "agility" refers to the skillfulness and ability to get things done. Mental and physical agilities "are dependent upon kidney qi being abundant, and marrow and essence being plentiful" (Wiseman and Feng 1998: 327).

In short, the HEART AS RULER metaphor is merely part of the GOVERNMENT metaphor system in traditional Chinese medicine. This metaphor system, which is fundamentally conceptual in nature, is only a manifestation of the more general outlook in Chinese thought – the Chinese cosmological vision, according to which the human is an integral part of nature, and the human body corresponds to the external world as its replica. Holding such a cosmological view, the theorists and practitioners of traditional Chinese medicine would look into the body by comparing it with the world in which they live. It is not surprising that they would see many "parallels" between the internal structure of the human body and the political and social structure of the external world when they were looking for such parallels between them.

3.3. The heart as the grand master of the internal organs

As shown in the definition of theory of the internal organs at the beginning of the previous section, the human body as an organic whole has a central operating system composed of the five zang organs. The very core of that system, however, is the heart. As the dominant part of the body, the heart is conceptualized as the "ruler" of a country, whereas other organs, both zang and fu ones, are conceptualized as the "officials" of the central government. The GOVERNMENT metaphor system has been demonstrated in the previous section. In this section, I will focus on the conceptualization of the heart with a leading role among the five zang organs that constitute the central operating system of the body with the assistance of the six fu organs. This conceptualization is again metaphorical in nature, based on the metaphor THE HEART IS THE GRAND MASTER OF THE INTERNAL ORGANS, manifested in the literature of traditional Chinese medicine.

As suggested earlier, the reason why the heart is assigned such a leading role is that it is perceived to possess the supreme mental power, or the "spiritual light", with which to command the whole body. Wang et al. (1997: 87), applying the HEART AS RULER metaphor, summarize its dominant role in one's thought and emotion as follows:

> 人的神志活动与心的关系最为密切，这是因为心为君主之官，神明之府，是精神活动产生和藏附的中心。
> The mental and emotional activities of humans are most closely related to the heart. This is because the heart is the organ of monarch, and the palace of the spiritual light. It is the center for generating mental power and hosting mental activities.

This passage mixes traditional and modern terminology for a medical characterization of the heart. In traditional terms, the reason why the heart "holds the office of monarch" is that it is "the palace of the spiritual light", and in contemporary terms, the heart is “the center for generating mental power and hosting mental activities”. “The heart spirits dictate life activities” (心神是生命活动的主宰), commanding and regulating the activities of the internal organs and other parts of the body (p. 53). The functional activities of all the organs and parts, such as the liver storing the blood, the lungs governing respiration, the spleen governing transformation, the kidneys storing the essence, are uniformly accomplished under the mastership of the heart.

In fact, the heart’s supreme role as the leader and commander of the central operating system was already established in the earliest existent medical text in China, the *Magic Pivot*. It is said there:

> 心者，五脏六腑之大主也，精神之所舍也。《灵枢》(Ji 1995, vol. 65: 129)
> The heart is the grand master of the five zang and six fu organs, and is the residence of the spirits. *The Magic Pivot.*

The heart is qualified to be the “grand master” of the five zang and six fu organs because it is the “residence of the spirits”. Being the “residence of the spirits”, or having the function of “governing the spiritual light”, distinguishes it from, and raises it above, the other four zang organs. As Wang et al. (1997: 3) point out, the zang and fu organs, in the conceptions of Chinese medicine, do not merely refer to the entities of these organs, or the “organs of blood and flesh”, but also to the five systems of physiological functions headed by the five zang organs of the living body. However, it is the heart as the commander in chief of the central operating system that commands, coordinates, and regulates its activities. It does that by virtue of its “supreme power” or “spiritual light”.

In the next two subsections (3.3.1 and 3.3.2), I discuss how the heart acts as the “grand master” of the internal organs pertaining to its roles of governing and regulating the “spirits” and “emotions”.

3.3.1. The “grand master” and the spirits

According to traditional Chinese medicine, the heart has two main functions. First, it “governs the blood and vessels” (主血脉 *zhu xuemai*), moving the blood through the channels and vessels in its constant circulation throughout the body. Second, it “takes charge of storing the spirits” (主藏

神 *zhu cangshen*),[51] dictating the spiritual and mental activities of a person (Wang et al. 1997). Here, the first function is carried out by the physical heart or the center of a physiological system, whereas the second function refers to that of the mental heart or the center of a mental system. It is the conception of this second function, namely the heart as the center of the mental system, that is probably unique to traditional Chinese medicine.

In Chinese medicine, the term 神 *shen* 'spirits' has two aspects of meaning (Wang et al. 1997: 43–44). The first refers to the spiritual and mental aspects of a person. When it is said that "the heart stores the spirits", or "the heart governs the spiritual light", it is this mental aspect of meaning that is activated. The second aspect refers to the external manifestation of physiological functions and pathological changes of the human body. This physiological aspect of meaning is summarized in the Chinese compound word 神气 *shenqi*, which literally means "spiritual qi", but really refers to the external manifestation of one's vigor and vitality in one's complexions, looks, airs, and manners. Generally speaking, the so-called "spirits" in Chinese medicine, or in Chinese culture at large, refer to the total manifestation of life processes and activities, both physiological and mental, of a human being. They are based on the nutritive substances of essence and blood in the body, and are the product of the interaction between the yin of blood and the yang of qi.

Specifically, the spirits in Chinese medicine are defined in both a broad and a narrow sense (Wang et al. 1997: 43–44). The spirits in the broad sense include the "spirit" (神 *shen*), which is the archetype of the spirits, the "ethereal soul" (魂 *hun*), which is the yang aspect of the spirits, and the "corporeal or animal soul" (魄 *po*), which is the yin aspect of the spirits.[52]

---

51 Note that, while the heart is "in charge of" storing the spirits, it does not mean that it is the only organ that "stores the spirits". In fact, the spirits may be stored separately in all five zang organs, as already alluded to in Chapter 2 and will be addressed here in 3.3.1.

52 I am following Wiseman and Feng (1998) in translating 魂 *hun* and 魄 *po* respectively as "ethereal soul" and "corporeal or animal soul". It is also common to use the *pinyin* transliterations for them (e.g., Larre and Rochat de la Vallée 1991, 1992, 1995, 1996). According to the *Magic Pivot*, the ethereal soul is "that which follows the spirits faithfully in their going and coming" (随神往来者谓之魂), whereas the corporeal or animal soul is "that which associates with the essences in their exiting and entering" (并精而出入者谓之魄). Readers are referred to La Larre and Rochat de la Vallée (1995: 37–43; 1996: 38–48) for a detailed discussion of the statement in the *Magic Pivot*.

Of these, the first type bears the same name as the "spirits" in general. That is, the "spirit" is one type, but the archetype, of the "spirits". This is because the "spirits" in general and the "spirit" in particular are both governed by the heart, just as the heart is simultaneously one of the five zang organs and their "grand master". In other words, the heart is both a member of the category, equal to the other four members, and the head of the category, superior to the other four. It has a dual identity. The spirits in the broad sense are congenital. They come into being in the conception of the fetus, as the product of the "essential qi". As is said in the *Magic Pivot*, "the spirits arise when the two essences encounter each other" (两精相搏谓之神), and the "two essences" here refer to the sperm and the egg (Wang et al. 1997: 43).[53] That is, the spirits are already there at the very beginning of the new life, and they will develop as the body grows.

The spirits in the narrow sense refer to mental activities and processes, which are acquired after birth, during the process of growth, and in the contact with the external world. Traditionally, five types are listed in this category. They are 意 *yi* 'intention; purpose', 志 *zhi* 'will', 思 *si* 'thought', 虑 *lü* 'reflection; contemplation', and 智 *zhi* 'wisdom'. As defined in the *Magic Pivot*, these five kinds of spirits form a chain, each one on the right growing out of the one to its left, but the whole chain grows out of the heart:

> 所以任物者谓之心，心有所忆谓之意，意之所存谓之志，因志而存变谓之思，因思而远慕谓之虑，因虑而处物谓之智。《灵枢》(Ji 1995, vol. 65: 91)
>
> That which takes charge of things is the heart. When the heart is utilized, there is intention. When intention is preserved, there is will. When will is maintained for changes, there is thought. When thought extends itself far and oriented, there is reflection. When reflection is applied in dealing with things, there is wisdom. *The Magic Pivot*. (Translation adopted with modifications from Larre and Rochat de la Vallée 1991, 1995, 1996)

The heart as the central faculty of cognition takes charge of dealing with things. The use of the heart results in intention. If the intention is prolonged, it becomes will. The maintenance of will for change will cause thinking.

---

53 In the macrocosm of nature, as in contrast to the microcosm of the human, the "two essences" can refer to those of Heaven and Earth. Heaven and Earth, the parents of the ten thousand things, represent respectively the yang and yin forces, the interaction of which "gives birth to" all things and beings. See also Larre and Rochat de la Vallée (1995: 30–35).

Deep and oriented thought is reflection. The application of reflection in dealing with things means wisdom. It is clear that these five types of "spirits" are all rooted in the heart. The heart is thus regarded as the locus of the cognitive agent from the holistic viewpoint of Chinese medicine.

As defined above in two aspects of meaning and in a broad and a narrow sense, the "spirits" in traditional Chinese medicine govern one's life processes and activities, such as thought, consciousness, and motion, and are manifested in one's look, manner, emotion, aspiration, intelligence, speech, and so on. In short, it can be said that the spirits govern and manifest life. No wonder the *Elementary Questions* says, "Those who obtain the spirits will prosper, and those who lose the spirits will die" (得神者昌，失神者亡).

In relation to the functions of the five zang organs, the spirits are also classified, in a way that combines the above two, into five types, known as the "five spirits" (五神 *wushen*). They are respectively called 神 *shen* 'spirit', 魂 *hun* 'ethereal soul', 魄 *po* 'corporeal or animal soul', 意 *yi* 'intention; purpose', and 志 *zhi* 'will'. What is unique to the theory of the internal organs are its conceptions reflected in a statement by the philosopher Wang Fuzhi (1619–1692): "What takes the critical position in the human body is the heart. The spiritual light of the heart, however, is stored separately in the five zang organs, and depends on the perception of the five sense organs" (人之身，居要者心也。而心之神明散寄于五脏，待感于五官 Cai 2000: 331). That is, the heart possesses and commands all the spirits but stores them separately in all five zang organs. The "spiritual light" also relies on the perception of the eyes, ears, nose, mouth, and body as a whole for its cognitive function. This Chinese view of the internal and external organs and of their interrelationship is a culture-specific version of the concept of "embodiment". One can say that it is a holistic characterization of the "embodied nature" of human cognition in the Chinese cultural context. The "spirits", ascribed to the heart but stored separately in the five zang organs, can work properly only with the help of the sense organs of the body. In other words, it is not just because the "mind" is located in the body, but because it arises from the body, from the internal zang organs and the external sense organs, that it is "embodied". So conceptualized, the five zang organs are all related to mental functions. This is because they produce and store essential substance (the "essential qi") of the body such as blood, qi, fluid, essence, which are taken as the physiological basis of mental vitality. The heart as the "grand master of the five zang and six fu organs" regulates and coordinates their functions and maintains a balanced state among them. If the heart's physiological functions are normal, the mind is lucid and sharp. Pathological changes of the heart will lead to disorder of psychological states and mental activities.

Because they all store the spirits, the five zang organs are thus called the "five spirits zang" (五神脏 or 五神藏 *wushen zang*). Each of them stores a particular type of spirit. Specifically, the heart stores the spirit (心藏神 *xin cang shen*) and "possesses" and "governs" all the spirits. The liver stores the ethereal soul (肝藏魂 *gan cang hun*), by which the ancients referred to the spirit that can exist independently of the body. Today, things such as sleepwalking, sleeptalking, illusion, and hallucination are ascribed to the function of the ethereal soul. The lungs store the corporeal or animal soul (肺藏魄 *fei cang po*), which is the type of spirit responsible for the instinctive feeling and bodily movement. For instance, the ability of the newborn to cry and take milk is understood as a manifestation of the corporeal soul (Wiseman and Feng 1998). For the remaining zang, the spleen stores the intention or purpose (脾藏意 *pi cang yi*), and the kidneys store the will (肾藏志 *shen cang zhi*). While the essential substances that the zang organs produce and store constitute the physiological foundation of mental vitality, mental processes and activities also affect the operation of the zang organs. The heart as the "grand master" of the internal organs, however, coordinates the functions of the five zang organs and regulates the activities of the spirits stored in them. If the regulation of mental activities goes wrong, the physiological functions of the five zang organs will go wrong as well. That is why the heart is said to "govern the spiritual light" while the spirits are stored separately in the five zang organs. Zhang (2001: 1083–1084) expounds and interprets the saying "the heart governs the spiritual light" as follows:

> …the heart has the function of controlling spirit, consciousness and thinking, which are the higher activities of the central nerves. This function plays an important role in regulating the functional activities of the other organs. As blood is the material basis of mental activities, sufficient heart-blood will appear as high spirit and clear mind, while insufficient heart-blood may cause disturbed mental activities, manifested as palpitation, amnesia, insomnia, etc. In addition, disturbance of the heart in controlling mental activities may also lead to functional disturbance of other zang and fu organs.

Apparently, if or how the heart fulfills its function of "governing the spiritual light" has important consequence on the functional activities of the other organs. The disturbance of the heart's function of controlling mental activities will cause other zang and fu organs to be functionally disturbed as well. This is when the emotional factors come into play.

3.3.2. The "grand master" and the emotions

In traditional Chinese medicine, the heart is the seat of emotions, as well as the "palace" of spirits. The conception of the heart as the seat of emotions is a widespread phenomenon, to say the least, but what is probably unique to Chinese medicine is the view that emotions, while centrally controlled and regulated by the heart, are related separately to the five zang organs, just as the spirits are separately stored in them. Also according to the theory of the internal organs, the five zang organs' functions of storing different types of spirits may produce different kinds of emotions (Wang et al. 1997: 45). As the *Elementary Questions* says, "Humans have five zang organs, and the five zang produce five qi, from which arise the emotions of joy, anger, sorrow, anxiety, and fear" (人有五脏，化五气，以生喜怒悲忧恐).[54]

That is, the five zang organs generate five qi, which result in five emotions or affects: anger (怒 *nu*), joy (喜 *xi*), overthinking (思 *si*), sorrow or anxiety (悲 *bei* or 忧 *you*), and fear or fright (恐 *kong* or 惊 *jing*).[55] They are each classified with a zang organ: anger with the liver, joy with the heart, overthinking with the spleen, anxiety with the lungs, and fear with

---

[54] It must be pointed out that here, as much as in 3.3.1 where I discuss the concepts of "spirits" in traditional Chinese medicine, the English emotion words that I use in the glosses and translations, though based on the Chinese-English dictionaries and the existing translations in the literature, are used in a loose sense. This is because categorizations and lexicons of emotion as well as others can be different to varying degrees across languages and cultures (see, e.g., Wierzbicka 1992, 1999). So, when I use an English emotion word X in the glosses, translations, or main text, it should be interpreted as "X is in some sense equivalent or similar to the Chinese original".

[55] In traditional Chinese medicine, there are two ways of labeling emotions: a spectrum consisting of "seven emotions" (七情 *qiqing*) (i.e., joy, anger, sorrow, anxiety, overthinking, fear, and fright), and a spectrum consisting of "five emotions" (五志 *wuzhi*) (i.e., joy, anger, sorrow, anxiety or overthinking, and fear). The latter conforms to the five-element schema as found in Table 4 in 3.1.1. There are variations in the English translations of the Chinese emotion terms. Readers are referred to Larre and Rochat de la Vallée (1996) for a study of emotions in traditional Chinese medicine.

the kidneys (肝在志为怒，心在志为喜，脾在志为思，肺在志为忧，肾在志为恐). While these emotions arise from the functions of their corresponding zang organs, their excessiveness will injure each of them accordingly. Thus, anger injures the liver, joy injures the heart, sorrow injures the lungs, overthinking injures the spleen, and fear injures the kidneys. Since emotions come from the qi, they emerge in various behaviors of qi. According to the *Elementary Questions*, the qi goes "up" in anger, "slow" in joy, "deflated" in sorrow, "down" in fear, "messed" in fright, and "knotted" in overthinking (怒则气上，喜则气缓，悲则气消，恐则气下，惊则气乱，思则气结). Specifically, when one is angry, one's qi will "rise up" with blood. When one is happy (and joy is the only positive emotion of all those listed above), one's qi, as well as one's blood, circulates smoothly and slowly, which is good for one's health. However, sudden excessive joy can injure the heart by making the spirits inside unsteady or dispersed so that the person can hardly concentrate on anything. The emotion of sadness will consume much qi, and that will lead to "qi deficiency". The emotion of fear will hurt the kidney qi, and that will cause the qi to "fall down". If one is caught in a fright, a shock, the circulation of qi will be in disorder. Finally, overthinking will injure the spleen, and that will likely impede the circulation of qi (Wang et al 1997: 45). All the emotions here are characterized as particular movements of qi. Chinese medicine believes that psychological causes of disease can lead to somatic effects and somatic diseases can lead to psychological effects (Larre and Rochat de la Vallée 1996). In other words, the circulation of qi affects the function of the zang organs, and vice versa. This is especially true of the heart as "the master of the network of communication and free circulation" among the zang and fu organs and throughout the body (p. 97). Since emotions are related to the zang organs, an excessive emotion will injure a zang organ to which the emotion is related. In return, the physiological malfunction of any zang organ will also exhibit psychological symptoms.

It needs to be noted that, although the heart is specifically related to the emotion of joy, it reacts to other emotions as well, because it is the "governor" of all psychological states and mental activities, and is the "sovereign" that moderates all the zang in their contradictory moods (Larre and Rochat de la Vallée 1996: 82). Of all the internal organs, in fact, the heart is the most sensitive to emotional changes. This is because emotional changes are believed to originate from the heart but impact other zang organs depending on their kinds. As Zhang Jingyue of the Ming dynasty (1368–1644) put it:

> 情志之伤，虽五脏各有所属，然求其所由则无不从心而发。《类经》(Wang et al. 1997: 87)
> The five zang organs all suffer from damages inflicted by their respective emotions. If, however, the causes of these damages are traced, all of them originate in the heart. *The Classified Canon*.

That is, while excessive emotions and affects injure the respective zang organs to which they belong, the causes of damage all stem from the heart. Zhang Jingyue explained how this is the case:

> 心为五脏六腑之主，而总统魂魄，并赅意志，故忧动于心则肺应，思动于心则脾应，怒动于心则肝应，恐动于心则肾应，此所以五志唯心所使也。《类经》(Wang et al. 1997: 87)
> The heart is the master of the five zang and six fu organs, presiding over the ethereal and corporeal souls, and directing intention and will. Therefore, when sorrow moves in the heart, the lung will respond, when overthinking moves in the heart, the spleen will respond, when anger moves in the heart, the liver will respond, and when fear moves in the heart, the kidney will respond. That is the reason why the five emotions are operated only by the heart. *The Classified Canon*.

Although the five emotions separately relate to the five zang organs, they "are all forged in the heart", and then affect the zang organs to which they relate. It is worth mentioning that emotions, as described in the above passage, "move" in the heart as a force. For this reason, it has been suggested that "whenever the symptoms of joy, anger, sorrow, fright, and overthinking are observed, it is always advisable to focus on the leveling of the heart fire" (五志所发，皆从心造，故凡见喜怒悲惊思之证，皆以平心火为主《儒门事亲》Wang et al. 1997: 181). Remember that the heart is the zang organ of fire. Here, however, the "heart fire" is a sort of pathological "fire" in the heart. Therefore, to "level the heart fire", that is, to reduce the "flaming of the heart fire" (心火上炎 *xinhuo shangyan*), is to get rid of the root cause of various emotional problems.

In short, traditional Chinese medicine asserts that emotions originate in the heart, which is the "grand master of the five zang and six fu organs". Their negative impact on the heart, however, will be transmitted to the other internal organs to which they belong. According to the *Yellow Emperor's Internal Classic*, "Sorrow, grief, worry and anxiety move the heart; when the heart is moved, the five zang and six fu organs are all rocked" (悲哀愁忧则心动，心动则五脏六腑皆摇).

Reflecting the influence of ancient Chinese philosophy, traditional Chinese medicine maintains that the heart also stores memory and knowledge and administers perception. For example, the *Magic Pivot* says, "One accumulates the spirits with the heart so as to know the past and present" (积神以心，以知往今 Wang et al. 1997: 181). As it seems, the heart is a container instrument with which one accumulates memory and knowledge so as to remember the past and know the present. The heart has this capacity because it presides over perception. As the *Classified Canon* says, "The ears are able to hear, and the eyes are able to see, all because of the heart" (是以耳之听，目之视，无不由乎心也 Wang et al. 1997: 181). The heart governs all the perceptual organs, and all things entering through them end up being stored in the heart for further processing.

In sum, the heart is "the grand master of the five zang and six fu organs" because of its two main functions. Physiologically, it "governs the blood and vessels". Mentally, it "governs the spiritual light". This second mental function of the heart has been the focus of our attention. The heart presides over mental processes and activities, which regulate and coordinate the functions of the other internal organs. Thus, as the *Elementary Questions* says, "If the master is lucid, all those beneath it will be at peace; if the master is not lucid, the twelve officials will be in danger" (主明则下安，主不明则十二官危).[56] Also, as one medical statement in ancient times summarizes it, "When the heart is in disorder, a hundred diseases will emerge; when the heart is in quiescence, ten thousand diseases will all disappear" (心乱则百病生，心静则万病悉去).

3.4. The heart or brain: Which one governs the spiritual light?

In traditional Chinese medicine, the "spiritual light" can refer to the life activities of the human body in general, but more specifically, it refers to the mental functions that guide the life activities of a living body. This "spiritual light" is traditionally ascribed to the functions of the heart, and therefore it is asserted that "the heart governs the spiritual light" (心主神明

56 The "twelve officials" here refer to the five zang and six fu organs, plus the pericardium of the heart. Again, the Chinese word 官 *guan* means both "organ" and "official". The meaning of "official" is selected to fit the obvious GOVERNMENT metaphor in the context.

xin zhu shenming). Specifically, as "the organ of monarch" (君主之官 *junzhu zhi guan*) with its mental power, the heart dictates all mental states, processes, and activities: carrying out thinking, storing memories, producing emotions, commanding intention and will, governing perception, and evolving dreams (Wang et al. 1997: 181). Now, the question is: If the heart fulfills all these mental functions, what does the brain do according to traditional Chinese medicine? Indeed, the brain takes a relatively peripheral position in this tradition, as will be discussed below.

In the theory of the internal organs, the brain is one of the so-called "extraordinary fu organs" (奇恒之腑 *qiheng zhi fu*), the others being marrow, bones, vessels, gallbladder, and uterus. These organs are distinguished from the zang organs for not producing essence, and from the fu organs for not decomposing food and conveying waste, and therefore are considered as less central than either the zang or the fu organs.

Nowadays, the brain is believed to have two main functions (Wang et al. 1997: 918–919). The first is to store the marrow and the second is to control and coordinate the movement of the four limbs. *The Magic Pivot* says, "The brain is the sea of marrow" (脑为髓之海 p. 917). The marrow derives from the essence stored in the kidneys, and travels up through the spinal cord to collect in the cranium. "If the sea of marrow is insufficient", says the *Magic Pivot*, "the brain turns and the ears ring, there is aching in the neck, dizziness, poor vision, and lethargy" (Wiseman and Feng 1998: 49). Secondly, the brain is related to the senses and control of physical movement. As the container of the "essential marrow" (精髓 *jingsui*), it is connected with the seven orifices in the head and contributive to their functions. The *Elementary Questions* says, "The head is the palace for the essential light" (头者，精明之府 Wang et al. 1997: 181). This statement recognizes the fact that the head hosts the sense organs that are in charge of perception, and contains the brain marrow that derives from the essence produced and stored in the kidneys, and that nourishes the sense organs to enhance their perceptual capability. The brain is also connected with all the marrow in the bones, coordinating the movement of the limbs and being responsible for their strength. However, as Wiseman and Feng (1998) point out, the main functions of the brain as perceived by Western medicine are ascribed in the theory of the internal organs to the heart and other zang organs.

In the Ming and Qing dynasties, however, the functions of the brain as the organ for mental processes and activities came to be recognized. For instance, Li Shizhen of the Ming dynasty (1368–1644), for the first time, proposed in his famous *Comprehensive Herbal Foundation* (《本草纲目》 *Bencao Gangmu*) that "The brain is the palace for the original spirit" (脑为元神之府), believing that consciousness and memory come from the brain (Wang et al. 1997: 930). His contemporary Jin Xizheng also suggested that "The memories of humans are all in the brain" (人之记性，皆在脑中 p. 181). Then, in the Qing dynasty, Wang Qingren explicitly argued that "Intelligence and memory are not in the heart, but in the brain" (灵机记性，不在心在脑 p. 181). He asked, "The heart is the pathway for the qi to exit and enter, and how can it produce intelligence and store memory?" (心乃出入气之道路，何能生灵机，贮记性 p. 931). He supported his argument with his observation on developmental changes over time in terms of memory. The newborns have no memory because their brain still does not have any marrow in it; the old people tend to lose their memory because their brain has gradually lost the marrow inside.

One ancient medical text of the Ming or Qing dynasty proposes that the treatment of forgetfulness is to enhance the interaction or coordination between the heart and the kidney (心肾相交 *xinshen xiangjiao*), which refers to the maintenance of balance between these two organs. The heart belongs to fire and the kidney to water. Their balance depends on the mutual restriction and mutual promotion of the heart fire and the kidney water. That is, the heart fire needs to go down to warm the kidney yang to prevent kidney water from overflowing, while the kidney water needs to go up to aid the heart yin to restrict heart fire's hyperactivity. As we can see from the statement below, the interaction or coordination of the heart and the kidney can supposedly treat not only physiological conditions, but also mental conditions.

> 治健忘者，必交其心肾，使心之神明，下通于肾，肾之精华，上升于脑，精能生气，气能生神，神定气清，自解遗忘之失。《类证治裁》(Wang et al. 1997: 29)
>
> To treat forgetfulness, one must interact and coordinate the heart and the kidney, so that the spiritual light of the heart is connected down to the kidney, and the essence of the kidney rises to the brain. The essence can produce the qi, and the qi can produce the spirits. When the spirits are settled and the qi becomes clear, forgetfulness is automatically dissolved. *Diagnosis and Treatment of Classified Symptoms*.

While the heart still governs the spiritual light, which commands and regulates other organs including the kidney, memory is located in the brain, which stores marrow derived from the essence produced and stored in the kidney. Thus, if the spiritual light of the heart is connected to the kidney, it will enhance the kidney's function of supplying the brain with essence that will turn into marrow in the brain. Sufficient essence (or marrow) in the brain will produce sufficient qi that will in turn enhance the spiritual light of the heart. The brain will benefit in such circularity of functional enhancement.

Today, the relationship between the heart and the brain is still under debate in the circles of Chinese medicine. There are three representative views, according to Wang et al. (1997: 180–182), as summarized below. One view argues that Chinese medicine should abandon the thesis that "the heart stores the spirit" simply because it is the brain, rather than the heart, that stores the spirit. The brain dictates the spiritual light. In the *Internal Classic*, the brain is said to be an extraordinary fu organ. In actuality, however, it "stores but does not discharge" (藏而不泻 *cang er bu xie*), and should be regarded as a zang organ.[57] Related to this view is the question why traditional Chinese medicine has attributed the intellectual function of the brain to the heart. The influence from ancient philosophy is cited as the most important contributing factor (p. 181–182). As we have seen in Chapter 2, ancient Chinese philosophy has a tradition of taking the heart as the "ruler" that "governs the spiritual light". Traditional Chinese medicine has borrowed and inherited that tradition. Also, since the ruler of the country is referred to as the "heart", the ruler's supreme political power is mapped onto the mental power which is attributed to the heart.

Another view, which is opposed to the first, believes that it is a misunderstanding to question the validity of the thesis that "the heart stores the spirit". The notion of "heart" in traditional Chinese medicine cannot be equated with the heart organ. Instead, it is a combination of heart and brain. According to the theory of the internal organs, the heart has two major functions: it governs the blood and vessels, and stores the spirit. To be more exact, these two functions represent the division of labor between the heart and the brain. That is, the heart governs the blood and vessels whereas the brain stores the spirits.

---

57 It is true that the brain "stores" marrow as those zang organs store essences. However, what this view has neglected is the fact that the brain itself does not produce essence as do the zang organs. As mentioned earlier, brain marrow derives from the essence produced by and stored in the kidneys. It goes upward through the spinal cord to converge in the cranial cavity (Wang et al. 1997).

Still another view points out that it is true that Chinese medicine differs from Western medicine in a fundamental way. That is, Chinese medicine believes that the heart stores and governs the spirits, whereas Western medicine ascribes the same functions to the brain. Both of them, however, emphasize the importance of blood transported from the heart to the brain through the channels and vessels that connect these two organs. This view makes a compromise between the two organs possible. Even if the brain is the real locus for all the mental processes and activities, it operates under the "mastership" of the heart, which commands the brain via the circulation of the qi and blood from the former to the latter. From the point of view of Chinese medicine, it makes better sense to say that "the heart governs the brain" than "the heart governs the spiritual light". This view, then, admits that "the brain governs the spiritual light" (脑主神明 *nao zhu shenming*), but it at the same time argues that the brain fulfills this function under the leadership of the heart. The heart, as the "grand master of the five zang and six fu organs", dominates the brain as well.

A slightly different version of this view argues that both the heart and the brain are responsible for the function of the spirits, but the heart takes the leading part whereas the brain plays a subordinate role. This view, as Wang et al. (1997: 182) point out, is actually derived from an argument in an early medical text by Zhang Xishun, the source of which is not identified:

> 神明之体藏于脑，神明之用发于心也。(Wang et al. 1997: 182)
> The substance of the spiritual light is stored in the brain, whereas the application of the spiritual light arises from the heart.

This view explicitly states that the brain stores the physiological substance of the "spiritual light", but the heart deploys and utilizes it.[58] The brain is a mere storehouse for it, and the heart has its ownership. In the statement below this view is further elaborated.

> 脑为元神，心为识神，脑中之神，体也，心中之神，用也。人欲用其神明则自脑达心，不用其神明，则仍由脑归心。(Wang et al. 1997: 182)

58 Traditional Chinese medicine attributes the "spiritual light" to the "essential qi" (精气 *jingqi*), which is regarded as the physiological substance or basis of the former and may include qi (气 *qi*), blood (血 *xue*), essence (精 *jing*), and so on.

> The brain is the original spirit whereas the heart is the cognitive spirit. The spirit in the brain is the substance, while the spirit in the heart is the application. When it is to be applied, the spiritual light will come to the heart from the brain. Even when it is not applied, the spiritual light in the brain still belongs to the heart.

As in this passage, the brain, or the spirit it stores, is called the "original spirit" (元神 *yuanshen*) whereas the heart, or the spirit it possesses, is called "cognitive spirit" (识神 *shishen*). The difference in labeling places the heart at a higher level than the brain. The brain houses the "original material", but the heart is able to manipulate it and make use of it for cognitive purposes. Specifically, the heart can deploy the spiritual light at its disposal whenever it needs to do so. Even if the heart does not need to use the spiritual light that stays in the brain, it still claims complete ownership of it from the brain. Thus, the brain is subordinate to the heart even though it actually "stores the spiritual light".

All these views, it is necessary to point out, are not original to traditional Chinese medicine. They are views put forth in the new light of modern development in both Chinese and Western medicine. The first view wants to accept the view of Western medicine as it is. The second and third views want to incorporate the Western view into the framework of traditional Chinese medicine in order to modernize it.

Today, as Wang et al. (1997: 101) conclude, Chinese medicine recognizes the close relationship between brain and mental activity. In practice, nevertheless, it still sticks to the traditional theory of internal organs and ascribes and subordinates the physiological function and pathological change of the brain to the central command of the heart, and to the separate functional subsystems of the five zang organs under the mastership of the heart.

3.5. Summary and discussion

The overall message that has emerged from the study presented in this chapter is that traditional Chinese medicine extensively shares the worldview of ancient Chinese philosophy. This worldview sees the human as an integral part of nature and as a replica of the universe, so that they correspond to each other in various ways. In this worldview, cosmological theories of yin-yang, the five elements, and the qi, which originate in ancient Chinese philosophy to explain the formation and transformation of the universe, are borrowed and incorporated into traditional Chinese medicine to account for the physiological functions and pathological changes of the human body. In return, these theories are enriched and consolidated in the medical context, and have become an important and valuable heritage of Chinese culture as a whole.

More specifically, the heart is conceptualized metaphorically as the ruler of the body in traditional Chinese medicine just as in ancient Chinese philosophy. "In the individual the heart is the son of Heaven, the image of Heaven, suggesting to man that he mold himself to Earth, to Heaven, and to Nature" (Larre and Rochat de la Vallée 1995: 46). According to the theory of the internal organs, the human body has a central operating system composed of five functional subsystems represented by the five zang organs. While the heart is one of the five zang organs, it takes a unique position with its supreme mental power. It is the ruler of the whole body. As listed in Chapter 2, the metaphor THE HEART IS THE RULER OF THE BODY has the following mappings:

THE HEART IS THE RULER OF THE BODY

Country	→	Body
Ruler	→	Heart
Central government/court	→	Central physiological system
Political power	→	Mental power
Governmental activities, processes, and states	→	Mental activities, processes, and states
Governmental officials	→	Bodily organs
Governmental functions, operations	→	Physiological functions, operations
Political situations of the country	→	Physiological conditions of the body

These mappings apply in traditional Chinese medicine as well. In this context, however, the mapping BODILY ORGANS ARE GOVERNMENTAL OFFICIALS consists of further mappings from governmental officials to internal organs. According to the *Elementary Questions*, the further mappings include the following, which I have cited as examples in 3.2.2. The mapping from the ruler to the heart is added to the list, too, since the heart is also one of the internal organs even though it is considered as superior to the rest of them.

INTERNAL ORGANS ARE GOVERNMENTAL OFFICIALS

Ruler	→	Heart
General	→	Liver
Justice	→	Gallbladder

Official of the Granaries	→	Spleen
Official of the Granaries	→	Stomach
Assistant	→	Lung
Labor Minister	→	Kidney

As is shown, the GOVERNMENT metaphor system is a complex and intricate one that looks into the human body for the interrelationship among its internal organs by comparing it with its macrocosm, the political and social entity of a country, the "body politic", with a structure widely known. It brings into relief the predominant worldview mentioned above.

In accordance with the theories of yin-yang and the five elements, traditional Chinese medicine also conceptualizes the heart metaphorically as the sun and the fire. The SUN and FIRE metaphors both entail the features of "heat" and "light" associated with the sun and fire. The "heat" is related to the physiological function of the heart. The heart pumps blood, with qi, around the body providing it with necessary energy and heat. The second feature, the "light", characterizes the mental function of the heart. With the "spiritual light" that it governs and houses, the heart "enlightens", as the "light source", not only the whole body by commanding and coordinating its activities, but also the whole world by understanding and changing its patterns. No wonder it is said that the ten thousand things grow out of the heart and the heart dictates the ten thousand things.

Another metaphor that is synonymous to that of HEART AS RULER is HEART AS MASTER. The heart is the "grand master" of the five zang and six fu organs. Being one of the five zang organs, the heart is in a unique position of mastering the rest of the internal organs because it governs the "spiritual light" or mental power. Although the heart commands all five types of spirits, it stores them separately in the five zang organs, with itself storing the "spirit", the archetype of all spirits. When the roots of various kinds of mental processes and activities are traced, they all come down to the heart. By the same token, various emotions, while belonging separately to the five zang, all originate from the heart.

Thus, metaphorically, the heart is both the "heart monarch" (心君 *xinjun*) and the "heart master" (心主 *xinzhu*). The monarch is an emperor or a king who is the "heart" of a state, while the master is the one who has the ownership of or authority over others. In the theory of the internal organs, the heart is distinguished from, and superior to, the rest of internal organs in that it is the "palace" or "residence" of the spirits. That is, it is also conceptualized metaphorically as a container that holds the supreme power over the other internal organs and the body as a whole. As Larre and

Rochat de la Vallée (1992: 2) have observed, "The heart is essentially a void because the void is the only possible dwelling place for the spirits". That is, the mental function of the heart lies in its quality of being "void", "empty", or "vacuous" as a container to hold the spirits. It may sound paradoxical that "For the heart, the fullness of life is emptiness" (p. 44). The mental function of the heart as the source of the enlightening radiance of the spirits is, however, fulfilled through its physiological function, namely, the circulation of blood. The "spiritual light" is radiated as blood is circulated, both from the heart. The circulation of the blood under the heart's authority carries "the double maintenance of life, which is both nutritive and spiritual" (p. 174).

Traditionally, Chinese medicine assigns little or no mental role to the brain. That role is attributed to the heart. The brain is merely an "extraordinary fu organ" that stores a special kind of essence – the brain marrow – and is thus called the "sea of marrow". It has been suggested that the real recognition of the important mental function of the brain did not happen until the introduction of Western medicine (see Wang et al. 1997: 182). Today, there are still different views regarding the relationship between the heart and the brain. One view believes that the brain, rather than the heart, governs the spiritual light. Another view believes that the heart governs the spiritual light, but the mental function of the heart includes that of the brain. A third view believes that the heart governs the brain, which houses the spiritual light. The second and third views represent the mainstream opinion in Chinese medicine today, which subordinates the mental function of the brain to the domination and supervision of the heart. As is said, there is new evidence in transplant surgery that suggests the validity of the thesis "The heart governs the spiritual light". That is, after a successful heart transplant, the organ receiver tends to display a similar mental and emotional state and linguistic behavior as the organ donor.[59]

At this point, I would like to present a Western perspective on one of the most remarkable differences between Chinese and Western medicine, namely, the difference in their views on which organ "governs the spiritual light", the heart or the brain. This difference highlights a more fundamental difference between "holism" and "dualism" in terms of the mind-body relationship that may distinguish between Chinese and Western philosophies and cultural models underlying the conceptions of body and mind. Judith Farquhar (1998), a medical anthropologist in America, discusses this difference by addressing the culture-specific characterization of the function

---

59 See Ouyang Qi's preface to the section of medicine in Ji (1995, vol. 65).

of the brain in Chinese medicine in her article entitled "Chinese medicine and the life of the mind: Are brains necessary?" She begins her article by asking a number of questions that suggest that the activities of the brain, unlike those of other organs, cannot be felt or experienced so easily:

> Think about it. In the everyday life of your body, how do you experience the activity of your brain? Is it like your heart, which can be felt in the pulse or as a beating in the chest in moments of tension or quietness? Is it like your stomach or intestines or urinary bladder, which can intrude on a perfectly taken-for-granted existence with sometimes embarrassing reminders of their functions? Of course, we do think on a daily basis. And we think that thinking is a function of the brain. But the connection between mind (thinking) and brain, though a widely shared feature of Western common sense, remains a very difficult subject for either science or philosophy to theorize about. The very fact that Western tradition has worked so hard to conceptualize the relationship between anatomical brain and living thought suggests that "brain" itself is not a self-evident experience in the life of the body.[60] (Farquhar 1998: 188)

Farquhar points out that Western medicine accords the central nervous system (CNS), associated with the brain, a powerful role in orchestrating the functions of all the organs, whereas "contemporary literature of Chinese medicine accords the brain a rather unimportant place in the dynamic system of the living body" (p. 188). The Chinese medical tradition, built on a heritage from the profound metaphysical thought of ancient Chinese philosophy, "emphasizes five great systems of function in the human body, centering on five organs: the heart, lungs, liver, spleen, and kidneys (no brain in this list!)" (p. 188). Apparently, Farquhar was surprised to note that the brain was not on the list of the most important organs, namely, the zang. On the contrary, as she finds, "the brain is one of the most passive sites known to Chinese medicine", as the "reservoir of marrow" (p. 189). Instead, the Chinese vision of the heart "seems rather closer to our biomedical un-

---

60 Of course, to say that the activity of the brain is not as obvious to us as that of the heart and some other internal organs does not mean that it is completely absent from our bodily experience. In fact, when one thinks long and hard, for instance, one may feel tension in the head, a heavy head, or even a headache. Today's cognitive science studies the central role of the brain in human cognition on the basis of brain science and it has greatly enriched the understanding of the brain as the real organ for thinking, knowing, understanding, feeling, as well as controlling movement and processing language (see, e.g., Lakoff 2006).

derstanding of CNS function than to our vision of the classically mechanical circulatory system" (p. 189). She notes, "Medical people of the great Chinese tradition were not ignorant about the contents of bodies, but they directed their attention elsewhere. They were more interested in the life of the human body than in its architecture" (p. 189). This interest in the life, rather than the architecture, of the body becomes manifest in the "holism" of Chinese medicine, which represents "an entirely different way of understanding and experiencing the body" (p. 190):

> Doctors practicing traditional Chinese medicine make no radical divide between disorders of the body and those of the mind. Every disorder biomedicine would call "psychiatric" is analyzed in Chinese medicine as a whole body problem, usually stemming from debility or hyperactivity of one of the five great systems centering on the heart, lungs, liver, spleen, and kidneys. Serious disorders of thought or language are usually traced to the heart, liver, or kidney, since these systems are especially involved with the more volatile and rapidly transforming substances of the body (spirit, energy, and seminal essence).

That is why, Farquhar (1998: 190) suggests, Chinese medicine, with a reputation for its "holism", may be appealing to many people in the West "in an era when it has become common to trace the shortcomings" of Western civilization to "the mind-body divide". Godwin (2001: 66–67) also characterizes the differences between Chinese and Western medicine as follows:

> Chinese medicine is a holistic and *wholehearted* approach to the human organism with all its mental, emotional, behavioral, social, and spiritual complexities. More and more Western doctors are finding it a rich addition to their traditional diagnostic tools. Whereas Western medicine has up until now tended to address the various systems separately (cardiovascular, gastrointestinal, musculoskeletal, neurohumeral, endocrinological, lymphatic, reproductive, urinary, respiratory, metabolic, sensory) and to develop theories about the diseases related to those organs, Chinese medicine looks for connections and movements between the systems and posits theories about mind-body health. The doctor studies and treats the person (looking for that person's special imbalance), and not just the disease.

It is obvious that Chinese and Western medicine, as different medical traditions, hold differing views on the "mind" and its relation to, or its locus inside, the body. Western medicine originates from classic Greek medicine that seems to have undergone the interaction between "cardiocentrism" and "cerebrocentrism" in early antiquity, although the interaction has led to the domination of the brain as the locus of the mind in modern time (see Clarke and O'Malley 1968; Crivellato and Ribatti 2007; Erickson 1997; Foolen 2008; Jager 2001; Marti 1991; Sharifian et al. 2008b; section 6.2). In contrast, Chinese medicine seems to have quite steadily centered on the heart as governing the "spiritual light".

Kuriyama (2002: 55), who studies the divergence between Chinese and Greek medicine, notes that such "divergence was as much a matter of experience as it was of theory". "Greek and Chinese doctors *knew* the body differently because they *felt* it differently" (p. 55), and the converse is also true: "they felt it differently because they knew it differently" (p. 60). Here are, for instance, some passages where he sees how divergences in their perception and conception of the body arose:

> Doctors in China missed much of the detail observed by Greek dissectors and incorporated invisible features that dissection could never justify. This especially is what makes the acupuncture man seem a mystery – the blind indifference to the claims of anatomy.
>
> Yet indifference to anatomy didn't mean a slighting of the eyes. Not at all: ancient Chinese doctors evinced great faith in visual knowledge. Like their Greek counterparts, they scrutinized the body intently. Only they somehow saw it differently. (p. 153)

> Overall, anatomical inspection left only faint impressions on the ancient Chinese conception of the body. Nonetheless, the exception reinforces an important lesson … namely, that there is more than one way to cut open the body and look, that what we habitually call anatomy is just *one kind* of anatomy. When dissectors inspected the body in ancient China they didn't see the nerves and muscles that Greek anatomists found so arresting. They lingered instead on measurements that Galen and his predecessors entirely ignored.[61] (p. 159)

> Greek pulse takers ignored the local variations that their counterparts in China found so richly telling; Chinese doctors saw nothing of muscular anatomy. This is how conceptions of the body diverge – not just in the meanings that each ascribes to bodily signs, but more fundamentally in the changes and features that each recognizes *as* signs. (Kuriyama 2002: 272)

---

61 For some of the detailed measurements of the parts of the body that appear in ancient Chinese medical texts, see Kuriyama (2002: 158) and Wang et al. (1997: 8–9).

Different perceptions and conceptions of the body in its structure and function have led to two major medical traditions in the world, which are so divergent from each other that they resort to very different approaches to and resources for treatment. While Western medicine has advanced and flourished in the modern world propelled and supported by modern sciences, Chinese medicine, on the other hand, has been relatively quiet and relegated to a secondary position in modern China. In the past decade or two, however, the West seems to have seen some growing interest in Chinese medicine's herbal medication, acupunctural treatment, and the more holistic view on mind and heart and mind and body.

To end this chapter, I would like to discuss Chinese people's current perceptions of Chinese medicine. I want to do this because an evaluation of the popular perception of, and attitude toward, Chinese medicine may bear cultural implications for the current status of the traditional conceptualization of the heart characterized in this chapter. Traditional Chinese medicine boasts a recorded history of several thousand years. In modern China, however, it has been nudged aside by modern Western medicine. To what extent does it still hold on to the belief and faith of average Chinese people? Or, reversely, to what extent do average Chinese people still believe or hold faith in traditional Chinese medicine?

It so happened that the year of 2006 witnessed a heated and massive debate on the Internet, involving thousands upon thousands of participants, about the status and fate of Chinese medicine in China's state medical system.[62] It all started with an article published in *Medicine and Philosophy* in April 2006 entitled "Bid Farewell to Chinese Medicine and Herbal Medication", in which the author Zhang Gongyao, a university professor of science history, summarizes his views voiced in his earlier articles published on his personal blog. He argues that there are "sufficient reasons to bid farewell to Chinese medicine and herbal medication in the name of cultural progress, science, maintenance of biological diversity, and humanity" (Chinesenewsnet 2006d). The article stirred up immediate controversy in medical circles. After that, in "An open letter to the Internet readers nationwide" dated June 10, Zhang claims that his earlier article "destroyed the myth that Chinese medicine is sacred and inviolable" and asserts that

---

62 The review provided here is based on the eight articles collected from the Chinese language DWNEWS.COM: Chinesenewsnet 2006a, 2006b, 2006c, 2006d, 2006e, 2006f, 2006g, and 2006h. These, listed according to their dates of publication, are collected in a short period between October 14 and November 6, 2006.

"Chinese medicine will exit the palace of science and return to where it started". He continued to post on the Internet a series of articles, which were then reposted by professional medical websites. At this point, both sides of the debate had already been engaged in a furious verbal battle.

On October 7, Zhang posted a public announcement to launch a drive to collect signatures of supporters for the withdrawal of Chinese medicine and herbal medication from the state medical system, and for their return to the handling by nongovernmental organizations. Within days, over ten thousand people, among whom many are medical professionals and Ph.D. students studying Chinese medicine, signed up (Chinesenewsnet 2006c). Ironically, words had broken out a few days before the drive that Korea would apply for the "World Cultural Heritage" status for Korean medicine, which shares a common origin with Chinese medicine (Chinesenewsnet 2006d). The news heated the ongoing debate to a new level of intensity, which would now concern the "revival of tradition and national dignity" as well.

In short, three views were expressed. The first is for the elimination of Chinese medicine. This view asserts that Chinese medicine is "a hotch-potch comprising philosophy, metaphysics, superstition, folk medicine and witchcraft", and "a pseudoscience" with "no experimental basis at all" (Chinesenewsnet 2006c), and it "has very little scientific value although it does have cultural value" (Chinesenewsnet 2006d). One prominent figure in this group is He Zuoxiu, a well-known outspoken physicist and an academician of the Chinese Academy of Sciences, who years ago uttered a very controversial statement: "90% of traditional Chinese culture is dregs, and you know that by just looking at Chinese medicine" (Chinesenewsnet 2006f). At a recent media interview, he insisted that "Chinese medicine's theories of yin-yang and the five elements are typical pseudoscience", in sharp contrast to Western medicine. He gave Western medicine a score of 90 points in contrast to merely 10 given to Chinese medicine.

The second view, which is neutral, insists on the parallel development and combination of Chinese and Western medicine in the state medical system.[63] This has actually been the governmental policy sine 1949, when the People's Republic of China was founded. However, it has not been particularly successful. In order to modernize or Westernize Chinese medicine,

---

[63] A recent successful example is the protocol that combines Western medicine with Chinese medicine in the treatment of SARS in Guangzhou in 2003 that resulted in a death rate of 3.6% in comparison with that of 17% in Hong Kong, where only Western medicine is used (Chinesenewsnet 2006c).

96% of those who graduate from colleges of Chinese medicine have received Western medicine training (Chinesenewsnet 2006a). Meanwhile, their training in Chinese medicine is less rigorous and many of them do not even want to read classical Chinese medical texts such as the *Yellow Emperor's Internal Classic*. It is said that, in diagnosing, many doctors of Chinese medicine now rely too much on modern medical equipment rather than on the traditional practice of "seeing, hearing, asking, and feeling" (Chinesenewsnet 2006b). As a result, Chinese medicine has been more and more marginalized in the state medical system.

The third view, which represents the majority, insists that "Chinese medicine should be protected and promoted" as "the national treasure and pride". It denounces the idea of eliminating Chinese medicine from the state medical system and regards it as "sheer nonsense" (Chinesenewsnet 2006f). It is said that more than 80% of the participants in the online debate is against this idea. The Chinese government also publicly responded to the drive that had garnered within days the signatures of over ten thousand supporters. The spokesperson of the Ministry of Health recently indicated that the Ministry is diametrically and determinedly opposed to the idea and the drive, and that they stemmed from "the ignorance of history and the ignorance and denial of the important role that Chinese medicine and herbal medication play in real life". At the same time, however, the spokesperson also admitted that "it is undeniable that Chinese medicine is faced with a difficult journey ahead of it" within the larger context of the commercialized operation of hospitals (Chinesenewsnet 2006b). On a different occasion, the spokesman of the National Bureau of Chinese Medicine Administration pointed out that those advocators of the signature-collecting drive, or "a farce that should soon end", "are ignorant of the history of their own country" or "have forgotten their own origins" (数典忘祖 *shudian wangzu*). They are said to be "anti-science in the name of science" (Chinesenewsnet 2006g).

It is interesting to note that a recent poll conducted by the publisher of *China Youth Daily* on 14,677 participants shows that 87.8% of the interviewees said they believe in Chinese medicine; however, only 27.7% said Chinese medicine is their first choice for treatment when they are ill. A different poll conducted by the "Sina.Com" on 20,219 people shows that 74.2% of them are supportive of Chinese medicine. When asked why they believe in Chinese medicine, 74.4% said because "Chinese medicine can indeed cure many diseases"; 41.8% said because "Chinese medicine is a national treasure"; and 31.0% said because "the theories of Chinese medicine are very convincing". It is suggested that, although Chinese medicine has never lacked its supporters in China, this does not mean that it has "an easy life" in its place of origin. Only 27.7% of the people first think of Chinese medicine for treatment when being sick and 61.3% of the people believe that Chinese medicine is confronted with a less and less optimistic future. *China Youth Daily* reports that 55.9% of the people are concerned that the current teaching model at colleges of Chinese medicine, which has been Westernized considerably, can hardly train good doctors of Chinese medicine, and this is exactly the dilemma that Chinese medicine faces. "As older doctors of Chinese medicine pass away, how many real 'masters' of Chinese medicine still remain", sighed a professor of Chinese medicine (Chinesenewsnet 2006e).

The review presented here suggests that as a heritage of Chinese culture Chinese medicine still enjoys popular support in China, but as a medical science it is on decline, overshadowed by the expanding influence of modern Western medicine. As many Chinese people believe today, Chinese medicine is to "nurture people" (养人 *yangren*) with a holistic view on the connections between body parts, between body and mind, and between body and environment, whereas Western medicine is to "cure diseases" (治病 *zhibing*) with an anatomical focus on the disease so as to get rid of it with the help of right medication or operation. Therefore, when one falls ill, especially with an acute illness, one should seek for Western medical treatment; but when one does not feel good in any part(s) of the body, one should see a doctor of Chinese medicine for advice and take herbal medication to "nurse or regain one's health".

In sum, the review of the current debate in China on Chinese medicine shows a very interesting phenomenon of a paradoxical nature. At the scientific level, Chinese medicine is in real crisis now, confronted by the strongest opposition ever, but at the cultural level, it still has its popular support of the majority in China. For instance, one poll showed that approximately 88% respondents still support Chinese medicine, but only about 28% would have Chinese medicine as their first choice when they fall ill. These numbers show the distinction between scientific knowledge and cultural conceptualization. We may hypothesize that people have a "scientific mind" and a "cultural mind", or a "scientific level" and a "cultural level" within a single mind, which do not necessarily overlap and may operate separately and alternatively in different contexts under different circumstances, resulting in views of an apparently paradoxical nature.

All in all, it is fair to say that Chinese medicine, as part of Chinese culture, still plays an active role in the minds of Chinese people when they try to understand various aspects of physiological conditions of the human body and natural and societal phenomena of the external world. It constitutes part of the cultural model shaping the cognition of Chinese people at the cultural level. This cultural model certainly also underlies the Chinese language as part of Chinese culture.

How the heart is conceptualized as manifested in the Chinese language is the topic of study for the next chapter.

Chapter 4
The HEART in present-day Chinese language

4.1. Introduction: A cognitive semantic study

In general, a language reflects its underlying conceptual systems and cultural models (e.g., Holland and Quinn 1987; Kövecses 1990, 2005, 2006; Lakoff 1987a; Lakoff and Johnson 1980, 1999; Palmer 1996; Sharifian and Palmer 2007; Wierzbicka 1992, 1997a, 1997b). Having traced the historical conceptions of the heart in ancient Chinese philosophy and traditional Chinese medicine in the previous two chapters, I now turn, in this chapter, to a synchronic study of their counterpart in the present-day Chinese language, which is really the focus of the current study. As I will show, the conventionalized linguistic usages in present-day Chinese actually have deep "roots" in the historical conceptions of the heart in ancient Chinese philosophy and traditional Chinese medicine. The latter are essential elements of the historical and cultural "soil" from which the former has sprouted and grown. My studies of conceptions of the heart in both ancient Chinese philosophy and traditional Chinese medicine, which are two important aspects of Chinese culture, should set up the stage for a more thorough linguistic study within the theoretical framework of Cognitive Semantics.

Before I move on, however, I must point out again, as I already did in Chapter 1, that the English terms related to human experience (e.g. *soul*, *spirit*, *mind*, *heart*, and the various emotion terms) may very well be culture-specific (see, e.g., Wierzbicka 1992, 1999). When I use them in the analysis of Chinese, they should be interpreted with this awareness in mind.

4.1.1. Cognitive Linguistics

As mentioned earlier, Cognitive Semantics is a branch of Cognitive Linguistics (CL).[64] As a linguistic paradigm, CL displays a great tolerance towards internal variety and towards external interaction with major linguistic disciplines and subdisciplines (Ruiz de Mondoza Ibáñez and Peña

[64] For introductory overviews of Cognitive Linguistics, see Croft and Cruse (2004), Evans and Green (2006), Lee (2001), Ungerer and Schmid (1996).

Cervel 2005b; Dirven 2005). Geeraerts (1995: 111) defines CL as "an approach to the analysis of natural language that focuses on language as an instrument for organizing, processing, and conveying information". Considering language as a system of categories, it holds a primary interest in the analysis of the conceptual and experiential basis of linguistic categories: "The formal structures of language are studied not as if they were autonomous, but as reflections of general conceptual organization, categorization principles, processing mechanisms, and experiential and environmental influences" (p. 111). Dirven (2005: 17) defines CL as "a linguistic theory which analyzes language in its relation to other cognitive domains and faculties such as bodily and mental experiences, image-schemas, perception, attention, memory, viewing frames, categorization, abstract thought, emotion, reasoning, inferencing, etc.".

So defined, CL upholds one basic principle and four tenets (Geeraerts 2006c: 3–6). The foundational principle is that language, as something primarily semantic, is all about meaning; for this reason, a cognitive approach to language should focus on meaning. The four tenets that spell out this fundamental principle are as follows. First, linguistic meaning is perspectival. Meaning is not just an objective reflection of the outside world; instead, it is a way of shaping that world, construing the world in a particular way or projecting an embodied perspective onto the world. Second, linguistic meaning is dynamic and flexible. Meaning has to do with shaping our world, and in dealing with a changing world, meanings change accordingly. Third, linguistic meaning is encyclopedic and nonautonomous. Since linguistic meaning reflects our overall experience as human beings, it is not separate from other forms of knowledge of the world that we have, but involves knowledge of the world that is integrated with our other cognitive capacities. There are two main aspects to the experiential grounding of linguistic meaning. On the one hand, we are embodied beings and the biological, organic nature of our experience is, in one way or another, reflected in the language we use. On the other hand, we also have a cultural and social identity, and languages embody the historical and cultural experience of groups of speakers. Fourth and last, linguistic meaning is based on usage and experience. That is, meaning is experientially grounded and the experience of language is an experience of actual language use.

Importantly, CL holds that there is no clear distinction between lexical and grammatical categories, with lexicon and grammar forming a continuum (Taylor, Cuyckens, and Dirven 2003). As Geeraerts (1995) suggests, if linguistic categorization is a major focus of CL, then studying the lexicon is the plausible first step to take. The lexicon is studied as a methodological point of departure for the study of the grammar at large, and the grammar of the language is studied along the same lines as its lexicon (see, e.g., Langacker 1987, 1990, 1991, 1999; Cuyckens, Dirven, and Talyor 2003). In fact, a central concern of CL is that lexical items, as well as grammatical constructions, symbolize conceptual categories, which have to be studied and investigated with respect to their cognitive function, rather than reflect purely formal linguistic principles and, as such, lexical and grammatical categories constitute a repository of world knowledge (Taylor, Cuyckens, and Dirven 2003). Within the paradigm of CL, Cognitive Lexical Semantics has directed its attention to the following three research areas in the past two decades (p. 2):

> (i) the internal structure of lexical categories (prototype structure, family resemblance structure, radial network structure); (ii) the polysemous nature of lexical items and the cognitive principles (e.g., metaphor, metonymy, image-schema transformations) motivating the relations between the different senses of lexical items; (iii) larger conceptual structures (e.g., metaphor research, frame semantics).

When larger conceptual structures that combine several individual categories are studied in relation to their cultural environment, the investigation is then broadened to the study of cultural models (Geeraerts 1995; see also Holland and Quinn 1987; Palmer 1996; Sharifian and Palmer 2007; Sharifian et al. 2008a).

The study of the lexicon of a language can reveal a great deal about its cultural environment. At this point, it is particularly relevant to refer to Wierzbicka's work in this research area. In her book *Understanding Cultures through Their Key Words* (1997a), Wierzbicka argues that linguistic semantics can make a unique contribution to cultural analysis. This is because there is "a very close link between the life of a society and the lexicon of the language spoken by it" (p. 1). She points out that to show that a particular word is of special importance in a given culture, one has to make a case for it (pp. 16–17):

> How can one justify the claim that a particular word is one of a culture's "key words"? To begin with, one may want to establish … that the word in question is a common word, not a marginal word. One may also want to establish that the word in question … is very frequently used in one particular semantic domain, for example, in the domain of emotions, or in the domain of moral judgments. Furthermore, one may want to show that this word is at the center of a whole phraseological cluster…. One may also be able to

> show that the proposed "key word" occurs frequently in proverbs, in sayings, in popular songs, in book titles, and so on.
>
> …
>
> A key word … is like one loose end which we have managed to find in a tangled ball of wool: by pulling it, we may be able to unravel a whole tangled "ball" of attitudes, values, and expectations, embodied not only in words, but also in common collocations, in set phrases, in grammatical constructions, in proverbs, and so on.

Following Wierzbicka's insights, in this chapter, I will focus on the semantic analysis of the Chinese word *xin* 'heart' as such a "key word". In the previous two chapters, I have shown that the traditional Chinese conceptualization of the heart as encoded by the word *xin* 'heart' is multi-faceted. The heart is conceptualized as the organ of thought, reason, and moral judgment as well as the seat of emotions, feelings, and desires. As such, it is perceived as the central organ of the person (with the former being microcosmic or synecdochic of the latter) and the central faculty of cognition that stands at the core of the relationship between the human and the universe as microcosm and macrocosm of each other. Thus, the Chinese notion of *xin* 'heart' is all-inclusive, extending into various domains of human experience. In this chapter I will demonstrate how this is true from a semantic point of view, analyzing linguistic evidence from the present-day Chinese language. Before I do so, however, I will first outline the kind of linguistic data I will be examining.

4.1.2. Linguistic data: Conventionalized expressions

In this chapter, I will provide a detailed study of conventionalized expressions in present-day Chinese pertaining to the heart as a part of the body and the most important organ of the person. Culture-specific ethnotheories of the person have important implications for the phraseology of a language because they motivate conventionalized expressions of that language (Goddard 2003). It is hoped that a thorough and systematic study of lexicalized concepts in everyday Chinese vocabulary will shed further light on the global cultural conceptualization of the Chinese "heart", "mind", and "person".

The conventionalized linguistic expressions that I study mostly take two forms in Chinese, compound words (复合词 *fuheci*) and set phrases (成语 *chengyu*), all containing *xin* 'heart' in them. In this sense, the study in this chapter belongs to the field of lexical semantics. Such studies could pave the way for broader and more integrated studies at higher levels such as grammar and discourse (Wierzbicka 1997b; see, e.g., Ch. 5).

In his characterization of compounding as a linguistic phenomenon, Palmer (1996: 248) suggests that naming is "attaching words to images" and names "provide us with some of our best clues to linguistic cognition". Although many of the things that we name are complex entities, naming typically, in the interest of efficient communication, "avoids descriptive detail of the base entity to be named and instead picks out and profiles one or more salient parts or aspects of its imagery" (p. 248). As long as the term is conventional or the context is known, the "name is sufficient to evoke the unspoken remainder of the imagery" with the help of semantic frames. For example, *pumpkin bus*, when referring to a tour bus that will take tourists to a pumpkin farm, evokes a schematic image with a semantic frame that includes *visit*, *travel*, *road*, *passengers*, *driver*, *farm*, and *countryside*, as well as *bus* and *pumpkin*. Thus, a compound word "is like an abbreviation of a longer possible description of the situation" (p. 251). In different contexts, for instance, the term *topless bar* can mean either "a bar counter that lacks a top" or "a commercial establishment where women are employed to dance naked to the waist for the sexual titillation of patrons who drink at a counter called a 'bar'". Usually consisting of two parts, compound words have a grammatical schema (e.g., [noun noun] or [noun verb]) between their two components, but their specific meanings are not predictable from syntax. With an abstract semantic schema (e.g., [modifier modified]), compounds are motivated by semantic connections, their two elements playing a variety of semantic roles (e.g., goal-instrument, instrument-goal, location-instrument, location-process, goal-process, goal-agent, part-whole). Importantly, compounds are often formed on the cognitive principles of metaphor and metonymy.

In present-day Chinese, compound words, which mostly consist of two constituents (represented by two characters), make up the vast majority of its lexical items. Li and Thompson (1981: 45–84) present a detailed study of Chinese compounds, on which the following brief discussion is based. As they point out, there is a great deal of disagreement over the definition of *compound* in Chinese due to a lack of clear demarcation between compounds and noncompounds no matter what criteria are applied. However, roughly, polysyllabic units that have certain properties of single words and that can be analyzed into two or more meaningful elements (i.e. morphemes) are considered as compounds in Chinese. For instance, a very common type is the subject-predicate compound, composed of two elements (e.g. a noun plus a verb or an adjective),[65] whose relation is one in which the first nominal element is the subject of the second verbal element. How is a subject-predicate compound distinct from a simple subject-predicate sentence when the Chinese language lacks morphological inflection? Here are some of the characteristics of the subject-predicate compound that make it distinct from a simple sentence: functioning as a single word (usually a verb and occasionally a noun), having idiomatic meanings, or containing a bound morpheme that cannot occur in isolation as a word. The major difference between a compound and a simple sentence lies, however, in the various syntactic properties that a sentence has. For example, a sentence can be negated by placing the negative morpheme between the subject and the predicate (e.g., *Tou bu teng.* [head not ache] 'The head does not ache.'), can be changed into an A-not-A question by using the predicate as the A element (e.g., *Tou teng bu teng?* [head ache not ache] 'Does the head ache [or not]?'), or can have a time adverb inserted between the subject and the predicate (e.g., *Tou wanshang teng.* [head at-night ache] 'The head aches at night'). A compound, being a word, is not able to undergo these processes. A few subject-predicate constructions, however, can function either as compounds or as simple sentences. It happens that *tou-teng* 'headache' is one of them (e.g., *Wo bu tou-teng.* [I not head-ache] 'I don't have a headache.' *Ni tou-teng bu tou-teng?* [you head-ache not head-ache] 'Do you have a headache [or not]?' *Ta changchang tou-teng.* [he often head-ache] 'He often has headaches.').

Other than the subject-predicate compound, another type, the verb-object compound, composed of two constituents having the syntactic relation of a verb and its direct object, also needs to be distinguished from a verb-object phrase. Any one of the following three properties will render a verb-object construction a compound: (i) one or both of the constituents being bound morphemes; (ii) idiomaticity of the meaning of the entire unit; and (iii) inseparability or limited separability of the constituents (p. 73). Besides, verb-object compounds are generally intransitive verbs that do not take a direct object, with some exceptions. In general, however, the verb-object compounds do not form a uniform group with respect to these properties; instead, their behavior forms a continuum, with any specific compound falling at some point on the continuum (p. 80):

---

65 In Chinese, an adjective can usually function independently as the predicate of a sentence without a copular or linking verb and, for that reason, is also called a stative or adjectival verb in Chinese grammar. See, e.g., Li and Thompson (1981).

> This continuum can be seen as a result of the fact that verb-object compounds are historically formed from verb-plus-object phrases: that is, certain verb-plus-object phrases have fused together through time to become compounds either as the verb or the object or both have lost their independent free morpheme status, or as the construction developed idiomatic meaning. Since such fusing processes in a language are never abrupt but are instead gradual, occurring over a long period of time as a verb-plus-object phrase develops into a completely fused word that is inseparable and completely idiomatic in meaning …, different verb-object compounds may be at different points along this path.

To summarize, the behavior of Chinese compounds, as characterized above, conforms to the claim that a clear demarcation does not exist between lexicon and grammar, which should form a continuum.

As mentioned earlier, Chinese compounds mostly have two elements. In this study, one of the two elements is the body-part term for "heart", 心 *xin*, which can take the first or the second position. When it takes the first position, it combines with the element following it to form either of the two constructions. When the second constituent is nominal too, the compound has the noun-noun construction (N-N). When the second constituent is verbal or adjectival, the compound takes up the subject-predicate construction (S-P). When *xin* 'heart' occupies the second position, it can be preceded by a nominal element, and the result is a noun-noun compound (N-N), When it is preceded by a verbal or adjectival element, the internal relationship between the two being, respectively, verb-object (V-O) or adjectival-noun (A-N). Sometimes, however, the verb-noun construction could be interpreted as being predicate-subject (P-S) in relation, that is, the two elements can be seen as in a reversed order from the subject-predicate construction (S-P). Chinese idiomatic phrases, or *chengyu* (成语) 'set phrases', are usually composed of four constituents (i.e., four characters in writing). Quite often, however, they are two compounds in juxtaposition. In this case, they sometimes involve two body-part terms. The conventionalized expressions to be analyzed include proverbs too, which "are generally regarded as repositories of folk wisdom" (White 1987: 151). They are provided where appropriate, either in the main text followed by their English translations in single quotes or in the parentheses following their English translations in double quotes.

In this chapter, some sentential examples, in which compounds are used in sentential contexts, are also cited for the purpose of illustration. Due to the great number of relevant compounds and the limited space, however, the examples of this kind have to be cited with restraint while a vast majority of them has to be left out. These examples are taken from dictionaries (DDHYCD 2001; H-YCD 1995; HYCYYCD 1996; H-YDCD 1993; XDHYCD 1980, 1996; XDHYCDBB 1989) and from actual discourse (e.g. newspapers, the Internet, TV dramas). They are provided with a word-by-word gloss (except some longer ones) and an English translation. In the gloss the following abbreviations are used: CL = classifier or measure word, COM = complement marker, PER = perfective, DUR = duration, MOD = modifier marker, PRT = particle, Q = question marker, and SUF = suffix. To simplify the gloss, I use PRT in an all-inclusive manner, to include various grammatical or functional particles, since these grammatical features are not so crucial to my analysis.

Having laid out the introductory information for my semantic analysis, I now turn to show how the Chinese cultural conceptualization of the *xin* 'heart' is manifested linguistically in the Chinese language. I will, in the following sections, analyze the Chinese conceptualization of the heart as a physical entity (4.2), as the locus of one's inner self (4.3), and as the locus of one's mental life (4.4) and emotional life (4.5). I will conclude this chapter with a summary of my semantic analysis and a discussion of its significance.

4.2. The heart as a physical entity

This section attempts to draw a very general outline of how the Chinese *xin* 'heart' is conceived to look and function, with details to be furnished in the subsequent sections. I will first provide an overview of the source domains of the *xin* 'heart' as it is conceptualized in metaphorical terms. I will then delineate the shape and structure of the *xin* 'heart' as it is modeled on the metaphorical conceptualization.

4.2.1. The source domains of the *xin* 'heart'

Given below in (1) is a group of words listed in HYDCD (2000: 1127–1130) that primarily refer to the heart, or more exactly to the mental heart, although they vary with regard to how commonly they are used in present-day Chinese. Each of these is a compound composed of two morphemes in the construction "heart + X", where *X* is a noun. All these compounds express the metaphorical formula HEART IS X, where HEART represents the target domain while *X* represents the source domain.

(1)
a. 心君 *xin-jun* (heart-ruler) 'heart'
b. 心灯 *xin-deng* (heart-lamp) 'heart; mind'
c. 心镜 *xin-jing* (heart-mirror) 'clean heart'
d. 心房 *xin-fang* (heart-house/room) 'heart; interior of heart'
e. 心窝 *xin-wo* (heart-nest) 'heart; deep down in one's heart'
f. 心田 *xin-tian* (heart-field) 'heart; intention'
g. 心地 *xin-di* (heart-land) 'heart; mind; character; moral nature'
h. 心苗 *xin-miao* (heart-seedling) 'heart; innermost being; intention; thought; idea'
i. 心源 *xin-yuan* (heart-source) 'heart, nature, disposition; temperament'
j. 心弦 *xin-xian* (heart-string) 'heart; heartstrings'

Most of these compounds reflect, in one way or another, the conceptualizations of the heart in ancient Chinese philosophy and traditional Chinese medicine studied in Chapters 2 and 3. In (1a), the heart is the "ruler" (emperor, king, monarch, sovereign, etc.). This is because, as explained in HYDCD (2000: 1128), the "ancients thought that the heart is the master of the whole body". The studies presented in Chapters 2 and 3 have already shown how and why this is the case. According to HYDCD (2000), both (1b) and (1c) originate as Buddhist terminology for the heart. It is said that Buddhism holds that the heart radiates its "spiritual thought" (神思 *shensi*) like a brilliant and bright lamp (p. 1128), and it is "clear and clean" (清净 *qingjing*) like a shining mirror (p. 1130). However, as I have shown in the previous chapters, the conceptualizations and images of the heart as a "radiating lamp" and a "shining mirror" already existed in early Confucianism and Daoism, where the ideal kind of heart had been conceptualized as the source of the "spiritual light", the "still water", and the "clear mirror", long before Buddhism was introduced into China in the mid Han dynasty (206 BC – 220 AD) from central Asia.[66] "Light", "clarity", and "brightness", con-

---

[66] See, e.g., Zhang (1993: 196). In Buddhism, the notion of *xin* 'heart' is also a central construct as the cognitive agent. It is suggested that the *xin* 'heart' should be cultivated (修心 *xiuxin*) or regulated (治心 *zhixin*) so that it will remain "clear" and "empty" (豁如太虚 *huo ru taixu*) and will not be "moved" by the ten thousand things in the material world (无心万物 *wuxin wanwu*) (pp. 196–200). After it was transplanted into China, Buddhism was transformed in the soil of Chinese culture and localized to some extent; it became one of the three major trends (Confucianism, Daoism, and Buddhism) in the flow of Chinese thought (see Ge 2001).

ceptually associated with human intelligence and wisdom, are ideal qualities of the heart as the central faculty of cognition that is capable of thinking and reasoning, and of knowing and understanding the external world.

In (1d) the "heart is a house or room", which is a special kind of container, a dwelling place. The previous two chapters have shown that the heart is conceptualized in ancient philosophy and traditional medicine as a "dwelling place" for the "spirits". Thus, it could be a "palace", a "mansion", a "residence", a "house", or a "room". The compound in (1d) is exemplified in (2).

(2) 主题公园正逐步敲开世界各地游客的心房。

Zhuti	*gongyuan*	*zheng*	*zhubu*	*qiao-kai*	*shijie*
theme	parks	PRT	step-by-step	knock-open	world
gedi		*youke-de*	***xin-fang*.**		
various-places		tourists'	heart-house		

'The theme parks are gradually knocking open the hearts (lit. heart-houses) of the tourists from all over the world.'

The tourists from all over the world are "falling in love" with the entertainment and attraction that the theme parks have to offer. While the love feeling comes from the inside of their "heart-house", the attraction of the theme parks is a force that is "knocking" at the door of their "heart-house" and is about to enter it after its door is opened.

As shown in (3) below, the "heart-house" has a "door" with a "threshold", which is the entrance of the "heart-house", the inmost being of a person or the innermost of the self. Whereas both (3a) and (3b) mean "the door of one's heart", (3a) is more commonly used than (3b).

(3)
a. 心扉 *xin-fei* (heart-door leaf) 'the door of one's heart'
b. 心门 *xin-men* (heart-door) 'the door of one's heart'
c. 心坎 *xin-kan* (heart-threshold) 'the bottom of one's heart'

Houses and rooms have doors for people to get in and out. Our "heart-house" also has a door for things to get in and out. When something is appealing to us, it would "knock at the door of our heart" (叩人心扉 *kou ren xinfei*). When we want to accept certain things, we would "open the door of our heart" (敞开心扉 *changkai xinfei*) to let them in. When we want to keep certain things out, we would "close our heart's door" (关闭心门 *guanbi xinmen*) to prevent them from entering. By the same token, we can open or shut the door of our heart when we want to let the contents of our heart out or keep them in.

(4) a. 我愿意敞开自己的心扉，向你倾诉一切。
Wo yuanyi chang-kai ziji de ***xin-fei,*** *xiang ni*
I willing widely-open self MOD heart-door to you
qing-su yiqie.
pour-tell all
'I wish to open my heart (lit. I'm willing to open the door of my heart widely), and tell you every thing (inside in a pouring manner).'

b. 我们依然紧锁心扉，死守界线，而且彼此伤害。
Women yiran jin-suo ***xin-fei,*** *si-shou*
we still tightly-lock heart-door defend-to-death
jiexian, erqie bici shanghai.
boundary-line also each-other hurt
'We still keep tightly locked the doors of our own hearts, defending to death our own boundary line, and we even want to hurt each other.'

In (4a), the narrator is willing and eager to "pour out" her inmost thoughts and feelings stored inside her heart to someone she loves or trusts. To do that, she of course needs to "open the door of her heart" first. When the door of their hearts is widely open, people are ready for a "heart-to-heart" talk. Example (4b) presents an opposite case. The two persons, because they do not love or trust each other, try to keep each other from "intruding into their own heart", by "locking the heart's door tightly". In such a case, neither of them can "enter" the other's heart.

Old-fashioned Chinese houses usually have a high threshold at the front door, and even at the door of each room. The Chinese heart has a "threshold", too, which is metaphoric of the inner self or the inmost being of a person.

(5) a. 字字句句在我心坎上打下了深深的烙印。
Zizi juju zai wo ***xin-kan*** *shang*
each-word each-sentence at my heart-threshold on
daxia-le shenshen de laoyin.
stamp-PER deep-deep MOD brand
'Each word stamped a marked brand on the threshold of my heart.'

b. 我从心坎里感谢您。
Wo cong ***xin-kan*** *li ganxie nin.*
I from heart-threshold inside thank you

'I thank you from the bottom of my heart (lit. from inside the threshold of my heart).'

The words in (5a) not only hit the "threshold" of the heart, but are also deeply imprinted on it so that they will stay there forever. As can be seen, the functions of remembrance and memory are ascribed to the heart. In (5b) the thanks that come from inside the "threshold of the heart", i.e. from one's true self, are sincere and "heartfelt". Communication is most effective when words said and heard go across the "thresholds of people's hearts".

The compound in (1e) refers to the heart as a different kind of container, a "nest", which is more akin to the heart in shape and size. A synonymous compound is 心窠 *xinke* (heart-nest/burrow) 'deep down in one's heart'. A nest and a house, however, have a similar function in that they are both "dwelling places" for animals or humans.

(6) a. 他的话句句都说进了大家的心窝里。
Tade *hua* *juju* *dou shuo* *jin le*
his words every-sentence all said into PER
dajia-de ***xin-wo*** *li.*
everybody's heart-nest inside
'His words all struck a chord in everybody's heart (lit. The words he said all went into everybody's heart-nest).'

b. 他第一次把掏心窝的话都和她说了。
Ta *diyi-ci* *ba* *tao* ***xin-wo*** *de* *hua*
he first-time PRT scoop heart-nest MOD words
dou he *ta* *shuo-le.*
all to her say-PER
'For the first time he told her all his inmost thoughts and feelings (lit. he said to her all the words scooped out of his heart-nest).'

In (6a), all the words said have entered the "heart-nests" of the people. That means what is said "echoes" the inmost thoughts and feelings stored in there, so it really "strikes home". In (6b), the words said are all "scooped out of the heart-nest", expressing the inmost thoughts and feelings from the depth of innermost self. Interestingly, a common way of describing people ignoring what others say is to say that words "went in one ear and came out of the other" (一只耳朵进一只耳朵出). Those who choose to ignore others' words are said to have taken others' words as "wind past their ears"

(耳边风 *erbian feng*). In both cases, other people's words have never reached their heart.

The heart is understood not only as a container, but also as a location. In (1f), the "heart-field" is a linguistic instantiation of the SOIL metaphor, which often appears in combination with the PLANT and WATER metaphors, all belonging to the semantic domain of agriculture. According to HYDCD (2000: 1128), (1f) is originally a Buddhist term for the heart. Buddhism maintains that the heart stores the seeds of good and evil that would grow under suitable circumstances, just like a field in which both crops and weeds would grow. It is said that Buddha taught the disciples that the heart is a piece of land where you will get fruits in return for whatever seeds you have sowed. Here are some sentential examples.

(7) a. 我把环保种子播撒在他的心田里。
Wo ba huan-bao zhongzi bosa zai tade
I PRT environment-protection seeds sowed at his
xin-tian *li.*
heart-field in
'I sowed the environment-protection seeds in his heart (lit. heart-field).'

b. 有时她那短暂的微笑，真会令我的心田开出温暖的花朵呢！
Youshi ta na duanzan de weixiao, zhen hui
sometimes she that transient MOD smile really would
ling wode ***xin-tian*** *kai-chu wennuan de*
make my heart-field bloom-with warm MOD
huaduo ne!
flowers PRT
'Sometimes that transient smile of hers would really make my heart (lit. heart-field) bloom with warm flowers!'

c. 她那无助的感觉一波又一波地涌进我的心田。
Ta na wu-zhu de ganjue yi bo you yi
she that no-help MOD feeling one wave again one
bo de yong jin wode ***xin-tian****.*
wave MOD surge into my heart-field
'That hopeless feeling of hers surged wave after wave into my heart (lit. heart-field).'

In (7a), ideas or thoughts are "seeds", and to communicate ideas or thoughts to other people, or to educate them, is to "sow the seeds" into their "heart-field". The seeds sowed into the field will grow, blossom, and bear fruits (of earlier education). Thus, (7a) involves some metaphorical mappings from the source to the target: Sower → Educator; Seeds → Ideas/thoughts; Sowing → Communicating; Field → Heart of the educated; Expected harvest → Expected result. In (7b), the heart is the seat of feelings or emotions. Happy and warm feelings are "flowers" grown in the "heart-field". In Chinese, the idiom 心花怒放 *xinhua nufang* (heart-flowers wildly-blossom) is a common metaphorical expression of happiness (see Yu 1995, 2002). In this case, the cause for the instant bloom of the "flowers", i.e. the "transient smile of hers", is the much-needed "nourishment" for the plants. Example (7c) describes the state of empathy, i.e., the sharing of one's feeling with another person. Here, one person's feeling of helplessness is the "water" that "surges" into the "heart-field" of another. It shows that true understanding and sympathy are established upon the connection of the two hearts through which feelings and thoughts in one person's heart can "flow" into that of another. The example involves various metaphorical mappings: Field → Heart; Water → Feeling; Way of water moving → Way of feeling experienced; Force of water → Strength of feeling; Water flowing from one field into another → Empathy. The metaphor here is structured by multiple image schemas such as CONTAINER, LINK, FORCE, and SOURCE-PATH-GOAL.

(8) a. "静"是心地最佳的风光。

"Jing"	*shi*	***xin-di***	*zui-jia*	*de*
"stillness/quiescence"	is	heart-land	the-best	MOD
fengguang.				
scenery/landscape				

'"Quiescence" is the best scenery of the heart (lit. heart-land).'

b. 现在最需要的是清净你的心地。

Xianzai	*zui*	*xuyao*	*de*	*shi*	*qingjing*	*nide*	***xin-di***.
now	most	needed	MOD	is	cleanse	your	heart-land

'Now what is needed most is to cleanse your heart (lit. heart-land).'

In (1g), the heart is a piece of "land", which is again a location. As illustrated in (8), the ideal condition of this land is that it is "quiescent", "still", "clear", "clean", and "pure". In (8a), a frame of mind (i.e. a peaceful and quiet mind) is the "landscape" or "scenery" of that "heart-land". This example reminds us of the ancient philosophical view that the heart should remain "still" or "quiescent" so that it can reflect the external reality accurately like still water or a mirror (see 2.2.4). The metaphor here involves the following mappings: Land → Heart; Landscape → Mental state; Physical quiescence → Mental peace. When water is still, it is clear and clean and its surface is level. Example (8b) again reflects a view in ancient Chinese thought, namely, the heart is the locus of morality and moral character (see 2.3). To be moral and ethical means "to have a pure and clean heart". This metaphor entails the following mappings: Land → Heart; Heart-land being clean and pure → Being moral; Heart-land being dirty and contaminated → Being immoral; To cleanse the heart-land → To become moral.

In (1h), the heart is a "seedling" of plant that needs special care and cultivation for its growth and maturity. This is one of the AGRICULTURE metaphors that have existed ever since the time of Mencius (see 2.3.3). In (1i), the heart is a "source" of water. According to HYDCD (2000: 1130), this word again originates in Buddhism, which regards the heart as the "source" of all things and laws. Particularly, the heart is the "source" of thoughts, ideas, feelings, emotions, and so forth, which are conceptualized as "water" in or from that source. Thus, in Chinese there are the following compounds:

(9) a. 心泉 *xin-quan* (heart-spring) 'thinking; feeling; intention; purpose'
b. 心波 *xin-bo* (heart-wave) 'thinking; feeling'
c. 心潮 *xin-chao* (heart-tide) 'a tidal surge of emotion; surging thoughts and emotions'

In (9a), the heart is a "source" from which thoughts, feelings, etc., come like water flowing out of a spring. In both (9b) and (9c) the heart contains a gigantic body of "water" that is "rippling" or "surging" inside. According to HYDCD (2000: 1129), (9b) has a Buddhist origin, where ideas and thoughts are conceptualized as rolling up and down like waves. In (9c) thoughts and emotions are in much more furious motion. These compounds are exemplified respectively by the sentences below.

(10) a. 干涸了的心泉又从胸中飞迸。
Ganhe-le *de* ***xin-quan*** *you* *cong* *xiong* *zhong* *feibeng.*
dry-PER MOD heart-spring again from chest inside gush
'The heart spring (i.e. thinking/feeling) that had been dry gushed again from inside the chest.'

b. 他振动着往日的心波。
Ta *zhendong-zhe* *wang-ri* *de* ***xin-bo***.
he vibrate-DUR bygone-days MOD heart-wave

'He was vibrating the heart-waves of (i.e. thinking of) the bygone days.'

c. 她心潮翻滚，无法入睡。
Ta ***xin-chao*** *fan-gun, wu-fa ru-shui.*
she heart-tide turn-roll no-way fall-asleep
'Her mind being in a tumult (lit. her heart-tides turning and rolling), she could not fall asleep.'

In (10a), the "heart-spring" had been dry until, all of a sudden, it "gushed" again with thoughts and emotions. It is a common metaphor in Chinese that the heart without thoughts and feelings is a "dried well" (枯井 *kujing*). In both (10b) and (10c), thoughts and emotions are in motion in the heart, like rolling waves and surging tides in the sea. The heart being rocked with surging thoughts and emotions, one is too excited to sleep (10c). In stark contrast with the "still water" image, the "surging water" metaphor highlights the emotional turmoil that should affect people's rational thinking, sober reasoning, and keen understanding. To do all this one needs to "calm down" emotionally.

The compound in (1j) is somewhat different from the rest in (1). It is open for two different interpretations. First, we can say that the "heart" and the "string" hold a whole-part relation between them, i.e., the "heart" as a musical instrument possesses "strings" as its parts. That is, the underlying metaphor is HEART IS A MUSICAL INSTRUMENT (WITH STRINGS). Second, the "heart-string" can also be seen as containing a metonymy or synecdoche (i.e., STRING FOR INSTRUMENT or PART FOR WHOLE). In this way, the mappings involved, both metonymic and metaphoric, can be expressed by means of this formula: HEART IS STRING (FOR INSTRUMENT). Since STRING STANDS FOR INSTRUMENT, the metaphor is HEART IS INSTRUMENT (WITH STRINGS). The "heart" is a "stringed musical instrument" because it would "resonate" when its "strings" are "moved" (动人心弦 *dong ren xinxian*) or "struck" (扣人心弦 *kou ren xinxian*). That is, the heart reacts and responds to the impacts of external reality when its strings are "touched" or "shaken", as the examples in (11) show.

(11) a. 生活中能触及心弦的每一个画面都是他创作的源泉。
Shenghuo zhong neng chu-ji ***xin-xian*** *de*
life in can touch-on heart-strings MOD
meiyi-ge huamian dou shi ta chuangzuo de yuan-quan.
every-CL frame all are he compose MOD source-spring

'Every scene in life that touches his heartstrings is the source of his creation and composition.'

b. 在撼人心弦的节奏中，我们找到了自我。
Zai han ren ***xin-xian*** *de jiezou zhong,*
at shaking people's heart-strings MOD rhythms in
women zhaodao-le ziwo.
we find-PER self
'We discovered our self in the rhythms that shook our heartstrings.'

Indeed, the heart produces sounds, not only in the physical sense of its beating, but also in the abstract sense of mental states and activities. The "sounds" from the heart are one's true feelings, thoughts, wishes, and aspirations, as illustrated by the following compounds.

(12) a. 心曲 *xin-qu* (heart-music/song/tune/melody) 'innermost being; mind; sth. weighing on one's mind'
b. 心声 *xin-sheng* (heart-sound/voice) 'heartfelt wishes; aspirations; thinking'
c. 心音 *xin-yin* (heart-sound/note) 'cardiac sound; heartfelt wishes; aspirations; thinking'

The following example elaborates on the images evoked by these compounds, i.e. the heart as a musical instrument with strings.

(13) 我的心都快跳出来了，砰砰的声音象音乐中的重低音，让我的身体的每一部分都随着它一起跳动，被它震撼。
Wode ***xin*** *dou kuai tiao chulai le, pengpeng*
my heart almost about jump out PRT thumping
de shengyin xiang yinyue zhong de zhong di-yin,
MOD sounds like music in MOD heavy low-bass
rang wode shenti-de mei-yi bufen dou sui-zhe ta
make my body's every part all follow-DUR it
yiqi tiaodong, bei-ta zhenhan.
together jump-move by-it shaken
'My heart was about to jump out, thumping and banging like the heavy and low bass in music, making every part of my body jump with it, shaken by it.'

This sentence describes the narrator's feelings of elation and excitement. The heart is beating so wildly that it feels as if it is about to "jump out". Metonymic for this forceful movement of the heart are the "thumping sounds" like the "heavy and low bass in music" that affect the whole body in a "shaking" way. It is the kind of impact, physical or psychological, that the "heart-string" is capable of producing. The more complicated image of the heartbeats compared to the "heavy and low bass in music" that "shakes" every part of the body is expanded and elaborated on the simple conceptual metaphor HEART IS A MUSICAL INSTRUMENT conveyed by the "heart-string" compound in (1j).

In summary, the heart is conceptualized in terms of various source domains, as illustrated by the compound words in (1). Thus, it is a "person" with supreme power, i.e. a "ruler" that commands the whole body. It is special kinds of object, a "lamp" that enlightens or a "mirror" that reflects. As a container, the heart is either a "house" or a "nest", the dwelling place for humans or animals. As a location, it is either a "field" where plants grow or a "land" with a particular landscape. The heart is a plant, too, but a "seedling" that needs special care and cultivation for its growth and maturation. While the heart can be a "light source" such as a "lamp", it is at the same time a "water source" from which water flows or in which water surges. Finally, the heart is also a "sound source", with "strings" that can produce musical notes responding to external factors. All these mappings, diversified as they are, are unified by the fact that the heart is conceptualized as the central faculty of both cognitive and affective mechanisms, which controls the mental power and regulates the emotional force of a person. In the following list of metaphors, I give one major entailment beneath the metaphorical mapping from the source to the target.

THE HEART IS A RULER

Ruler	→	Heart
Political power to control the state	→	Mental power to control the body

THE HEART IS A LAMP

Lamp	→	Heart
Physical light to illuminate	→	Mental ability to think, reason

THE HEART IS A MIRROR

Mirror	→	Heart
Physical capability of reflecting	→	Mental capability of knowing, understanding

THE HEART IS A HOUSE

House	→	Heart
Dwelling place for humans	→	Dwelling place for thoughts, feelings

THE HEART IS A NEST

Nest	→	Heart
Dwelling place for birds, etc.	→	Dwelling place for thoughts, feelings

THE HEART IS A FIELD

Field	→	Heart
Place for botanic growth	→	Place for mental and moral growth

THE HEART IS A LAND

Land	→	Heart
Landscape	→	Character, personality, moral nature

THE HEART IS A SEEDLING

Seedling	→	Heart
A plant needing cultivation to grow	→	A faculty needing cultivation to mature

THE HEART IS A WATER SOURCE

Source	→	Heart
Emerging or surging water	→	Emerging or surging thoughts, emotions

THE HEART IS A MUSICAL INSTRUMENT

Musical instrument with strings	→	Heart
Capability of producing sounds	→	Capability of producing thoughts, feelings

As this list confirms, each mapping connects a different source domain to the same target domain, the heart. That is, the mappings converge on one and the same target from different angles or different source domains, each mapping one specific aspect or function onto the "blended space" of global conceptualization of the heart, and each also placing it in a new light. While the source domains are all different and are not necessarily consistent with each other, there is some sort of coherence among them. For instance, they are centers of some sort: the ruler as the center of power, and the lamp as the center of light. They are objects that enlighten (lamp, mirror) and that serve as dwelling places (house, nest). They are sources of power, light, water, or sound (ruler, lamp, mirror, water source, musical instrument), they are associated with agriculture (field, land, water source, seedling), and they are responsive to changes or forces (mirror, musical strings). The conception of the heart rests on all of them, as well as on each of them. None of them offers a complete picture away from the rest of them, but each of them is a piece of a puzzle that contributes to the whole picture in combination with the others.

4.2.2. The shape and structure of the *xin* 'heart'

From the list of compounds in (1) we can see that the Chinese heart is understood through a variety of metaphorical mappings based on different spatial image-schemas: three-dimensional objects, three-dimensional containers, two-dimensional locations, and one-dimensional strings (see also Wang 2001). The linguistic evidence showing that the heart is conceptualized as having different image-schematic shapes – roundish, flat and thin, and narrow and long – also comes from the classifiers (known as measure words too in Chinese) that the Chinese word *xin* takes. There are three of them:

(14) a. 颗 *ke*: classifier primarily for things roundish, e.g. planet, satellite, pearl, tooth, bullet, bean.
b. 片 *pian*: classifier primarily for things flat and thin, e.g. a slice of bread, a leaf, a stretch of land, a vast expanse of water (surface).
c. 条 *tiao*: classifier primarily for things long and narrow or thin, e.g. a thread, a leg, a fish, a cucumber, a street.

In the following are three examples that illustrate how these three classifiers are used in sentences:

(15) a. 姑娘哭了，她知道，这一点感觉是被那颗灼热的心唤醒的。
Guniang ku-le, ta zhidao, zhe yidian ganjue shi bei
girl cry-PER she know this bit feeling is by
*na-**ke** zhuo-re de **xin** huanxing de.*
that-CL scorching-hot MOD heart awaked PRT
'The girl cried. She knew that this bit of feeling had been awaked by that warm (lit. scorching hot) heart.'

b. 他对那姑娘真是一片痴心，可是姑娘却看不上他。
*Ta dui na guniang zhen shi yi-**pian** chi-**xin**, kesh*
he to that girl really be one-CL crazy-heart but
guniang que kan-bu-shang ta.
girl on-the-other-hand not-think-much him
'He is infatuated with / crazy about (lit. really a stretch of silly-heart to) the girl, but she doesn't think much of him.'

c. 三人一条心，黄土变成金。

San	*ren*	*yi-**tiao***	***xin,***	*huang*	*tu*	*biancheng*
three	people	one-CL	heart	yellow	earth	become
jin.						
gold						

'When three people have one heart (i.e. are of one mind/heart), even yellow earth will turn into gold.'

In (15a), the girl in despair and hopelessness was moved by another "scorching hot heart". Here the heart is an "object" that looks more or less like the actual organ of heart. In (15b), the emphasis is on a certain abstract quality of the heart based on a metonymic relation. In this case, it is infatuation contained by or associated with the heart. The respective metonymy is CONTAINER FOR CONTAINED or OBJECT FOR QUALITY. That is, the "heart" stands for something it contains or some quality it possesses. Here are some more examples of this kind: 一片冰心 *yi-pian bingxin* (one-CL ice-heart) 'in all moral purity'; 一片真心 *yi-pian zhenxin* (one-CL true-heart) 'in all sincerity'; 一片诚心 *yi-pian chengxin* (one-CL sincere-heart) 'in all sincerity'; 一片好心 *yi-pian haoxin* (one-CL good-heart) 'with the best of intentions'; and 一片苦心 *yi-pian kuxin* (one-CL bitter-heart) 'troubles and pains taken for a good cause; with great pains'. All these examples suggest a great amount of X (e.g. moral purity, sincerity, good intention, pains) associated with the heart, so it seems appropriate to interpret the classifier as having the implication of "stretch" rather than "slice". This interpretation is consistent with the metaphorical image of the heart as a location, such as a field (1f) or a land (1g). It is on this image that the following more novel metaphorical expression is based (from Wang 2001):

(16) 我的心是一片荒芜的原野，没有播种的愿望，没有收获的喜悦。

Wode	***xin***	*shi*	*yi-**pian***	*huangwu*	*de*	*yuanye,*	*mei-you*
my	heart	is	a-CL	waste	MOD	land	not-have
bozhong	*de*	*yuanwang,*		*mei-you*	*shouhuo de*		*xiyue.*
sowing	MOD	wish		not-have	harvest MOD		joy

'My heart is a stretch of waste land, which has no wish for sowing, and no joy of harvest.'

Here the hopeless and desperate heart is a stretch of wasteland, flat, barren, and desolate. In (15c), the classifier suggests something thin (or narrow) and long. This time, the emphasis is on the "line" of thought, which is again conceptualized as being contained by or associated with the heart (i.e.

HEART FOR THOUGHT or, more abstractly, CONTAINER FOR CONTAINED). Each heart has its own "line" of thoughts and ideas that differs from those of others. Thus, 'A hundred people have a hundred (different) hearts (or minds)' (百人百条心). In (15c), a proverb, the unity of "three people having one heart", i.e. sharing the same line of thoughts, is valued as great strength that is able to turn earth into gold.

The following list of compounds provides more details about the conceptualization of the Chinese heart as a special kind of entity. They literally refer to various parts of the heart, which may have different roles to play as the heart hosts thoughts and emotions.

(17) a. 心头 *xin-tou* (heart-head/top) 'mind; heart'
b. 心底 *xin-di* (heart-bottom) 'the bottom of one's heart'
c. 心尖 *xin-jian* (heart-tip) 'heart; innermost being'
d. 内心 *nei-xin* (inner-heart) 'heart; innermost being'
e. 深心 *shen-xin* (deep-heart) 'innermost heart; innermost being'

As we can see, the heart has a "top" (17a) and a "bottom" (17b). It also has a "tip" (17c), which should be located at the very bottom of the heart, considering the shape of the heart organ. As a container, the heart also has an interior, the inner space (17d). The bottom of the container is "deep" in the heart (17e). The "bottom", the "tip", the "interior", and the "depth" of the heart all represent the "innermost being" of the self. The "top" of the heart, however, seems to be the place where mental and emotional processes and activities take place in their most active form. Look at the following examples.

(18) a. 这个问题一直压在她的心头。
Zhe-ge wenti yizhi ya zai tade ***xin-tou.***
this-CL question constantly weigh on her heart-top
'This question has always been weighing on her mind (lit. heart-top).'

b. 她根本没把他的宣示放在心头。
Ta genben mei ba tade xuanshi fang zai ***xin-tou.***
she absolutely didn't PRT his declaration put at heart-top
'She absolutely didn't pay any attention to his declaration at all (lit. She absolutely didn't put his declaration on the top of her heart).'

c. 一把火猛然袭上心头，他也火大起来。

Yi-ba	*huo mengran*	*xi*	*shang*	***xin-tou,***	*ta*	*ye*
one-CL	fire suddenly	charge	up-onto	heart-top	he	also
huo da-qilai.						
fire grow-start						

'A flame of fire suddenly rose in his heart (lit. charged up onto the heart-top), and he was also flying into a rage (lit. his fire was also starting to flame up).'

In (18a), the question has always been bothering her, or she has been constantly pondering upon it. This question, which is an active one in her mind, has been lying on the "top of her heart" awaiting a solution. In (18b), the lady paid absolutely no attention to the declaration (of love) from the man, that is, she never placed his declaration on the "top of her heart" for any serious consideration. Example (18c) has to do with the emotion of anger, which is "fire" that flames up to scorch the "top of the heart". Obviously, it is an instantiation of the ANGER IS FIRE metaphor.[67] As this example shows, inactive emotions or feelings are located "deep in the heart". When they are activated, they go up, toward the "top of the heart". Thus, the "heart-top" receives the most impact from the emotional forces.

(19) a. 一抹怀疑在他心底浮现。

Yi-mo	*huaiyi*	*zai*	*tade*	***xin-di***	*fuxian.*
one-CL	suspicion	at	his	heart-bottom	emerge

'A touch of suspicion emerged from the bottom of his heart.'

b. 亡国之恨，丧家之悲，败身之辱尽埋心底。

Wang-guo	*zhi*	*hen,*	*sang-jia*	*zhi*	*bei,*	
conquered-nation	MOD	hatred	lost-home	MOD	sorrow	
bai-shen	*zhi*	*ru*	*jin*	*mai*	***xin-di.***	
ruined-body	MOD	shame	all	bury	heart-bottom	

'The hatred of a conquered nation, the sorrow of a lost home, and the shame of a ruined reputation (lit. body) are all buried beneath the bottom of the heart.'

67 Readers are referred to Yu (1995, 1998) for more detailed studies of Chinese expressions of anger and happiness. There I point out that Chinese seems to place more emphasis on the heart as the container of emotions than does English, for which the container is often the body. See, also Kövecses (2000, 2002) for detailed discussions of the ANGER IS FIRE metaphor.

c. 我从心底里佩服他。
Wo cong ***xin-di*** *li peifu ta.*
I from heart-bottom in admire him
'I admire him from the bottom of my heart.'

In contrast to the "top of the heart", the "bottom of the heart" is where things, mental or emotional, are less active. As in (19a), when one starts to have a little feeling of suspicion, this feeling initially "emerges" from the "bottom of the heart". It can be expected that this feeling may expand and rise, under certain circumstances, to the "top of the heart". When people want to suppress their bad feelings and thoughts, they "bury" these feelings and thoughts "beneath the bottom of their heart", as in (19b), which involves mixed feelings of hatred, sorrow, and humiliation. Feelings and thoughts so buried are not really "dead"; they are just "dormant" in storage and can burst out again under the right circumstances. Example (19c) shows that the "bottom of the heart" is the "innermost being" of the self, the seat of one's inmost thoughts and feelings. Feelings and thoughts that arise from this location are sincere and true of that self.

(20) 她第一眼就从小伙子清澈的目光中看到了他内心的真诚。
Ta diyi-yan jiu cong xiaohuozi qingche de
she first-glance then from young-man's limpid MOD
mu-guang zhong kandao-le ta ***nei-xin*** *de zhencheng.*
eye-light in see-PER his inner-heart MOD sincerity
'At the first glance, she saw, from the young man's limpid eye (lit. eye-light), the sincerity of his inner heart.'

The "interior", as well as the "bottom", of the heart-container is the "innermost being" of the self. People often talk about their inmost feelings or thoughts in the "depth of the inner-heart" (内心深处 *neixin shenchu*), and by that they probably refer to both "interior" and "bottom" of their heart. What is stored in the "inner-heart" represents the true nature of the self. Since the eye is the "window" of the "inner-heart", it is possible to "see", through the eye, what is stored in the "inner-heart" (20). This, of course, is not always the case because people can "open or close up their inner-heart" (敞开或关闭内心) as they choose to. Each "inner-heart" is a small "world" (内心世界 *neixin shijie*). The heart, the central faculty of cognition, has Heaven and Earth and the ten thousand things all in it. Little wonder it is traditionally seen as microcosmic of the universe (see Ch. 2).

(21) a. 这是发自深心的喜悦。
Zhe shi fa zi ***shen-xin*** *de xiyue.*
this is arise from deep-heart MOD joy
'This is the joy that has arisen from the depth of the heart (lit. the deep heart).'

b. 从这个作品中我们可以看出作者的深心。
Cong zhe-ge zuopin zhong women keyi
from this-CL literary-work in we may
kanchu zuozhe-de ***shen-xin.***
see author's deep-heart
'From this literary work we can see the author's innermost being (lit. deep heart).'

The joy that arises from the "depth of the heart" is true joy (21a), since the "deep heart" is the locus of the true self. In (21b), the writer has projected his or her "deep heart", the innermost being that is normally invisible to others, into his or her literary work so that readers can "see" it from within this work.

The compounds listed in (22) provide further information on how the Chinese heart may look and work according to its conceptualization in Chinese culture.

(22) a. 心窍 *xin-qiao* (heart-aperture/orifice/hole) 'hole in the heart; capacity for clear thinking'
b. 心孔 *xin-kong* (heart-hole) 'hole in the heart; capacity for clear thinking'
c. 心眼 *xin-yan* (heart-eye/hole) 'heart; mind; intention; intelligence; cleverness; unfounded doubts; unnecessary misgivings; tolerance'
d. 心目 *xin-mu* (heart-eye) 'mind; inward eye; mental view; mind's eye'

As in (22a) and (22b), the Chinese heart has a "hole" in it, through which thinking and reasoning are conducted, as ancients believed (HYDCD 2000: 1129; cf. relevant passages in Chs. 2 and 3). Through metonymic extension, this "heart-hole" also refers to the "capacity for clear thinking". In Chinese, another compound 开窍 *kaiqiao*, which literally means "open the hole or orifice", is used to refer to the point in the developmental process at which a child "begins to know things" (H-YCD 1995: 543) because of a certain degree of mental maturity. Apparently, the folk theory attributes this "sudden change" in mental development to the "opening of the hole" in the heart. That is, little children do not have this "hole", or do not have it opened up yet. At certain point during their developmental process, they will have the "hole" in the heart opened up, which will lead to the "sudden change" in mental maturity. The age at which this "sudden change" takes place varies from individual to individual. Those who "do not know as well" or who "should know better" are said to "have not yet opened up their hole (in the heart)" (没开窍). Even adults do not necessarily have their "heart-hole" open all the time, simply because it can be "blocked up" for various reasons. Once that happens, people lose their "capacity for clear thinking". It is then appropriate to say that they "do not open up their hole (in the heart)" (不开窍), which means that they need to "have their thinking straightened out". Given below are two sentential examples of (22a).

(23) a. 他让金钱迷住了心窍。
Ta rang jin-qian mi-zhu-le ***xin-qiao****.*
he let gold-money enchant-stop-PER heart-hole
'He was obsessed by lust for money (lit. He let the desire for money cloud the hole of his heart).'

b. 他的话打开了我的心窍，知道该怎么办了。
Tade hua da-kai-le wode ***xin-qiao****, zhidao gai*
his words open-up-PER my heart-hole know should
zenme ban le.
how do PER
'What he said cleared up my thinking (lit. opened up my heart-hole) and then I knew what to do next.'

When the "heart-hole" is blocked, say, by the desire for money, people cannot think or reason (23a). When the "heart-hole" is opened up, people "see light" and they know what to do and how to act, guided by their heart (23b).

The compounds in (22c) and (22d) literally mean "heart-eye". In (22c), however, the morpheme *yan*, although it is the word primarily meaning "eye" in Chinese, can also mean "small hole". As is judged from how it is used in the context, the morpheme *yan* in (22c) is likely to mean "hole". If that is the case, then *yan* in (22c) is similar to, but not exactly the same as, *qiao* in (22a) and *kong* in (22b). Given below are some sentential examples:

(24) a. 长点儿心眼儿，别上人家的当。
Zhang dianr ***xin-yanr****, bie shang-renjia-de-dang.*
grow a-little heart-hole don't be-deceived-by-others

'Smarten up (lit. Have your heart-hole grow a little) and don't be taken in.'

b. 他有心眼儿，什么事都想得周到。
Ta you ***xin-yanr,*** *shenme shi dou xiang de*
he has heart-hole whatever things all think COM
zhoudao.
thoroughly
'He is alert (lit. has heart-hole) and thoughtful.'

c. 他人不错，就是心眼儿太多。
Ta ren bu-cuo, jiu-shi ***xin-yanr*** *tai duo.*
he person not-bad only-that heart-holes too many
'He isn't a bad person (or is quite a good person), but just a little oversensitive (lit. has too many heart-holes).'

d. 他心眼儿窄，受不了委屈。
Ta ***xin-yanr*** *zhai, shou-buliao weiqu.*
he heart-hole narrow cannot-bear feeling-wronged
'He is narrow-minded (lit. his heart-hole is narrow) and intolerant.'

Given that thinking and reasoning are conducted through the "heart-hole", if one can "get one's heart-hole grow a little", one will become a little smarter (24a). Also, if one's "heart-hole is good" (心眼儿好), then all the thoughts, ideas, senses that come through it tend to be good as well. That means this person is good by character, namely, good-natured or kind-hearted. If someone's "heart-hole is bad" (心眼儿坏), this person is then wicked or ill-natured. People who are up to no good "haven't installed a good heart-hole" (没安好心眼儿). Whereas thoughtful and considerate people all "have heart-holes" (24b), those who are not thoughtful or considerate are usually said to "have no heart-hole" (没心眼儿), and those who are slow-witted "lack heart-holes" (缺心眼儿). It is not clear how many "heart-holes" one should have, but it is certain that having too many of them is no good (24c). In that case, one is oversensitive and has many unnecessary misgivings. If the "heart-hole" is too narrow, as in (24d), it is then not an easy passage for thinking, reasoning, etc., to go through. This is what is known in English as being "narrow-minded". The "heart-hole being small" (小心眼儿) is a synonymous expression of the "heart-hole being narrow". One's "heart-hole can be as small as a needle's eye" (心眼跟针眼那么大), which of course represents a very negative character.

The morpheme *mu* in (22d) is another word primarily meaning "eye" in Chinese, and in this case it should be taken literally as such. However, "heart-eye" is subject to two differing interpretations in terms of the internal grammatical relationship between the two morphemes. It can mean "heart and eye", which stands in coordinative relationship, or it can mean "heart's eye", which forms a possessive relationship. The second case, which seems to be a more reasonable interpretation, is similar to the English phrase the "mind's eye". That is, the "eye" does not refer to the external sense organ, but to the "inward eye", through which mental images are "seen". Here are two examples.

(25) a. 在我的心目中，他还是个孩子。
Zai wode ***xin-mu*** *zhong, ta hai shi ge haizi.*
at my heart-eye in he still is a child
'To my mind (lit. In my heart-eye), he is still a child.'

b. 动人情景犹在心目。
Dong-ren qingjing you zai ***xin-mu***.
moving-people scene still at heart-eye
'The moving scene remains (or is still) fresh in my memory (lit. in my heart-eye).'

In (25a) the speaker has a mental view of the person under discussion though there may be a discrepancy between this subjective image, which could be imaginary or biased, and reality. In (25b) the speaker can "see" the moving scene vividly through the "heart's eye", which means it is deeply imprinted in the memory stored in the heart.

The compounds in (26) consist of the morpheme for "heart" and a so-called "localizer" in Chinese grammar. Defined loosely, the function of Chinese localizers, as their name suggests, is to locate things in relation to other things. They are similar to English prepositions in function, but occur after the nominal in collocation, and are more noun-like in terms of how they behave in Chinese syntax.

(26) a. 心里 *xin-li* (heart-in) 'in the heart; at heart; in the mind'
b. 心中 *xin-zhong* (heart-inside) 'in the heart; in the mind'
c. 心间 *xin-jian* (heart-inside) 'in the heart; at heart; in the mind'
d. 心上 *xin-shang* (heart-upon) 'in the heart; at heart'

The compounds in (26a–c) all suggest that the heart is a container with a void interior. As in (26d), the heart is either a two-dimensional location or a three-dimensional object with a top. The compound in (26a) is illustrated by the sentences below.

(27) a. 他看在眼里，痛在心里，急在眉间。
Ta kan zai yan li, tong zai ***xin-li,*** *ji zai mei*
he saw at eyes in felt-pain at heart-in worried at brows
jian.
between
'He saw with his eyes, felt pain in his heart, and his worry showed between his eyebrows (lit. and worried between his eyebrows).'

b. 可是这件事他也只能放在心里想，不敢说出来。
Keshi zhe-jian shi ta ye-zhi-neng fang zai ***xin-li***
however this-CL matter he can-only put at heart-in
xiang, bu gan shuo chulai.
think not dare speak out
'However, he can only think about this matter (lit. put this matter in his heart to think about), but dare not speak it out.'

c. 他那番话让我在心里铭记一辈子。
Ta na-fan hua rang wo zai ***xin-li*** *mingji*
he that-CL word make me at heart-in always-remember
yi-beizi.
whole-life
'Those words of his will be remembered (lit. Those words of his made me bear them firmly in my heart) for the rest of my life.'

d. 我们说了不入耳的话，你可千万别往心里去啊！
Women shuo-le bu-ru-er de hua, ni
we say-PER intolerable-to-the-ear MOD words you
ke-qianwan-bie wang ***xin-li*** *qu a!*
should-never to heart-in go PRT
'If we have said anything intolerable to the ear (i.e. anything bad), you should never take it to heart (lit. let it go into your heart).'

Three body-part terms appear in (27a). The person saw something distressful with his eyes. Since the distressful information was processed in the heart, it caused the heart to feel the pain, while his worry was shown on his face, between his eyebrows, where the frown was displayed.[68] In (27b) the person can only "put the matter in his heart to think about" but "dare not speak it out". Apparently, the heart is the container in which thoughts and ideas are processed. The sentence in (27c) has to do with remembrance. In the Chinese original, 铭记 *mingji* 'always remember' literally means "engrave or inscribe and remember". That is, if people want to remember something forever, they "engrave" or "inscribe" it in their heart. In (27d), the heart is the "information processing and storing center". Even if the ears have received information "intolerable to the ear", as long as this information is not let into the heart, it will not be "processed" and "saved" as such. In other words, as long as people do not "take it to heart", as the English idiom goes, they will not take anything offensive as it is and remember it as such.

(28) a. 他却只能压抑心中的感觉。

Ta que zhi neng yayi ***xin-zhong*** *de ganjue.*
he however only can suppress heart-in MOD feeling
'He, however, can only suppress the feeling in his heart.'

b. 进城几年了，乡亲们的嘱托他一直记在心间。

Jin cheng ji nian le, xiangqinmen-de zhutuo
enter city several years PER fellow-villagers' advice
ta yizhi ji zai ***xin-jian.***
he always remember at heart-inside
'Having lived in the city for several years, he always bears in mind (lit. inside his heart) the fellow villagers' advice.'

The two examples in (28) illustrate (26b) and (26c) respectively. The sentence in (28a) shows again that people's feelings are in their hearts. In this case, the person is not hopeful that he will get love from someone whom he loves. As a result, he can only suppress his feeling inside the heart. The sentence in (28b) has to do with remembrance or memory again. When the advice is remembered, it is actually stored inside the "heart-container".

---

68 In Yu (2002: 355–357) I argued that eyebrows take a very prominent position in conceptualization and expression of emotions and looks in Chinese. While the face, as a whole, is the barometer of emotions (see Yu 2001), its focus seems to be located around the eyes and brows. The eyes and brows are paired together not only physically but also conceptually, as is demonstrated by many compounds and idioms in the Chinese language.

(29) a. 一点小事，别放在心上。
Yi-dian xiao-shi, bie fang zai ***xin-shang***.
a-bit small-thing don't put at heart-on
'It's such a petty thing. Don't let it weigh on your mind (lit. Don't place it on your heart).'

b. 小事一桩，不必挂在心上。
Xiao-shi yi-zhuang, bu bi gua zai ***xin-shang***.
small-thing one-CL no need hang at heart-on
'It's a trifling matter. Forget it (lit. Don't hang it on your heart).'

The sentential examples in (29a) and (29b) illustrate (26d). These two sentences can be said when other people are, for instance, apologizing to you for something that they have done wrong, or expressing their thanks for a favor that you have done them. Although they are synonymous to each other, they evoke somewhat different images of the thing talked about. In (29a), the thing is an object placed on the top of the heart. In (29b), it is a long soft thing that can be hung on the heart. Either way, when the thing is kept on the top of the heart, the person is thinking about it and will not stop doing it until the thing is removed from the top of the heart.

The compounds in (17), (22) and (26) are different from those in (1) in terms of how they contribute to the conceptualization of the heart. Those compounds in (1) project onto the heart the features of other concrete things: ruler, lamp, mirror, house, etc. On the other hand, the compounds in (17), (22) and (26) furnish some image-schematic information concerning the heart as a container, which is a special kind of object with a void interior. They provide fragments of information about the shape and structure of the heart as a physical entity. We know that the heart as a container has certain important parts: the top, the void interior, the bottom with a tip, the hole(s), and the eye(s). It seems that the top is the initial landing place for things coming from the outside, say, through the sense organs. Thoughts and ideas are often "placed" on the top of the heart for mental processing, and feelings and emotions usually "charge toward the top" of the heart when they are activated. Both the interior and the bottom represent the "innermost being of the self", namely, the true nature and character of the self. However, they also have different functions in their division of labor. The interior is where more active thoughts and emotions are "stored" and "processed", whereas the bottom is where more dormant thoughts and emotions are "settled" or "buried". That is, thoughts and emotions that are activated go up toward the top, and those that are deactivated go down to the bottom. If people want to suppress feelings and thoughts that are rising to the top of the heart, they need to "press" them down, or even "bury" them beneath the bottom. The heart-container has at least one "hole" through which thinking and reasoning are conducted. If the hole is blocked, one cannot think or reason well. We do not know exactly where the hole is located in the heart, but probably it is in the top part. The heart also has "eyes". In some cases, the "eyes" may just refer to the "holes" for thinking, reasoning, etc. In others, they may be the so-called "eyes" for mental visions, that is, the "eyes" through which mental images are "seen". In short, what we have here is a very rough image-schematic sketch of how the Chinese heart, as a physical entity, may look and work.

In this section, it has already become clear that the Chinese *xin* 'heart' is the innermost being of the self and the site of both cognitive and affective activities. It is the seat of inmost thoughts and feelings, where thoughts and emotions are stored, processed, and manipulated. In the next few sections, I will further analyze the linguistic data to show how richly the cultural conceptualization of the Chinese *xin* 'heart' is manifested in the Chinese language.

4.3. The heart as the locus of one's inner self

Lakoff and Johnson (1999: Ch. 13) point out that the study of the self concerns the structure of our inner lives and who we really are. As demonstrated in the previous section, the Chinese *xin* 'heart' is conceived of as the locus of the inner self, i.e. the true self, of a person. It is believed to be the innermost being where the depths of one's "soul" and "spirit" are located. For that reason, it is regarded as "holy" and "sacred". This conceptualization is consistent with the cultural characterization inherent in ancient Chinese philosophy and traditional Chinese medicine that "the heart governs the spiritual light" (心主神明), where the "spiritual light" commonly refers to the totality of spiritual and mental aspects of a person. In the broad sense of the term, as defined in traditional Chinese medicine, the "spirits" (神 *shen*) include the "spirit" (神 *shen*), which is the archetype of the spirits, the "ethereal soul"(魂 *hun*), which is the yang aspect of the spirit, and the "corporeal or animal soul" (魄 *po*), which is the yin aspect of the spirit. The "spirits" in the broad sense are congenital, coming into being in the conception of fetus. Though the three types of spirits are said to be separately stored in the heart, liver, and lung, they are all governed by the heart, the "grand master of the five zang and six fu organs". In other words, the heart is the innermost being in which people's "spirits" and "souls" are rooted. In the Chinese language, as illustrated below, the terms for the three types of spirits are all attached and attributed to the "heart", their "governor", in compound words referring to mental and spiritual aspects of a person.

(30) a. 心神 *xin-shen* (heart-spirit) 'mind; state of mind'
b. 心魂 *xin-hun* (heart-ethereal soul) 'mind; state of mind; heart; soul; spirit'
c. 心魄 *xin-po* (heart-corporeal soul) 'heart; soul; spirit'

In various ways, these words can mean "mind; state of mind; soul, spirit" as well as "heart". If people look restless, it is because their "spirit" in the heart is unstable or unsettled (心神不定 *xinshen buding*). Such a state of mind is traditionally described as "the spirit departing from its abode" (神不守舍 *shen bu shou she*), especially in Chinese medicine, where "abode" refers to the heart, the "residence" of the spirit. People's "ethereal soul" and "corporeal soul", both being associated with the heart as types of spirits, can be "awed" (慑人心魂 *she ren xinhun*) or "moved" (动人心魄 *dong ren xinpo*) by external factors. When such processes take place, one's innermost being is shaken. The compounds in (30) manifest the folk belief in Chinese culture that the heart is the "abode" of spiritual and mental aspects of a person.

The fact that the heart is regarded as the inner self of the person is also seen from the linguistic manifestation of a conceptual metaphor A HUMAN IS A PLANT. While a human being is a plant, the human heart is the root of that plant. The root is the part that stems immediately from the seed that contains the true identity of the plant. Growing underground into the soil, the root is crucially responsible for the wellbeing of the plant above the ground. The metaphorical analogy between the human and the plant and between the heart and the root is attested by these proverbs: (a) 树长根，人长心 'As much as trees need roots, humans need hearts'; (b) 人靠好心，树靠好根 'Humans depend on good hearts, just as trees depend on good roots'; (c) 浇树要浇根，知人要知心 'When watering trees, one should water their roots; when getting to know people, one should get to know their hearts'; and (d) 人怕伤心，树怕伤根 'People suffer the most if their hearts are hurt, just as trees suffer the most if their roots are wounded'. The heart is the root of the human being (a). If the root of a plant is good, this plant will grow well; in the same vein, if the heart of a human being is good, this human being will be good-natured (b). Both (a) and (b) suggest that the heart is the locus of people's true nature and real character. That is, the heart embodies the true self. This is why when we get to know people, we need to know their hearts, just as when we water trees, we need to water their roots (c). Unless we know their hearts, we do not really know other people well. If people's heart is hurt, as we will commonly say, for instance, that they are "heartbroken" or "brokenhearted", the damage to them, not just emotionally, but physically as well, is similar to damages to trees when their roots are wounded (d). A "scar" in the heart is difficult to heel.

Another aspect of the conceptual metaphor A HUMAN IS A PLANT lies in the mapping between the face and the bark, as illustrated by the proverb 人活面子树活皮 'Humans live for their face whereas trees live for their bark'. What this proverb really means is: "Save your face because it is all the purpose of your life". It reflects an important value in traditional Chinese culture where the concept of "face" is central to the understanding of human interaction and relationship, especially in terms of dignity and prestige (see Yu 2001). After all, the face is the focus of the "outer self" in contrast with the heart as the core of the "inner self". No wonder people who want to reform or redeem themselves thoroughly have to "change their face and wash their heart" (革面洗心 *gemian xixin*).

4.3.1. The heart and one's innermost being

The heart is people's innermost being where the inmost thoughts and secrete feelings are stored. Unless people want to "open their hearts" to others, it is difficult, if not impossible, for others to know what thoughts and feelings they have "in their hearts". Little wonder the Chinese have the following proverbial sayings: (a) 人心隔肚皮 'Human heart is hidden behind (or inside) the chest (lit. Human heart is separated by the belly skin)'; (b) 人心难测水难量 'It is difficult to fathom one's heart, just as it is difficult to measure water'; and (c) 泥鳅难捉，人心难摸 'It is difficult to catch loaches, and it is difficult to fathom (lit. touch) human hearts'. Since we cannot "see" other people's heart as is "separated by the belly skin", it is therefore difficult to "fathom" or "touch" it. This is why such dimension concepts as "deep", "bottomless", "innermost", "inmost" are associated with the heart even though, as a bodily organ, it is only "inches long" (寸心 *cunxin* [inch-heart]). However, people's true self will be likely disclosed over the passage of time: "As distance can test a horse's strength, so will time reveal a person's heart" (路遥知马力，日久见人心).

Since the heart is the inner self, words coming from and actions motivated in the depth of one's heart represent one's true self. Therefore, as shown in (31), such concepts as sincerity, cordiality, honesty, loyalty, and piety are all attributed to the "heart" as its qualities.

(31) a. 诚心 *cheng-xin* (sincere/honest-heart) 'sincere desire; sincerity; whole-heartedness; sincere and earnest; devout'
b. 衷心 *zhong-xin* (inner-heart) 'heartfelt; wholehearted; cordial'
c. 真心 *zhen-xin* (true-heart) 'wholehearted; heartfelt; sincere'
d. 实心 *shi-xin* (actual-heart) 'sincere; honest; solid'
e. 忠心 *zhong-xin* (loyal-heart) 'loyalty; devotion'
f. 虔心 *qian-xin* (pious-heart) 'with a pious heart; earnestly and sincerely'
g. 素心 *su-xin* (undyed-heart) 'one's real intention; one's true will; clean and honest; pure in heart'

In the following are some examples in which the compounds in (31) are used in sentences:

(32) a. 我们诚心向你求教。
Women ***cheng-xin*** *xiang ni qiujiao.*
we sincere-heart from you ask-for-advice
'We sincerely (lit. with a sincere heart) ask you for advice.'

b. 我衷心感谢你的帮助。
Wo ***zhong-xin*** *ganxie nide bangzhu.*
I inner-heart thank your help
'I thank you for your help from the bottom of my heart (lit. from my inner heart).'

c. 我知道你是真心对我好。
Wo zhidao ni shi ***zhen-xin*** *dui wo hao.*
I know you are true-heart to me good
'I know your affections for me are genuine (lit. I know you are nice to me with a true/real heart).'

d. 他对朋友的一片忠心从来没受到怀疑。
Ta dui pengyou de yi-pian ***zhong-xin*** *conglai-mei*
he toward friends MOD one-CL loyal-heart never
shoudao huaiyi.
was in-doubt

'His loyalty (lit. All his loyal heart) to his friends was never in doubt.'

e. 他是一个素心人。
Ta shi yi-ge ***su-xin*** *ren.*
he is a-CL undyed-heart person
'He is a simple and honest (lit. an undyed-heart) person.'

When people are sincere, they have a "sincere heart" (32a). Such people are capable of achieving things that are otherwise improbable or impossible: "If one's heart is sincere, even rocks can blossom" (心诚石头都能开花). As in (32b), the "heartfelt" thanks come from the "inner heart". Genuine affections originate in a "true heart" (32c). A "true heart" is of tremendous value in human interaction and relation. "When a true heart matches another true heart, even rocks will turn into gold" (真心对真心，石头变黄金). Since loyalty is a quality of the heart, people who are loyal have a "loyal heart" (32d). A simple and honest person is one who has an "undyed heart" or "heart with its original color" (32e). That is, whatever this person shows is true of the real and original heart.

The heart is the locus of one's true self. When two persons form an interpersonal relationship, this relationship is defined by the degree to which they know each other's true self and, in other words, each other's hearts. Whereas the face is the focus of interpersonal communication (Yu 2001), the heart is the locus of interpersonal relationship. When "two hearts are linked" (心连心), it is the best interpersonal relationship. The tie connecting and "plugged" into two hearts is the "wire" of communication, and successful communication is the "connection between the hearts" (心的沟通), in which the "traffic" of thoughts and feelings is not jammed or impeded. Via interpersonal communication of various kinds and means, thoughts and feelings in one heart are transferred to and processed by another, and vice versa.[69] That is the understanding of each other's hearts upon which a close or intimate interpersonal relationship is built. Here is a group of com-

[69] The image here derives from a "conduit metaphor" (Reddy 1993, see also Kövecses 2002: 73–74, Lakoff and Johnsn 1980: 10–13). In a conduit metaphor, ideas or thoughts, packed in linguistic expressions, go through a pipe in communication. Here is an example in Chinese (from Yu 1998: 201): 有关意见和控告的投诉管道将更为顺畅 'The pipe for lodging relevant criticisms and complaints will be more smooth and unimpeded'.

pounds, based on the CONTAINER FOR CONTAINED metonymy, which define interpersonal communication and relationship.

(33)
a. 谈心 *tan-xin* (talk-heart) 'heart-to-heart talk'
b. 会心 *hui-xin* (meet/understand-heart) 'understanding; knowing'
c. 知心 *zhi-xin* (know-heart) 'intimate; understanding'
d. 对心 *dui-xin* (suit/match/get along-heart) 'suit; be to one's liking/taste; be to each other's liking/taste'
e. 掏心 *tao-xin* (scoop out-heart) 'from the bottom of one's heart'
f. 交心 *jiao-xin* (hand over-heart) 'lay one's heart bare; open one's heart to'
g. 换心 *huan-xin* (exchange-heart) '*dial.* intimate; understanding'

An important means of communication is having sincere and candid conversations and dialogues, through which thoughts and feelings are communicated from one heart to another. This kind of "heart-to-heart talk" is literally called "talk-heart" in Chinese (33a). Sometimes, people can get to know and understand others' thoughts and feelings without oral communication. That is when their hearts "meet the hearts" of others (33b). When two persons' hearts meet each other, they will have the chance to "see" the true self of each other. Since KNOWING IS SEEING (see Kövecses 2002: 158, 218–219; Lakoff and Johnson 1999: 53–54; Yu 2004), they will get to "know the heart" of each other (33c). That is when they start to form an intimate relationship between them. Two friends who really know the true self of each other are called "know-heart friends" (知心朋友 *zhixin pengyou*), known in English as "bosom friends". Such friends find their hearts "suit", "match", and "get along" well with each other (33d). People who have established, or would like to establish, an intimate relationship between them are willing and ready to "scoop out their hearts" or "scoop thoughts and feelings out of their hearts" so that it will be easier for others to "see" their inner self (33e). They will not mind "handing over their hearts" to other people whom they love or trust (33f). They may even want to "exchange their hearts" with such people (33g). After all, the best way to understand people is to "compare your own heart with others' hearts" (将心比心 *jiang xin bi xin*), i.e. to "put oneself in somebody's shoes". The only way to "win others' hearts" is to "give them your own heart in exchange" (将心换心 *jiang xin huan xin*), meaning "to win other people's hearts by one's sincerity". In human interaction and relation, "It's fair to exchange a heart for another heart, as fair as to exchange eight *liang* for half *jin*" (八两换半斤，人心换人心).[70] Here are two sentential examples of (33a) and (33b).

(34) a. 他经常深入群众，和工人们促膝谈心。
Ta jingchang shenru qunzhong, he
he often delve-deep-into masses with
gongrenmen ***cu-xi*** ***tan-xin***.
workers near-knee talk-heart
'He often goes into the masses and has a heart-to-heart talk (lit. knee-to-knee and heart-to-heart talk) with the workers.'

b. 对于他的眼色她报以会心的微笑。
Duiyu tade yan-se ta bao yi ***hui-xin***
to his eye-color she answer with meet-heart
de weixiao.
MOD smile
'She answered his wink (lit. eye-color) with an understanding (lit. heart-meeting) smile.'

In (34a), *cu-xi tan-xin* is an idiom that literally means "have a knee-to-knee and heart-to-heart talk" with someone. The image is that of two persons sitting so close to each other that their knees almost touch when they are "talking heart". In (34b), the understanding without oral communication between two persons is the "meeting of their hearts". Given below are two proverbs containing (33c): (a) 朋友遍天下，知心能几人？'One's friends may spread all over the world, but how many of them can be intimate/bosom (lit. heart-knowing) friends?'; and (b) 知人知面不知心 'In getting to know people, you get to know their faces but not (necessarily) their hearts'. These sayings are about difficulty and importance of making "heart-knowing" friends. A person cannot have many "heart-knowing friends" because usually one only get to know others by their faces, but not by their hearts, and judging people by their faces and words can be quite unreliable, as illustrated by the following idioms:

(35) a. 面善心恶 *mian-shan xin-e* (face-kind heart-wicked) 'a kind face but a wicked heart'

---

70 In this saying, *liang* and *jin* are units in an old Chinese weight system, where one *jin* is equal to 16 *liang* (therefore eight *liang* and half *jin* are equal in weight). This system has been discarded for the current one where one *jin* equals 10 *liang*. One Chinese *jin* is equivalent to half kilogram.

b. 面善心诈 *mian-shan xin-zha* (face-kind heart-cheating) 'have an honest appearance but be full of cunning and deceit'
c. 面从心违 *mian-cong xin-wei* (face-follow heart-oppose) 'comply in appearance but oppose in heart'
d. 心口不一 *xin-kou bu-yi* (heart-mouth not-one) 'do not say what one thinks'
e. 口是心非 *kou-shi xin-fei* (mouth-yes heart-no) 'say yes and mean no; say one thing and mean another; do not say what one means'
f. 口甜心辣 *kou-tian xin-la* (mouth-sweet heart-peppery) 'sweet words but a wicked heart'

All these idioms characterize the discrepancy between how one looks and what one says on the one hand, and what one thinks on the other. The former (i.e. faces and mouths) represents the surface self whereas the latter (hearts) represents the inner self. In (35a) and (35b), the "kind faces" are really deceptive, covering the true nature of evil supposedly located in the heart. The face is after all an external body part. It can only stand for people's outward appearance, in contrast to the heart that represents their true self. The example in (35c) characterizes an interpersonal relationship that is maintained only on the surface. Again, the face contrasts with the heart as they represent, respectively, one's outside and inside (see also Yu 2001). The three idioms in (35d–f) denote the difference between people's words and thoughts. When people's "heart and mouth are not one", what they say is different from what they think (35d). People can also "say yes but think no", i.e. to speak with "an insincere heart" (35e). As a proverb goes, "The human heart is hidden behind the mouth" (人心藏在嘴后边), i.e., what one says may not reveal what one really thinks. In (35f), a person can have "a sweet mouth but a peppery (i.e. wicked) heart". One saying describes some people as having "a white-sugar mouth and a white-arsenic heart" (白糖嘴巴砒霜心), i.e. they have "a sweet mouth but a poisonous heart". On the other hand, a sharp-tongued person may have a soft-heart, and this person is then said to have "the mouth of knife but the heart of bean curd" (刀子嘴，豆腐心).

The opposite of (35d) is 心口如一 *xinkou ruyi* (heart-mouth like-one), meaning "say what one thinks; speak from the heart; be frank and forthright". This is what one should be like when having a "heart-to-heart talk". Of course, there are frank and forthright people who tend to speak "out" what they actually think "in" their heart, and such people are said to "have their heart growing on their mouth" (心在嘴上长着), i.e., they "don't save words in their heart, but speak out whatever is there (in the heart)" (心里不存话，有什么说什么). Besides, straightforward and outspoken people are also said to have "their heart straight and their mouth quick" (心直口快 *xinzhi koukuai*). When the heart is "straight", whatever is inside comes out more readily and easily. Of course, sometimes people also say something, especially something bad, which they do not really mean. In Chinese this is said as "having the mouth but not having the heart" (有口无心 *youkou wuxin*). In short, the heart is where one's inmost thoughts and feelings are stored, and therefore it is utterly important that people get to know others' hearts when making friends (33c), as important as the fact that, when watering trees, one should water their roots rather than other parts of them.

(36) a. 她不贪富，不恋贵，只想找个对心的人。

Ta bu tan fu, bu lian gui, zhi xiang
she not seek riches not long-for honor only want
zhao ge ***dui-xin*** *de ren.*
find a suit-heart MOD person
'She doesn't seek riches, or long for honor; she only wants to find someone to her liking (lit. a heart-suiting person).'

b. 说句掏心的话，你真不该发那么大脾气。

Shuo ju ***tao-xin*** *de hua, ni zhen*
speak CL scoop out-heart MOD words you really
bu-gai fa-name-da-piqi.
shouldn't-have flown-into-such-a-rage
'To be frank (lit. speaking some scooped-out-of-heart words), you shouldn't have lost your temper like that.'

c. 通过交心，他们相互间加深了了解。

Tongguo ***jiao-xin,*** *tamen xianghu jian*
through hand over-heart they mutually between
jiashen-le liaojie.
deepen-PER understanding
'Through opening their hearts to each other (lit. Through handing over each other's hearts), they have deepened their understanding of each other.'

d. 他是我的换心朋友。

Ta shi wode ***huan-xin*** *pengyou.*
he is my exchange-heart friend
'He is my bosom (lit. heart-exchanging) friend.'

The above sentences exemplify (33d–g). An ideal lover is one that "suits the heart" of another (36a). A good couple consists of two persons whose hearts "suit", "match", and "get along" well with each other. That is, the two hearts form a good pair. In (36b), the expression "scooped-out-heart words" is subject to two interpretations. First, people can "scoop words out of their heart", and "words scooped out of their heart" express their true thoughts and feelings. Secondly, people can also "scoop their heart out" directly, and in so doing they let others "see" what is in their heart. Either way, other people get to "see" the true and inner self of those who do the "scooping". Here is another example that illustrates the second interpretation explicitly: 我把我的心都掏出来给你了，你还是不相信我 'I've scooped out my heart and given it to you, but you still don't believe me'. In general, however, when people "scoop their hearts out" and "hand them over" to each other, they will for sure deepen their understanding of each other (36c). Friends who do this are called "heart-exchanging friends" (36d). In Chinese, it is said that 交朋友是交心 'To make friends is to exchange hearts'. Otherwise, they may simply be "wine-and-meat friends" (酒肉朋友), meaning "friends who only drink wine and eat meat together". Friends of this kind are likely to be "fair-weather friends", as is known in English.

(37) a. 贴心 *tie-xin* (stick to-heart) 'intimate; close'
b. 碰心 *peng-xin* (touch/bump-heart) '*dial.* be of one mind/heart; to each other's taste'
c. 合心 *he-xin* (fit/unite-heart) 'be of one mind/heart; be to one's liking/taste'
d. 离心 *li-xin* (depart-heart) 'be at odds with the community or the leadership'
e. 隔心 *ge-xin* (separate-heart) 'with estrangement or misunderstanding'

The compounds in (37) show that interpersonal relationship, such as intimacy and estrangement, is expressed in terms of spatial distance between the hearts. The conceptual metaphors are INTIMACY IS CLOSENESS (BETWEEN THE HEARTS) and ESTRANGEMENT IS DISTANCE (BETWEEN THE HEARTS).[71] Thus, in (37a), an intimate or close relationship means "two

71 For further discussions of the metaphors such as INTIMACY IS CLOSENESS, AFFECTION IS CLOSENESS and FRIENDSHIP IS CLOSENESS, see Kövecses (2000: 92; 2002: 74). According to Kövecses (2000: 92), these metaphors seem to derive

hearts sticking to each other". A "bosom friend" in Chinese is also called a "sticking-to-heart friend" (贴心朋友 *tiexin pengyou*). Such a friend is one to whom you can speak "sticking-to-heart words" (贴心话 *tiexin hua*), i.e. words spoken in confidence. People who like and please each other are those whose hearts "touch" or "bump" each other (37b), or whose hearts "fit to" each other or "are united with" each other (37c). On the contrary, when people are at odds with the community or the leadership, their "hearts depart" from the community or the leadership (37d). People who are estranged from each other are those whose "hearts are separated" from each other (37e).

(38) a. 他既是群众的带头人，又是群众的贴心人。

Ta	*ji*	*shi*	*qunzhong*	*de*	*daitou*	*ren,*	*you*
he	both	is	masses	MOD	leading	person	and
shi	*qunzhong*	*de*	***tie-xin***	*ren.*			
is	masses	MOD	stick to-heart	person			

'He is both a leader and a close friend (lit. sticking-to-heart person) of the masses.'

b. 他们两人谈得挺碰心。

Tamen	*liang*	*ren*	*tan*	*de*	*ting*	***peng-xin.***
they	both	persons	talk	COM	rather	bump-heart

'They talked to each other rather congenially (lit. with their hearts bumping each other) / They both had a rather agreeable (lit. heart-touching) chat.'

The sentences in (38) exemplify (37a) and (37b). Leaders are virtuous when they are also close friends of the masses, i.e. their "hearts stick to those of the masses" (38a). In (38b), the two persons were having such a congenial and agreeable chat that their "hearts touched or bumped each other". An intimate relationship between people, after all, is spatial closeness between their hearts.

---

from the "high level metaphor AN EMOTIONAL RELATIONSHIP IS A DISTANCE BETWEEN TWO ENTITIES (like two people), which applies primarily to love and affection and an absence of these". In English, therefore, there are these expressions: *They are close friends*, *We are attached at the hip*, *They are inseparable*. It is interesting to note that in Chinese, as demonstrated in (37), the distance between "two entities" is oftentimes that between "two hearts", although the CLOSENESS metaphor is applicable to people as well.

(39) a. 只要大家合心干，任务定能完成。

Zhiyao	*dajia*	***he-xin***	*gan,*	*renwu*	*ding*
as-long-long	everyone	unite-heart	work	task	certainly
neng	*wancheng.*				
can	be-accomplished				

'As long as everyone works with one heart (lit. with a united heart), the task will for sure be accomplished.'

b. 咱俩不隔心，有什么事你别瞒我。

Zan-lia	*bu*	***ge-xin,***	*you*	*shenme*	*shi*
two-of-us	not	separate-heart	have	any	thing
ni	*bie*	*man-wo.*			
you	don't	keep-me-in-the-dark			

'The two of us are very close to each other (lit. don't have our hearts separated between us). If there is anything bad, you shouldn't keep me in the dark.'

The sentence in (39a) illustrates (37c) in the sense "unite the hearts (into one)". When people are intimate with each other, their "hearts are not separated from each other", as is shown in (39b), which exemplifies (37e). That is, estrangement between people is spatial and physical separation of their hearts.

4.3.2. The heart and one's personal disposition

Another aspect of the heart as the true self lies in the fact that one's disposition, temperament, and character are ascribed to the nature of one's heart. As discussed earlier, the heart is traditionally taken as the "innermost being", the "true self", of a person in Chinese culture. Since the kind of heart determines the "nature" of a person, it is then the locus of the personality traits of that person. If a person's heart is good, this person is "good-natured". If a person's heart is bad, then this person is "ill-natured".

(40) a. 心性 *xin-xing* (heart-nature) 'disposition; temperament'
b. 心影 *xin-ying* (heart-shadow) 'a person's mind; character; moral nature'

The compound in (40a) shows that a person's disposition and temperament consist in the nature of that person's heart. In (40b) a person's character and moral nature are the "shadow" of this person's heart. That is, the kind of heart one has determines the kind of personal and moral character one has. Since the heart guides the behavior, what kind of heart one has determines how one acts in a particular situation.

(41) a. 粗心 *cu-xin* (thick-heart) 'careless; thoughtless'
b. 细心 *xi-xin* (thin-heart) 'careful; attentive'
c. 心粗 *xin-cu* (heart-thick) 'be careless or thoughtless by nature'
d. 心细 *xin-xi* (heart-thin) 'careful; scrupulous'

In (41) there are two pairs of antonymous compounds, of which (41a) and (41b) have an adjective-noun construction whereas (41c) and (41d) have a subject-predicate construction. The compounds in (41a) and (41c), and those in (41b) and (41d), are synonymous, but those with the subject-predicate structure in (41c, d) seem to refer only to a lasting characteristic of the personality while those with adjective-noun structure in (41a, b) can refer to a one-time mental state as well.

(42) a. 粗心的驾驶员对于公众是一种危险。
Cu-xin *de* *jiashiyuan* *duiyu* *gongzhong* *shi* *yi*
thick-heart MOD driver to public is a
zhong *weixian*.
kind danger
'A careless (lit. thick-hearted) driver is a danger to the public.'

b. 她做什么事都很细心。
Ta *zuo* *shenme* *shi* *dou* *hen* ***xi-xin***.
she does any thing all very thin-heart
'She is meticulous (lit. thin-hearted) in whatever she does.'

As shown by the examples in (42), the diameter of the heart seems to be an important distinguishing factor: a "thick heart" means "carelessness" and "thoughtlessness" while a "thin heart" means "meticulousness" and "cautiousness". Here are two more idioms containing (41a): 粗心大意 *cuxin dayi* (thick-heart big-thought) 'negligent; careless; inadvertent'; 粗心浮气 *cuxin fuqi* (thick-heart flighty-qi) 'not thoughtful and rash'. In the former, "thick-heart" is coordinated with "big thought".[72] Here, the "big thought"

[72] It needs to be noted in passing that the Chinese word 意 *yi* is polysemous with a number of related meanings, including "meaning; idea; thought; wish; desire; intention; suggestion; hint; trace" (H-YCD 1995: 1214).

in one's "thick heart" actually suggests "negligence", i.e. the "overlooking" of things that may be less than "big". However, it is the heart, not the eyes, to blame given that the former is the "ruler" of the latter. As in the latter, a "thick heart" is the "container" of "flighty qi", i.e. the "restless and reckless qi" that will disturb the "stillness" of the heart and cripple its thinking, understanding, and reasoning capacity. It is worth mentioning that differences in spatial dimensions of the heart do not always entail consistent metaphorical conceptualizations of the heart. For instance, a "small heart" (小心 *xiaoxin*) mainly suggests "carefulness" and "cautiousness" in modern Chinese (see 103a below), but according HYDCD (2000: 774) it can also mean "having misgivings or fears" or "being narrow-minded". Similarly, a "big heart" (大心 *daxin*), which is not so commonly-used in present-day Chinese, can mean both "having great aspiration and ambition" and "being arrogant and self-conceited" (HYDCD 2000: 739).[73]

(43) a. 耳软心活 *er-ruan xin-huo* (ear-soft heart-movable) 'soft ears and lively mind; easily influenced by others; ready to believe anything'

b. 冷眼热心 *leng-yan re-xin* (cold-eye hot-heart) 'outward indifference but inward fervency; affected indifference'

c. 眼大心肥 *yan-da xin-fei* (eye-big heart-fat) 'be proud and arrogant'

d. 眼高心傲 *yan-gao xin-ao* (eye-high heart-haughty) 'be proud and haughty; having a haughty look and a proud heart'

The set phrases in (43) involve the heart and the sense organs on and around the face. In (43a), people with "soft ears" and a "movable heart" are "easily influenced by others" because they are "ready to believe anything".[74] The idioms in (43b–d) involve the eyes as well as the heart. The

73 Readers are referred back to 2.3.3, where Xunzi compared and contrasted a "gentleman" with a "petty man". When the gentleman is "big-hearted", he reveres Heaven and follows its Way. When he is "small-hearted", he is awe-inspired by his sense of moral duty and regulates his conduct to accord with it. When a petty man is "big-hearted", he is haughty and irritable. When he is "small-hearted", he is wicked and crooked. Therefore, whether a man is a "gentleman" or a "petty man" depends not on the dimension, but on the disposition or nature, of his heart.

74 Apparently, things that are "soft" are more susceptible to external "force". In Chinese, for instance, the meaning of 脸软 *lianruan* (face-soft) is illustrated in this sentence: 他太脸软，总是不好意思拒绝别人的要求 'He is too soft-

eyes are our important organs of sight in particular, and of cognition in general (Yu 2004). With our eyes we see and read. Seeing and reading are important channels through which we expand our territory of knowledge and cognition. The eyes are important not only for what they do, but also for how they look. They are important physical features that constitute people's identity. While the face is the most distinctive part of a person, both physically and socially (Yu 2001), its focus is really where the eyes are (Yu 2002). The idiom in (43b) describes a situation in which the person has "cold eyes" but a "hot heart", and the outward and the inward do not match. Both (43c) and (43d) emphasize the close relationship between the eyes and the heart, and between seeing and thinking. "Big-eyed" and "fat-hearted" people are proud and arrogant (43c). Their eyes are so "big" and their heart is so "fat" that others appear very "small" in their eye or heart. It is interesting to note that in English, people who think too highly of their own importance have a "big head" whereas those who are "big-hearted" are generous people. In (43d), proud and haughty people have "high eyes" and a "haughty heart". Apparently, people with their eyes "high" either "look down upon" or "look over" other people (Yu 2004).

(44) a. 胆大心细 *dan-da xin-xi* (gallbladder-big heart-thin) 'bold but cautious; brave but not reckless; courageous and wise'
b. 心红胆壮 *xin-hong dan-zhuang* (heart-red gallbladder-strong) 'be sincere and courageous'
c. 琴心剑胆 *qin-xin jian-dan* (musical instrument-heart sword-gallbladder) 'have the soul of a musician and the courage of a warrior; the sentiments of the lute and the spirit of the sword – a cultivated mind animated with a chivalrous spirit'
d. 赤胆忠心 *chi-dan zhong-xin* (sincere-gallbladder loyal-heart) 'utter devotion; whole-hearted dedication; ardent loyalty'

The examples in (44) are idioms involving the heart and the gallbladder. While the heart represents the self and sincerity, the gallbladder is taken as the container of courage in Chinese culture (see Ch. 3; Yu 2003a). Therefore, people with "big gallbladders" are courageous, but it will be more desirable if they also have "thin hearts", thus striking the balance be-

faced, always finding it difficult to reject others' demands'. In contrast, 脸硬 *lianying* (face-hard) means "not easily persuaded to give in; not easily swayed by emotions; not sparing anyone's sensibilities" (Yu 2001: 7).

tween courage and caution. In Chinese, 胆大 *danda* (gallbladder-big) means "courageous; brave" whereas 胆小 *danxiao* (gallbladder-small) means "timid; cowardly". The bigger one's gallbladder is, and the more gallbladders one has, the more courage one has. For instance, these two lines are taken from two TV drama series: 你的胆可真够肥的 'Your gallbladder is indeed fat' or 'You are so bold'; 你就是借给我一个胆我也不敢做这事 'Even if you lend me a gallbladder, I still don't dare to do this'. In (44c), *qin* is a general term for certain musical instruments, such as those with strings. The "musical instrument" and "sword" that modify the heart and gallbladder respectively constitute a case of metonymy inside metaphor (see Goossens 1995). Those with "a heart of a musical instrument and a gallbladder of a sword" have "the soul of a musician and courage of a warrior".

(45) a. 心宽 *xin-kuan* (heart-broad/wide) 'not lend oneself to worry and anxiety'
b. 心窄 *xin-zhai* (heart-narrow) 'narrow-minded'
c. 心高 *xin-gao* (heart-high) 'have (too) high ambitions/aspirations'

The compounds in (45) involve some other spatial or dimensional terms. Both (45a) and (45b) refer to the inner space of the heart. It is better for the heart to be broad or wide than narrow since it is a "container" and its value is judged by its capacity. Furthermore, a broad passage inside the heart facilitates the circulation of qi and blood, which in turn should enhance the health of the whole body. Little wonder that Chinese has idioms such as 心宽体胖 *xinkuan tipang* (heart-broad body-plump) 'carefree and contented; fit and happy'. That is, if one has a "broad" heart, one will have a "plump body". A "plump body" is seen as the signs of health, happiness, and fortune in traditional Chinese culture. In (45c) the "heart-high" means that one has high ambitions or aspirations. However, if one's ambitions or aspirations are too high, it may mean that this person is not realistic or down-to-earth. Here are two idioms to these effects: 心高气盛 *xingao qisheng* (heart-high qi-vigorous/energetic) 'ambitious and proud or aggressive'; 心高气傲 *xingao qi'ao* (heart-high qi-proud/haughty) 'ambitious and proud; proud and arrogant; aim too high and arrogant'. The compounds in (45a) and (45c) are exemplified by the following sayings: (a) 心宽不在屋宽 'If one's heart is broad, it doesn't matter whether the house is spacious or not'; (b) 何劳问宽窄，宽窄在心中 'Why bother to ask if it is broad or narrow (i.e. if the house is spacious or not), since breath and narrowness exist in one's heart'; and (c) 心高如天，命薄如纸 'The heart is as high as the sky, but the fate is as thin as paper'. In (a), if one has a "broad heart", one will not care so much about the size of the house. This saying derives from a line in an ancient poem shown in (b), which says that one should not bother to ask if the house is spacious or not because it is up to the heart to interpret or define the concepts of "broad" and "narrow". The saying in (c) characterizes people who have lofty aspirations but do not have opportunities to display their talents.

(46) a. 心硬 *xin-ying* (heart-hard) 'hardhearted; stonyhearted; callous; unfeeling'
b. 心软 *xin-ruan* (heart-soft) 'be softhearted; be tenderhearted'
c. 心浮 *xin-fu* (heart-floating/flighty) 'flighty and impatient; unstable'

The compounds in (46) suggest the "substance" of the heart: something "hard" in (46a), "soft" in (46b), and "floating" in (46c). In a different context, however, (46a) and (46b) may have meanings different from those listed, such as in 腰软心硬 *yaoruan xinying* (waist-soft heart-hard) and 腰硬心软 *yaoying xinruan* (waist-hard heart-soft). The former means "physically weak but mentally strong" whereas the latter means "physically strong but mentally weak". As in (46c), 浮 *fu* in Chinese means primarily "float", but also "on the surface; superficial; temporary; shallow and frivolous; flighty; hollow; inflated". Thus, a person with a "floating" heart is unreliable and cannot do "solid" work.

(47) a. 不是我心硬，让孩子从小吃点儿苦没有坏处。

Bushi	*wo*	***xin-ying,***	*rang*	*haizi*	*cong*	*xiao*
not-that	I	heart-hard	let	children	from	childhood
chi	*dianr*	*ku*	*mei-you*	*huaichu.*		
eat	a-little	bitterness	there is-no	harm		

'It's not that I am hardhearted (or unfeeling); there is no harm in letting children go through some hardship (lit. eat a little bitterness) from their childhood.'

b. 他虽然说话硬，但是心软，同情心厚。

Ta	*suiran*	*shuohua*	*ying,*	*danshi*	***xin-ruan,***	*tongqing-xin*
he	though	talk	tough	but	heart-soft	sympathy-heart
hou.						
thick						

'Although he talks tough, he has a soft heart (lit. his heart is soft), with a strong sense of compassion (lit. and his heart of compassion is thick).'

c. 他这个人心浮得很，什么事情也做不下去。

Ta zhege	*ren*	***xin-fu***	*de-hen,*	*shenme*
he this	person	heart-floating	a-lot	whatever
shiqing	*ye zuo-bu-xiaqu.*			
things	all unable-to-keep-doing			

'He is very flighty and impatient (lit. heart-floating), unable to get anything done (lit. to keep, or focus on, doing anything).'

In (47b), the person "talks tough" but "has a soft heart" inside. That is, his "toughness" is merely a matter of appearance, and in essence he has a "soft" character with a "thick heart (i.e. strong sense) of sympathy". Note that in Chinese 厚 *hou* means "thick in height" while 粗 *cu* means "thick in diameter".

4.3.3. The heart and one's moral sense

One's moral character is an extension of one's personal character. The heart is both the "source" and the "container" of thoughts and ideas. If the source and container are good, their "products" and "contents" are also good, and vice versa. That is why the heart is traditionally held as the "organ of moral direction" of a person (Hansen 1992: 162), serving as the "behavior guiding mechanism" of that person (p. 20). As shown in 2.3, the heart is conceived of as the locus of moral sense and moral character in ancient Chinese thought. To foster and maintain a good sense of morality, it is crucial to "cultivate the heart" (修心 *xiuxin*), "nurture the heart" (养心 *yangxin*), "straighten (i.e., rectify) the heart" (正心 *zhengxin*), "cleanse the heart" (净心 *jingxin*; 清心 *qingxin*), "empty the heart" (虚心 *xuxin*) when it is filled with desires, "preserve the heart" (存心 *cunxin*) for its good nature, and "recover the heart" (求心 *qiuxin*) if it has been lost. It is interesting to note that this relationship between moral character and heart has been preserved in present-day Chinese.

The compounds in (48) provide examples showing that people's character, good or bad, rests with their heart. It is a quality of the heart.

(48) a. 良心 *liang-xin* (good-heart) 'conscience'
b. 慈心 *ci-xin* (virtuous-heart) 'with a kind heart; be tenderhearted'
c. 善心 *shan-xin* (kind-heart) 'mercy; benevolence'
d. 野心 *ye-xin* (wild-heart) 'wild ambition; careerism'
e. 狠心 *hen-xin* (ruthless/relentless-heart) 'cruel; heartless; merciless; pitiless; ruthless; callous'
f. 兽心 *shou-xin* (animal-heart) 'the heart of an animal – ruthless; relentless; callous'
g. 贪心 *tan-xin* (insatiable-heart) 'greed; avarice; rapacity; greedy; avaricious; voracious'

People's conscience is their "good heart" (48a). Thus, those who have a good conscience "have a good heart" (有良心 *you liangxin*), and those who are conscienceless or heartless "do not have a good heart" (没良心 *mei liangxin*). People with wild ambitions are those who have a "wild heart" (48d). A careerist is a "wild-heart specialist" (野心家 *yexin jia*), and a person of evil ambitions is a "wild-heart wolf" (野心狼 *yexin lang*).

(49) a. 他昧着良心做事。
Ta mei-zhe ***liang-xin*** *zuo shi.*
he hide-DUR good-heart do thing
'He's doing this (evil) against his conscience (lit. with his good-heart concealed).'

b. 你应该摸着良心想一想。
Ni yinggai mo-zhe ***liang-xin*** *xiang-yi-xiang.*
you should touch-DUR good-heart think-it-over
'You should think it over with your hand touching your good-heart (i.e. conscience).'

These two sentences illustrate (48a). If people do something evil against their conscience, they are doing it "with their good heart concealed" (49a), since it will not be able to "see" any more when covered up. Example (49b) is a piece of advice: Before you do anything evil, you should think about it with your hand touching your "good heart". That is, people should do things going with rather than against their conscience. Those conscienceless people do not have a "good heart" any more because, as sometimes said, it has been either "rotten" (良心烂了) or "eaten by a dog" (良心让狗吃了). Very often, people's "good heart" is replaced by a "greedy heart" (贪心 *tanxin*), as illustrated by two proverbs: (a) 人心不足蛇吞象 'A person with an insatiable heart is like a snake trying to swallow an elephant'; and (b) 万丈深渊有底，五寸心窝难填 'An abyss of ten-thousand *zhang* deep has a bottom, but a heart-nest of five-inch big is difficult to fill (i.e. greediness can never be satisfied)'.[75]

(50) a. 心毒 *xin-du* (heart-poisonous) 'wicked; vicious; malignant'
b. 心黑 *xin-hei* (heart-black) 'black-hearted'
c. 心狠 *xin-hen* (heart-ruthless/relentless) 'cruel; merciless'

The compounds in (50) show that evil people have their heart "poisonous", "black", or "ruthless". That is, one's moral character is ascribed to one's heart as its characteristics or qualities. The compounds below characterize a positive moral character.

(51) a. 爱心 *ai-xin* (love-heart) 'loving care'
b. 孝心 *xiao-xin* (filial-heart) 'filial sentiments; filial devotion'
c. 冰心 *bing-xin* (ice-heart) 'moral purity'

Examples (51a) and (51b) show that loving care and filial devotion both come from one's heart. To show loving care is to "dedicate or donate one's loving heart" (献爱心 *xian aixin*). In (51c), moral purity is the "ice-heart" that appears to be transparent and pure.

(52) a. 二心 *er-xin* (two-heart) 'disloyalty; half-heartedness; unfaithful; insincere'
b. 异心 *yi-xin* (different-heart) 'infidelity; disloyalty'
c. 外心 *wai-xin* (outside-heart) 'unfaithful intentions (of husband or wife)'
d. 变心 *bian-xin* (change-heart) 'change loyalties; break faith'
e. 负心 *fu-xin* (fail/betray-heart) 'ungrateful (esp. in love); fail to be loyal to ones' love'
f. 屈心 *qu-xin* (bend-heart) 'have a guilty conscience'
g. 昧心 *mei-xin* (hide/conceal-heart) '(do evil) against one's conscience'

The compounds in (52a–e) show that such concepts as disloyalty, unfaithfulness, insincerity, and infidelity are also hinged on the heart. If peo-

75 *Zhang*, a unit of length in traditional Chinese measure system, is equal to three and one third meters.

ple have "two hearts", it means that their heart is divided, not focused, on something or somebody (52a).[76] When the heart is "divided", there are "two different branches of the heart" (52b). The marriage is a bond with a moral boundary, and unfaithful thoughts and deeds "cross the line" and "fall outside the boundary", i.e., the unfaithful one has an "outside heart" (52c) when having an "outside encounter" (外遇 *waiyu*). Turning unfaithful or disloyal is to "change the heart" that is originally faithful and loyal (52d), or to "fail or betray the heart" of the other (52e). To have a guilty conscience is to "bend one's heart" (52f), and to do evil against one's conscience is to "hide or conceal one's heart" (52g; see 49a above).

(53) a. 她对丈夫有二心。

Ta	*dui*	*zhangfu*	*you*	***er-xin*.**
she	to	husband	has	two-heart

'She is disloyal (lit. has two hearts) to her husband.'

b. 我们要永远相爱，决不负心。

Women	*yao*	*rongyuan*	*xiang-ai,*	*jue-bu*
we	should	forever	mutually-love	never

***fu-xin*.**
betray-heart
'We should love each other forever, and never betray our love (lit. betray each other's heart).'

c. 这种屈心的事我不干。

Zhe zhong	***qu-xin***	*de*	*shi*	*wo*	*bu*	*gan.*
this kind	bend-heart	MOD	thing	I	not	do

'I wouldn't do a mean thing (lit. a thing that bends my heart) like that.'

As in (53a), people can be "two-hearted", as much as "two-faced", to their spouse.[77] A saying goes, "One should not be afraid of a tiger with three

---

[76] Readers are reminded of the relevant discussion on Xunzi's concepts of "unity" and "oneness" of the heart in 2.2.2. Xunzi argued that the world should not have two Ways, and the sage should not have two hearts (天下无二道，圣人无两心). That is, one's heart should remain as a "unified one" and maintain its "oneness" in focus.

[77] Another compound word that is quite popular in contemporary discourse is 花心 *hua-xin* (flowery-heart), which is often used to refer to people who tend to have extramarital affairs.

mouths, but one has every reason to be afraid of a person with two hearts" (不怕虎生三只口，只怕人怀两样心). In (53b), to remain loyal is "not to fail or betray the heart of the other". It would be ideal if two lovers would "never change their hearts even though the seas may run dry and the rocks may crumble" (海枯石烂，永不变心). In (53c), feeling guilty is to "feel one's heart being bent".

(54) a. 公心 *gong-xin* (fair/public-heart) 'public spirit; fairness'
b. 私心 *si-xin* (selfish-heart) 'selfish motives/ideas; selfishness'

In (54), the sense of fairness or selfishness, and public spirits or selfish motives, all originate in the heart as part of its moral predispositions. Selfish thoughts and considerations are "mixed" (私心杂念 *sixin zanian*) in the sense that they are not "pure" or "clean". That is why the heart needs clarification and purification, as in (55).

(55) a. 清心 *qing-xin* (clear-heart) 'empty one's mind of worries; have peace of mind; purify the heart; have a pure heart'
b. 净心 *jing-xin* (clean-heart) 'cleanse one's heart'

Two familiar idioms in ancient Chinese philosophy that contain (55a) and (55b) are 清心寡欲 *qingxin guayu* (clear-heart reduce-desire) 'purify one's heart and reduce the number of one's desires' and 净心修身 *jingxin xiushen* (cleanse-heart cultivate-body) 'cleanse one's heart and cultivate one's moral character'. Reflecting (55a) the old saying goes, "If one's desire is light, one's heart is clear; when one's heart is clear, one can see principles/reasons" (欲淡则心清，心清则理见). The desire, or too much of it, is what makes the heart "dirty". When the heart is "clean" and "clear" for not being filled with desires, it can make sound judgments based on right principles and good senses. As in (55b), it is important to "cleanse the heart" because "When the heart is clean, it shines forth as a solitary lamp" (心净孤明独照). That is, a "clean and pure heart" is a "shining lamp" that enables one to "see" in the "dark". The LAMP metaphor is another instantiation of the heart being the "governor of the spiritual light".

(56) a. 心肝 *xin-gan* (heart-liver) 'conscience; (a term of endearment mostly used with one's small children) darling; dear; sweetheart; honey'

b. 心肠 *xin-chang* (heart-intestine) 'heart; intention; *dial.* state of mind or mood'

In (56), *xin* 'heart' is combined with *gan* 'liver' and *chang* 'intestine' to mean "heart" in the sense of "conscience". The heart, the "fire" organ, and the liver, the "wood" organ, are two zang organs that are closely related. The heart and (small) intestine are also closely related to each other as a pair of zang and fu organs that stand in the interior-exterior relationship (see Ch. 3).[78] Here are some common collocations and set phrases: 没心肝 *mei xingan* (not have heart-liver) 'heartless', 好心肠 *hao xinchang* (good heart-intestine) 'kindhearted', 坏心肠 *huai xinchang* (bad heart-intestine) 'evil-minded', 热心肠 *re xinchang* (hot heart-intestine) 'warm-hearted', 心肠软 *xinchang ruan* (heart-intestine soft) 'be softhearted', 心肠硬 *xinchang ying* (heart-intestine hard) 'be hardhearted', 铁石心肠 *tieshi xinchang* (iron-stone heart-intestine) 'be iron-hearted; be heartless', and 心肠歹毒 *xinchang daidu* (heart-intestine bad-poisonous) 'wicked heart'. As we can see, the heart and intestine can be "good" or "bad", "soft" or "hard", depending on the moral character of the person. They can be "hot", but there seem to be no antonymous collocations or idioms that suggest that they can be "cold". However, when they are said to be "hard", their "coldness" is implied because "hardness" and "coldness" are correlative to some extent.

(57) a. 心毒手辣 *xin-du shou-la* (heart-poisonous hand-peppery/vicious) 'vicious and ruthless; callous and cruel; black-hearted and cruel'

b. 心狠手辣 *xin-hen shou-la* (heart-ruthless hand-peppery/vicious) 'cruel and ruthless; wicked and merciless; cruel and evil'

c. 心黑手辣 *xin-hei shou-la* (heart-black hand-peppery/vicious) 'black-hearted and cruel'

d. 心慈手软 *xin-ci shou-ruan* (heart-virtuous hand-soft) 'softhearted; faint of heart and hesitant in action; kindhearted and irresolute'

---

78 Readers are also referred to Yu (1995, 1998: Ch. 3, 2001) for further discussions of the "heart-liver" and "heart-(small) intestine" combinations in conventionalized expressions in Chinese. There, such combinations are discussed within the cultural schemas of the theories of yin-yang and the five elements.

The examples in (57) are four idioms involving the heart, our internal organ of moral sense, and the hand, our external body part with which we deal with the external world (see Yu 2003c). The heart thinks while the hands act. They represent, metonymically or metaphorically, two important aspects of a person: thought and action. The kind of heart one has affects how one acts. That is exactly why the heart is called "the behavior-guiding mechanism" and "the organ of moral direction".

(58) a. 心慈面软 *xin-ci mian-ruan* (heart-virtuous face-soft) 'kindhearted and obliging; kind heart and soft countenance; soft-hearted'
b. 面善心慈 *mian-shan xin-ci* (face-kind heart-virtuous) 'affable and kindhearted'
c. 心善面冷 *xin-shan mian-leng* (heart-kind face-cold) 'have a kind heart but a cold face – be kind-hearted but stone-faced'
d. 面善心狠 *mian-shan xin-hen* (face-kind heart-ruthless) 'be innocent in appearance but a very wolf at heart'

The idioms in (58) involve the heart and the face (cf. 35a–c above). The face is one of the most important parts of our body because it is the most distinctive part on the interactive side of our body capable of revealing our inner states (see Yu 2001). That is, the face and the heart form a special relationship. People sometimes judge others' character by their faces, although it is not reliable to do so. The English word *face* has two basic counterparts in modern Chinese: *lian* 'face' and *mian* 'face'. In the first two idioms (58a, b), "kindhearted" people also have "soft and kind faces". A "soft-faced" and "kind-hearted" person tends to "save other people's face" (留面子 *liu mianzi*) or "give other people face" (给面子 *gei mianzi*) (Yu 2001). In the last two idioms (58c, d), the faces are deceptive. A "stone-faced" person, who looks very "cold", may actually have a kind heart (58c). In contrast, a "kind-faced" person may also have a "wicked heart", covering up the true character (58d). The face is after all an external body part, only standing for people's outward appearance, in contrast to the heart that represents their inner state.

(59) a. 丹心 *dan-xin* (red-heart) 'loyal heart; loyalty'
b. 赤心 *chi-xin* (red/sincere-heart) 'sincere heart; genuine sincerity; whole-hearted devotion'
c. 红心 *hong-xin* (red-heart) 'red heart; loyal heart; true heart'
d. 黑心 *hei-xin* (black-heart) 'black heart; evil mind'

The original color of the heart is red, so the red is the "good" color whereas the black is the "evil" color, as in (59). The three modifiers in (59a–c) can all mean "red". The compounds in which they collocate with *xin* 'heart' all have a positive meaning in terms of moral values.

(60) a. 谁知道他的心是黑的是红的。
Shui zhidao tade ***xin*** *shi heide shi hongde.*
who knows his heart is black is red
'Who knows if his heart is black or red (i.e. if he is a bad or good person or if he has bad or good intentions).'

b. 好处他一个人独吞了，真黑心。
Haochu ta yi-ge-ren du-tun-le, zhen ***hei-xin****.*
profits he alone single-swallow-PER really black-heart
'He took exclusive possession of (lit. alone swallowed) all the profits; he is so evil-minded (lit. black-hearted).'

Since the heart is inside the chest, it is not easy to "tell" the actual color of a person's heart (60a). That is, one's moral character is not always obvious to other people. However, it is possible to infer it from that person's actions (60b). The color of the heart can change. A person who has developed an immoral character is said to "have eaten charcoal that has blackened his good heart" (吃了木炭，黑了良心). The desire to make riches is believed to be the source of evil, as the saying goes, "As much as white wine reddens the human face, yellow gold blackens the worldly heart" (白酒红人面，黄金黑世心). It is even said that "without a black heart one can never make riches" (心不黑发不了财).

The heart is the "organ of moral direction or behavior guidance". Therefore, people doing bad things are guided by their heart, and their wrong doings are called "mistakes of the heart" (心过 *xinguo*). "Mistakes of the heart are difficult to correct; if people can correct them, then they won't have mistakes any more" (心过难改，能改心过，则无过矣). Also, the heart is the "organ of moral sense". If people are mistaken in moral judgments, they are said to have contracted a "heart disease" (心病 *xinbing*).[79] It is therefore said, metaphorically, that "Human diseases are mostly heart diseases, and if one's heart has turned bad, then it is very dif-

[79] Note that in Chinese 心病 *xinbing* normally means "worry; anxiety", which are "illnesses" of the mind. See also (114b) and (115) and the relevant discussion in 4.5.3 below.

ficult to cure it" (人病多是心病，心坏了，就很难治好). Here, the word "disease" is not used in a physiological sense, but in a moral sense. Thus, it is not the physical heart that has gone wrong; what has turned bad is the moral character, whose locus is culturally believed to be the heart. Thus, small or petty men are usually characterized as having "the heart of small men" (小人之心). It is said that "A small man has many hearts (i.e. is over-sensitive), just as bamboos have many roots" (竹子根多，小人心多). This is another case in which "hearts" and "roots", and "people" and "plants" are paralleled and connected. Another proverb says "Just as the waters of the mountain brooks are easy to rise and recede, the heart of a small man is easy to chop and change" (易涨易退山溪水，易反易复小人心).

4.3.4. The heart and one's love

That the heart is the seat of the true self is also exemplified by the conception of love, which is a complex physical, emotional, and mental experience rooted deeply in one's spirit and soul. While true love is believed to be the expression and manifestation of the true self, it is located in the heart.[80] Therefore, the heart, as the container of love, is often referred to metonymically as love itself (i.e. CONTAINER FOR CONTAINED). For instance, here is an outdated traditional idea regarding women winning love from men: 要抓住一个男人的心一定要先抓住这个男人的胃 'In order to grab a man's heart, a woman must first grab his stomach'. That is, if a woman wants to gain the love (lit. control the heart) of a man, she must first be a good cook for him (lit. control his stomach). Here, the "heart" is metonymic for love and the "stomach" for appetite or taste.

Now, look at the following two examples related to romantic love.

(61) a. 她就那么重重地敲打着他的心扉，让他有种被电流击中的感觉。

Ta jiu name	*zhongzhong-de*	*qiao-da-zhe*			*tade*
she thus so	heavily	knock-pound-DUR			his
xin-fei,	*rang* *ta* *you*	*zhong*	*bei*	*dian-liu*	
heart-door	make him have	kind-of	by	electrical-current	
jizhong *de*	*ganjue.*				
struck MOD	feeling				

[80] In this chapter I treat "love" as a unique feeling that reflects and expresses one's true self, and therefore categorize it under the "inner self". I will, nevertheless, come back to "love" in 4.5.4 where I discuss positive feelings of the "emotional life".

'She thus kept knocking and pounding his heart (lit. heart-door), making him have the kind of feeling of being struck by an electrical current.'

b. 两颗年轻的心逐渐贴近了起来。
Liang-ke nianqing-de ***xin*** *zhujian tie-jin-le*
two-CL young hearts gradually stick-closer-PER
qilai.
start
'The two young hearts started getting closer (lit. stuck) to each other.'

In (61a), "she" is so appealing to "him" that her attraction keeps "knocking and pounding his heart door". It is expected that once the "heart door" is "knocked open", his heart will be filled with love for her. Note that her appeal to him is an "electrical current" striking him and going through his body. This is reminiscent of vogue expressions that speak of the feeling of romanic love in metaphorical terms of electricity; thus having "electricity coming or not" (来电、不来电) means "having or not having the feeling of romanic love for someone", and "electricity going through" (过电) means "experiencing the feeling of romantic love". In short, romantic love is the communication and interaction between two "hearts". The right communication and interaction will produce "magnetic force" that will eventually "pull the two hearts together" (61b; cf. 37 above).

(62) a. 他总是心不在焉，他的心已被隔着墙的姑娘"叼"走了。
Ta zongshi ***xin-bu-zai-yan,*** *tade****xin*** *yi bei*
he always heart-not-here his heart already by
ge-zhe-qiang de guniang "diao"-zou-le.
beyond-the-wall MOD girl carry-away-in-the-mouth-PER
'He was always absent-minded (lit. heart-not-here or absent-hearted), and his heart had been taken away (lit. "carried away in the mouth") by the girl beyond the wall.'

b. 这颗多年漂泊的心终于找到了属于自己爱的港湾。
Zhe-ke duo-nian piaobo-de ***xin*** *zhongyu zhaodao-le*
this-CL many-years drofting heart finally find-PER
shuyu ziji ai de gangwan.
belong-to self love MOD harbor
'This heart that had kept drifting for many years finally found the harbor of love that belonged to itself.'

c. 我骗你？我就是把心剜出来给你煮了吃了，你还当是吃白薯呢。
Wo pian *ni?* *Wo* *jiushi* *ba* ***xin*** *wan chulai* *gei* *ni*
I deceive you I even PRT heart cut out give you
zhu-le *chi-le,* *ni* *hai* *dang* *shi* *chi* *baishu*
cook-PER eat-PER you still think be eating sweet-potato
ne.
PRT
'I'm deceiving you? Even if I cut my heart out and let you cook and eat it, you would still think that you were eating a sweet potato.'

As we can see, "he" in (62a) did not have his heart in him any longer because it had been "carried away in the mouth" by the girl who lived on the other side of the wall. In Chinese, the verb 叼 *diao* refers to the action of an animal, such as a bird or a dog, holding or carrying something in the mouth. When one has "fallen in love" with some one else, one "loses one's heart" to the other. Since the heart is the "locus of the mind", and the "seat of the true self", therefore, after one has lost one's heart, one becomes "absent-minded" and "beside one's self". In (62b) the "heart" is conceptualized as a vessel that had been "drifting (on the sea)" (漂泊 *piaobo*) for many years and finally found the "harbor" (港湾 *gangwan*) to which it belonged. It is the "harbor of love". In plain words, this person had been searching for true love for many years and finally found the right person with whom she had fallen in love. We can see the "heart" as a metonymy, or synecdoche, for the person as a whole (PART FOR WHOLE). The "heart", as a part of a person, has this privilege because it is, again, the seat of the true self. In (62c), taken from a TV drama series, the speaker believes that her true love is not appreciated by the person she loves. The hopelessness on her part is that even if she let her lover "eat her heart", he would still think that he was "eating a sweet potato". The "sweet potato" is selected here probably because its shape resembles that of the physical heart.

When it is said that the heart is the seat of the true inner self, this part is then distinguished from the rest of the body, the other or outer self of the person. This conceptualization is illustrated by the following two examples, also taken from a TV drama series. They again concern love, this time between a husband and wife.

(63) a. 我可是拴得住他的人，拴不住他的心。
I can tether him the person to me, but I can't tether his heart to me.

b. A: 心不在，留住人有什么用？
When his heart is absent, what's the use of keeping him the person?

B: 可是只要人在，心慢慢是会回来的。
But, as long as he the person is here, his heart will gradually come back.

Here, the husband has engaged in an affair with another woman. The wife, saddened by this fact, is thinking of her divorce, because, as she believes, even if she is able to "tether her husband the person to her", she is unable to "tether his heart to her" (63a). When her husband's "heart", i.e. true love, is gone, what the point is of keeping him the person, she asks. As a saying goes, "When one's heart is gone, it is hard to retain the person, and even if the person stays, he or she will turn into a foe (against you)" (心去人难留，留下结冤仇). However, the wife's friend recommends a different approach to the problem. That is, the wife should try to keep her husband instead of divorcing him. As long as she can keep him, "his heart will gradually come back" (63b).

4.4. The heart as the locus of mental life

As analyzed in Chapters 2 and 3, the Chinese *xin* 'heart' has traditionally been conceptualized as the locus of the "mind", its mental functions including thought, reason, intellect, volition, memory, and so forth. This section will demonstrate that this predominant cultural conceptualization formulated in ancient times is still manifested pervasively in the Chinese language today. That is, the heart as part of the body, instead of being in contrast with the "mind", as is the case in modern English, is the locus of the "mind" in Chinese. It is in this sense that the "heart" is often used in contrast with the "body/person", as shown in the following two sentences:

(64) a. 你是人累还是心累？

Ni	*shi*	***ren***	*lei*	*haishi*	***xin***	*lei?*
you	are	person/body	tired	or	heart	tired

'Are you physically tired or mentally tired (lit. Are you tired in the person/body or in the heart)?'

b. 你只要心不老，人就不会老。

Ni	*zhiyao*	***xin***	*bu*	*lao,*	***ren***	*jiu*	*bu*	*hui*	*lao.*
you	as-long-as	heart	not	age	person	then	not	will	age

'As long as your mind (lit. heart) is not aging, then you the person (or your body) will not age.'

In these examples, 人 *ren* ‘person’ actually refers to the physical body of the person, in contrast to 心 *xin* ‘heart’, which actually refers to the “mind” of the person. This contrast is equivalent to that between 身 *shen* ‘body’ and 心 *xin* ‘heart/mind’, which means “body and mind” when used together (身心 *shenxin*). For instance, 身心健康 *shenxin jiankang* means “physically and mentally healthy” or “physical and mental health”.

The following compounds also show that in Chinese the “heart” is traditionally conceptualized as the locus of the “mind” :

(65) a. 心灵 *xin-ling* (heart-soul/spirit) ‘mind; heart; soul; spirit; psyche’
b. 心智 *xin-zhi* (heart-wisdom) ‘mind; noema’
c. 心理 *xin-li* (heart-reason/principle) ‘mind; mentality; psychology’
d. 心态 *xin-tai* (heart-state/condition) ‘mental state, mentality; psychology’

While the compounds in (65a–c) can all mean “mind”, each of them contains “heart” as one of its two constituents. Not only “soul” and “spirit” (65a) are ascribed to the “heart”, so are “wisdom” (65b) and “reason” and “principle” (65c). In (65c), the Chinese word for “mentality” or “psychology” literally means “heart-reason” or “heart-principle”. It is worth mentioning that in Chinese the study of the mind and the study of the heart are respectively called 心理学 *xinlixue* (heart-principle-study) ‘psychology’ and 心病学 *xinbingxue* (heart-disease-study) ‘cardiology’. In Chinese they both literally study the “heart”. Example (65d) shows that the “mental state” or “mentality” is actually a “state” or “condition” of the “heart”.

(66) a. 向前看，别回头，时间是医治心灵创伤的良药。
Xiang qian kan, bie hui-tou, shijian shi yizhi
to ahead look don’t turn back-head time is treat
xin-ling *chuangshang de liang-yao.*
heart-soul wound MOD good-medicine
‘Look forward and don’t turn back (your head). Time is the good medicine for treating the wound of the mind (lit. heart-soul).’

b. 她认为自己爱的不是他的财富，而是他可以创造财富的心智与能力。
Ta renwei ziji ai de bu shi tade caifu, er shi ta keyi
she think self love PRT not be his wealth but be he can
chuangzao caifu de ***xin-zhi*** *yu nengli.*
create wealth MOD heart-wisdom and ability

'She thinks that what she loves is not his wealth, but his mind (lit. heart-wisdom) and ability with which he can create wealth.'

The example in (66a) involves the basic conceptual metaphor TIME IS SPACE (see, e.g., Lakoff 1993; Yu 1998: Ch. 4). Thus, "look forward and don't turn back" means figuratively "look forward to the future and don't look back at the past". In other words, the advice made is not to dwell upon the past when the wound of the mind is inflicted. Instead, look to the future and let the wound of the mind be healed by time, which is the "good medicine" to cure such wounds. In (66b), wisdom is a quality of the heart, which is conceptualized as the seat of intellect, or the organ that embodies intellectual faculties.

In what follows in this chapter, I will examine the linguistic data that evidence the Chinese cultural conceptualization of the heart as the locus of one's mental life, which includes thought, intellect, intention, volition, and so forth.

4.4.1. The heart and thought

Traditionally, the heart is considered to be the center of thought in Chinese culture. This conceptualization is evidenced by the following group of compound words that all contain *xin* 'heart' as their first of the two morphological constituents:

(67) a 心思 *xin-si* (heart-think/thought) 'thought; idea; thinking; state of mind'

b. 心念 *xin-nian* (heart-think/idea) 'thought; idea; thinking; intention'

c. 心愿 *xin-yuan* (heart-hope/wish) 'cherished desire; aspiration; wish; dream'

d. 心期 *xin-qi* (heart-expect) 'expectation; hope; wish; aspiration; intention'

e. 心劲 *xin-jin* (heart-strength/energy) 'thought; idea'

f. 心象 *xin-xiang* (heart-image) 'thought; idea; thinking; state of mind; mood'

g. 心事 *xin-shi* (heart-matter/affair) 'something weighing on one's mind; a load on one's mind; worry'

In (67a) and (67b), as we can see, when people think, their "heart thinks", and thoughts, ideas, mood, etc. are attributed to the heart. In a line of a poem, the compound word 思念 *sinian,* which consists of the second constituents of (67a) and (67b) and means "think of; long for; miss", is characterized as the "common vibration and resonance between two hearts" (思念是心与心的共振共鸣). As in (67c) and (67d), people also hope, wish, desire, and expect with their hearts, and their aspirations, hopes, wishes, expectations, dreams, etc. come from their hearts. In (67e), one's thoughts and ideas constitute one's mental power comprising one's mental "strength" or "energy". The compound in (67f) suggests that thoughts and ideas, etc., are images in the heart. In (67g), whatever weighs on one's mind is actually weighing on the top of one's heart; it is therefore the "heart-matter". "A thing weighing on one's mind (lit. a heart-matter) is a mountain" (一件心事一座山).

(68) a. 我猜不透他的心思。

Wo *cai-bu-tou* *tade* ***xin-si***.
I guess-not-penetrate his heart-thought
'I can't read his mind (lit. his heart-thought) / I can't figure out what's on his mind (lit. what's his heart-thought).'

b. 他的话说出了大家的心念。

Tade *hua* *shuo* *chu le* *dajia-de* ***xin-nian***.
his words speak out PRT everyone's heart-thought
'His words expressed (lit. spoke out) everyone's thought.'

c. 这就了却了我的一桩心愿。

Zhe *jiu* *liaoque-le* *wode* *yi-zhuang* ***xin-yuan***.
this then fulfill-PER my one-CL heart-wish
'This serves to fulfill a cherished desire (lit. a heart-wish) of mine.'

d. 我们大伙儿是一个心劲，要尽快把事情办成。

Women *dahuor* *shi* *yi-ge* ***xin-jin***, *yao*
we all are one-CL heart-strength want
jin-kuai *ba* *shiqing* *ban-cheng*.
as-quickly-as-possible PRT things do-accomplish
'We all have only one thought (lit. one heart-strength/energy): to get the job done as quickly as possible.'

The sentential examples in (68) illustrate some of the compounds in (67). "Reading people's mind" is trying to figure out the thoughts in their heart (68a). When the mental effort leads to no result, it means that one has "spent one's heart-thoughts in vain" (白费心思 *baifei xinsi*). People may have a common thought that they each keep in their hearts. The right expression of that thought verbally will bring that thought out of their hearts (68b). People all have wishes and aspirations that they want to fulfill, and these mental states and activities again originate in the heart: They are what the heart wishes for (68c). When people all have "one thought", namely, the "strength" or "energy" of their hearts is directed and applied to one purpose, they are likely to achieve what they want to (68d). The heart is the "ruler" of the body. When the heart is determined to have something done, it will make the body do it.

(69) a. 心机 *xin-ji* (heart-mechanism) 'thought; idea; thinking; scheming'
b. 心数 *xin-shu* (heart-number/figure) 'calculation; scheming; planning'
c. 心计 *xin-ji* (heart-calculate/stratagem) 'calculating; scheming; planning'
d. 心术 *xin-shu* (heart-art) 'intention; design; calculation; scheming; planning'
e. 心裁 *xin-cai* (heart-cutting/planning) 'idea; conception; mental plan'

The compounds in (69) represent mental activities of calculating, scheming, planning, and designing, which all depend on thinking, reflecting, and contemplating deeply on the part of the heart. In (69e), the morpheme *cai* suggests a tailor's designing and cutting in the making of clothing. No matter what people want to design, original ideas always come from their heart, and originality in designing is often said as a "unique heart-cutting" (独出心裁 *duchu xincai*). Here are some sentential examples:

(70) a. 她年龄不大，但很有心机。
Ta nianling bu da, dan hen you ***xin-ji***.
she age not old but very-much have heart-mechanism
'Young as she is, she has a mind of her own (lit. has a lot of heart-mechanism).'

b. 他这个人工于心计。
Ta zhe-ge ren gong-yu ***xin-ji***.
he this-CL person adept-at heart-calculate
'He is adept at scheming (lit. heart-calculating) / This person is very calculating.'

c. 他这个人心术不正。
Ta zhe-ge ren ***xin-shu*** *bu zheng.*
he this-CL person heart-art not straight
'This person harbors evil intentions (lit. This person's heart-art is not straight, i.e. crooked).'

When people have a good mind, they have good "mechanisms of the heart" rather than the brain (70a). Calculating people primarily have a "calculating heart", i.e. they are good at "heart-calculating" (70b). In (70c), the "art of the heart" literally refers to the "art of cultivating one's heart" (cf. Ch. 2). It is important, however, that the "cultivation of the heart" is on the "right track". The practice of cultivating the heart on a "wrong path" will only lead to more evil thoughts and intents. A pair of conceptual metaphors involved in (70c) is MORAL IS STRAIGHT and IMMORAL IS CROOKED.

The compounds in (71) further illustrate that the heart conducts various mental activities.

(71) a. 心想 *xin-xiang* (heart-think) 'think to oneself; think'
b. 心领 *xin-ling* (heart-get/understand) 'understand; appreciate'
c. 心照 *xin-zhao* (heart-illuminate) 'understand without being told'
d. 心疑 *xin-yi* (heart-suspect) 'become or be suspicious'
e. 心服 *xin-fu* (heart-be convinced) 'be genuinely convinced; acknowledge (one's defeat, mistake, etc.) sincerely'
f. 心许 *xin-xu* (heart-praise/permit) 'tacitly consent to; acquiesce in; appreciate; think highly of'
g. 心甘 *xin-gan* (heart-willing) 'do sth. willingly; be ready and willing; be reconciled to; resign oneself to; be content with'

Note that (67a) above literally means "heart thinks", but it is used as a noun meaning "thought", "idea", "mood", etc. The compound in (71a) again means "heart thinks" literally, but this time it is a verb meaning "think to oneself" or "think" in general. The idiom 心想事成 *xinxiang shicheng* (heart-think things-accomplished) refers to the desirable situation where "things are accomplished as one hopes or wishes". Both (71b) and (71c) show that understanding is achieved by the heart. In (71b), for the understanding and appreciation of something the heart "gets" that thing. The verb *zhao* in (71c) is associated with the mirror (to reflect) and light (to illuminate), and for the understanding of something the heart "reflects" that thing like a mirror or "illuminates" it like light. When people become suspicious, they have questions and doubts in their heart (71d), i.e. their "heart suspects". The compound in (71e) shows that when people are genuinely convinced that they have lost or erred, their "heart is convinced". When people not only say they are convinced, but also really feel that way in their heart (心服口服 *xinfu koufu*), they are genuinely convinced. In (71f), acquiescence is "the heart giving permission" whereas appreciation is "the heart giving praise". As in (71g), if people are willing to do something, their "heart is willing".

(72) a. 我心想他早晚总会来的。
Wo ***xin-xiang*** *ta zao-wan zong hui lai de.*
I heart-think he sooner-or-later surely will come PRT
'I thought (lit. I heart-thought) he would turn up sooner or later.'

b. 您的美意，我心领了。
Ninde mei-yi, wo ***xin-ling****-le.*
your good-intention I heart-get/understand-PER
'I appreciate (lit. I heart-get/understand) your kindness (lit. good intention).'

c. 他的话前后不一，令人心疑。
Tade hua qian-hou-bu-yi, ling ren
his words front-back-not-one making people
xin-yi*.*
heart-suspect
'His words were self-contradictary, making people suspicious (lit. making people's heart suspect).'

d. 他心甘情愿当人民的勤务员。
Ta ***xin-gan*** *qing-yuan dang renmin-de qinwuyuan.*
he heart-willing feeling-willing be people's odd-jobman
'He is a willing servant of the people (lit. He is heart-willing to be a servant of the people).'

Given in (72) are some sentential examples. They all illustrate that the heart is the real agent of mental activities such as thinking, appreciating or suspecting. Thus, for instance, when people are suspicious, their "heart suspects" (72c). No wonder that, when having serious doubts, people will "draw a big question mark in their heart" (在心中打个大问号).

4.4.2. The heart and intellect

In the Chinese language, as already seen, the heart is the locus of the "mind", responsible for various mental functions, such as thinking, understanding, knowing, and reasoning. With all those mental activities that it does, naturally, the heart is conceived of as the seat of intellectual faculties. Look at the following three compounds.

(73) a. 慧心 *hui-xin* (intelligent-heart) 'wisdom'
b. 心灵 *xin-ling* (heart-quick/clever) 'clever; intelligent; quick-witted'[81]
c. 心秀 *xin-xiu* (heart-elegant/excellent) 'be intelligent without looking so'

As we can see, wisdom is the natural product of an "intelligent heart" (73a). Intelligence, cleverness, and quick-wit are qualities of the heart too (73b, c). Thus, those people who are clever, intelligent, or quick-witted all have an "clever or excellent heart".

(74) a. 劳心 *lao-xin* (work-heart) 'work with one's mind or brains'
b. 心得 *xin-de* (heart-obtain) 'what one has learned from work, study, etc.'
c. 心算 *xin-suan* (heart-calculate) 'mental arithmetic; do arithmetic in one's head'

The compound in (74a) was originally used by Mencius in his well-known saying in which he divided people into those who work with their "heart/mind" and those who work with their brawn (劳心者治人，劳力者治于人), as discussed in Chapter 2. The compound in (74b), illustrated in a sentence below, shows that learning is a process of obtaining knowledge by and storing it in the heart-container. In (74c), mental arithmetic, i.e. math-

[81] Note that (73b) and (65a) at the beginning of section 4.4 are usually listed in dictionaries as two separate entries, rather than two senses under one entry. However, they are not on a par with, say, *bank* as "land along the side of a river" and *bank* as "a financial institution where money is deposited or withdrawn". Apparently, (65a) and (73b) are somewhat related, with one referring to the "mind" and the other denoting a quality of the "mind". They both have to do with the "heart" in Chinese.

ematic calculation without the help of paper and pen or calculator etc. is done in the heart, instead of the head as in the English translation.

(75) 我想谈谈学习这篇课文的心得。
Wo xiang tantan xuexi zhe-pian kewen de ***xin-de***.
I want talk-about study this-CL text MOD heart-obtain
'I want to talk about what I have gained (lit. what my heart has obtained) from studying this text.'

It is well known that doing intellectual activities requires both intention and volition on the part of the doer. The relationships between the heart, on the one hand, and intention and volition, on the other, are the topics for the next two subsections.

4.4.3. The heart and intention

In the Chinese conceptualization, people's intent and will originate in, and arise from, their heart. According to the *Magic Pivot*, the ancient medical text, when the heart is utilized, there is intention; when intention is preserved, there is will (see 3.3.1). The compounds that respectively mean "intention" and "will" both contain *xin* 'heart', as shown below:

(76) a. 心意 *xin-yi* (heart-intention) 'intention; purpose; regard; kindly feelings'
b. 心志 *xin-zhi* (heart-will) 'will; resolution'

These two compounds are illustrated by (77a) and (77b). Literally, intention is "heart's intention" and will is "heart's will". It is difficult to "see" other people's intentions, unless expressed through words or actions, because intentions reside in their heart (77a). In order to be resolute, people should have "firm" will in their heart (77b).

(77) a. 你们不了解他的心意。
Nimen bu liaojie tade ***xin-yi***.
you not understand his heart-intention
'You don't understand his intention (lit. heart-intention).'

b. 人若有疑虑，则心志不坚，会时常犹豫。
Ren ruo you yilü , ze ***xin-zhi*** *bu jian, hui*
people if have doubts then heart-will not firm should

shichang *youyu.*
often be-irresolute
'If people have doubts, then their will (lit. heart-will) is not firm, and they should often be hesitant.'

In what follows, I will first focus on the data demonstrating the relation between the heart and intention. I will then turn to the relation between the heart and volition in the next subsection.

(78) a. 有心 *you-xin* (have-heart) 'have a mind to; set one's mind on; intentionally; purposely'
b. 无心 *wu-xin* (not-have-heart) 'not in the mood for; not intentionally; unwittingly; inadvertently'

Since intents or purposes are the "contents" inside the heart-container and, by conceptual metonymy CONTAINER FOR CONTAINED, *xin* 'heart' has come to mean "intention". Thus, "have-heart" in (78a) and "not-have-heart" in (78b) respectively mean "have the intention" and "not have the intention", as illustrated by the sentences in (79):

(79) a. 我有心去看看他，又怕打扰他。
Wo ***you-xin*** *qu* *kankan* *ta,* *you pa* *darao* *ta.*
I have-heart go see him but afraid disturb him
'I'd like (lit. have the heart) to go and see him, but I'm afraid to disturb him.'

b. 他说这话是无心的，你可别见怪。
Ta *shuo* *zhe-hua* *shi* ***wu-xin*** *de,* *ni* *ke*
he say this is not have-heart PRT you had-better
bie *jianguai.*
not take-offence
'Don't take offence. He didn't say it intentionally (lit. He didn't have the heart when he said this).'

The old saying goes, 'When you intentionally plant flowers, they won't blossom; but when you unwittingly insert willows, they will grow into big trees with large shades' (有心栽花花不开，无心插柳柳成荫). That is, when you intentionally do something, the result tends to be not good, but when you do something unintentionally, the result can be unexpectedly good. In Chinese, the idiom 有心无力 *youxin wuli* (have-heart no-strength) means "have the intention (of doing something) but lack the strength/ability (to do it)". Another popular saying, often said jokingly, goes: 我有那贼心也没那贼胆 (lit. I have that thievish heart but don't have that thievish gallbladder), meaning "Even if I have the intention to do it (i.e. something bad), I still don't have the courage to do it". That is, the "heart" represents intention whereas the "gallbladder" represents courage.

(80)
a. 好心 *hao-xin* (good-heart) 'good intention'
b. 邪心 *xie-xin* (evil-heart) 'evil thought; wicked idea; evil intention'
c. 歹心 *dai-xin* (vicious-heart) 'malice; malicious intent'
d. 初心 *chu-xin* (beginning-heart) 'one's original desire, aspiration, intention'
e. 本心 *ben-xin* (original-heart) 'original intention; true intention'
f. 素心 *su-xin* (white/undyed-heart) 'one's real intention; one's true will; clean and honest; pure in heart'

There are further examples in which "heart" refers to intention, as in (80). Thus, "good heart" represents good intention whereas "evil or vicious heart" represents "evil or vicious intention" (80a–c). One's "beginning heart", "original heart", or "undyed heart" is one's original or real intention (80d–f). The sentences below illustrate (80a, d–f).

(81)
a. 你这是好心当作驴肝肺。

Ni	*zhe*	*shi*	***hao-xin***	*dang-zuo*	*lü*	*gan*	*fei.*
you	this	is	good-heart	take-for	donkey	liver	lung

'You are taking an honest man's heart (lit. a good heart) for a donkey's liver and lungs (i.e. You are taking someone's goodwill for ill intent).'

b. 事虽如此，他不改初心。

Shi	*sui*	*ru*	*ci,*	*ta*	*bu*	*gai*	***chu-xin*.**
things	though	like	this	he	not	change	beginning-heart

'He will not change his original intention (lit. beginning heart) in spite of what has happened.'

c. 我本心想学医，结果学了文学。

Wo	***ben-xin***	*xiang*	*xue*	*yi,*	*jieguo*
I	original-heart	want	study	medicine	finally
xue-le	*wenxue.*				
learn-PER	literature				

'I originally (lit. original-heart) wanted to learn medicine, but learned literature instead.'

d. 这与素心相违。
Zhe yu ***su-xin*** *xiang-wei.*
this and undyed-heart mutually-violate
'This goes against my true intention/will (lit. undyed heart).'

The "donkey's liver and lungs" are no good (81a). The person addressed simply cannot tell good from bad, or distinguish between a good intention ("a good human heart") and a bad intention ("a donkey's liver and lungs"). In (81b), the person would not change his "beginning heart", regardless of the unexpected. In (81c), the speaker's "original heart" was to study medicine, but he or she learned literature instead. In (81d), one's true or real intention is the "undyed heart", i.e. the heart with its original color (cf. 32e in 4.3.1).

(82) a. 居心 *ju-xin* (store up-heart) 'harbor (evil) intentions'
b. 存心 *cun-xin* (preserve-heart) 'cherish certain intentions; intentionally; deliberately; on purpose'
c. 出心 *chu-xin* (exit-heart) 'harbor intentions; intention; purpose'
d. 生心 *sheng-xin* (give birth to-heart) 'harbor certain thoughts; be oversensitive; be suspicious'
e. 起心 *qi-xin* (get up-heart) 'cherish certain intentions'
f. 立心 *li-xin* (erect-heart) 'make up one's mind; be resolute; be determined; cherish certain intentions'
g. 发心 *fa-xin* (set out-heart) 'make up one's mind (to do sth.); have one's mind made up; be determined'
h. 成心 *cheng-xin* (establish-heart) 'intentionally; on purpose; with deliberate intent'

The compounds in (82) all have the verb-object construction, having the meaning of "harbor or cherish certain intentions", "make up one's mind", "with deliberate intent", or "on purpose". Note that (82b) represents an important concept in Mencius' philosophy (see 2.3.3). According to Mencius, human nature, embodied by the human heart, is originally good. Therefore, it is important for people to "preserve the heart", namely to preserve its good nature. The word, as is used in present-day Chinese, is different in meaning. Given below are some sentential examples:

(83) a. 我不是存心这么做的。
Wo bu shi ***cun-xin*** *zheme zuo de.*
I not be preserve-heart so do PRT
'I didn't do it on purpose (lit. do it with a preserved heart).'

b. 只要你发心去学，定会学成的。
Zhiyao *ni* ***fa-xin*** *qu* *xue,* *ding* *hui*
as-long-as you set out-heart to learn definitely will
xue-cheng *de.*
learn-it-successfully PRT
'As long as you make up your mind (lit. set out your heart) to learn, you will certainly succeed in learning it.'

c. 别生气，他不是成心的。
Bie *shengqi,* *ta* *bu* *shi* ***cheng-xin*** *de.*
don't be-angry he not be establish-heart PRT
'Don't be angry. He didn't mean it (lit. He didn't establish his heart on it).'

As in (83a), "to preserve the heart" simply means "to cherish or harbor certain intentions". In (83b), to make up one's mind is "to set out one's heart". People need to learn things with their "heart set out going". In (83c), the addressee is asked to not to get angry since "he" did not do it with an "established heart", i.e. "he" did it unintentionally.

Having laid out the data showing the relations between heart and intention, I now turn to the relationship between heart and volition.

4.4.4. The heart and volition

Volition refers to the act of using one's will and one's power to control, decide, or choose a course of action (LDCE 1979). In the Chinese conceptualization, volition originates in the heart, and there are extensive linguistic data to demonstrate that this is the case. As already seen in 4.4.3, "will" in Chinese is "heart-will" (76b). People's success depends not only on whether their heart-will is "firm" (心志坚), but also on "where their heart-will is oriented" (心志向何方), or in which direction people pursue their course of action. That is, making volitional efforts is to "utilize one's heart in a certain way".

(84) a. 用心 *yong-xin* (use-heart) 'diligently; attentively; with concentrated attention'
b. 一心 *yi-xin* (one-heart) 'wholeheartedly; heart and soul; of one mind; at one'
c. 专心 *zhuan-xin* (focus-heart) 'concentrate one's attention; be absorbed'

d. 悉心 *xi-xin* (all/entire-heart) 'devote all one's attention; take the utmost care'
e. 潜心 *qian-xin* (submerge-heart) 'with great concentration; devote oneself to sth.'
f. 分心 *fen-xin* (divide-heart) 'divert/distract one's attention'

The compounds in (84) characterize mental concentration, as they are exemplified respectively by the following sentences:

(85) a. 你应该用心做习题。
Ni yinggai ***yong-xin*** *zuo xiti.*
you should use-heart do exercises
'You should work hard at exercises (lit. use your heart to do problems).'

b. 他一心想上大学。
Ta ***yi-xin*** *xiang shang daxue.*
he one-heart want go-to college
'He is set on (lit. is one-hearted on) going to college.'

c. 如你不更加专心地工作，你将被解雇。
Ru ni bu gengjia ***zhuan-xin*** *de gongzuo, ni jiang*
if you not more focus-heart MOD work you will
bei jiegu.
be dismissed
'If you don't concentrate more on your work (lit. don't work with more focused heart) you'll be dismissed.'

d. 她悉心照料病人。
Ta ***xi-xin*** *zhaoliao bingren.*
she entire-heart take-care-of patient
'She takes the utmost care of the patient (lit. takes care of the patient with her entire heart).'

e. 她潜心研究科学。
Ta ***qian-xin*** *yanjiu kexue.*
she submerge-heart study science
'She applies herself to scientific study with great concentration (lit. with a submerged heart).'

f. 她学习起来，什么事也不能使她分心。
Ta xuexi qilai, shenme-shi-ye bu neng shi ta
she study start no-matter-what not can make her

fen-xin.
divide-heart
'Nothing can divert her attention (lit. divide her heart) once she starts studying.'

"To utilize one's heart" in (85a) simply means "to exert one's concentration in mental activities". It is believed that volition is a function of the heart and studying without "deploying or applying the heart" will likely end up learning little or nothing. To be "one-hearted" means to be "single-minded" on something (85b). A common idiom is 一心一意 *yixin yiyi* (one-heart one-intention) 'put one's whole heart into (something)'. It is important to "be bent on" the thing one is doing, especially if it is an intellectual activity because, as the old saying goes, 一心不能二用, meaning "One cannot run after two horses (lit. One heart cannot be used for two purposes or on two tasks) at the same time". In (85c) *zhuan-xin* literally means "to focus or specialize one's heart", and "focusing one's heart on, or specializing one's heart in, one's work" is what it takes to do it well. Here are two idiomatic expressions commonly used to that effect: 专心一意 *zhuanxin yiyi* (focus-heart one-intention) 'stick to one thing at a time'; 专心致志 *zhuanxin zhizhi* (focus-heart devote-will) 'with single-hearted devotion'. The example in (85d) is similar to (85b) and (85c) in that the person concentrates her "entire heart" on her job. In (85e), the person "submerges her heart" (i.e. buries herself) in her scientific research so that she will not be distracted by anything beyond it, and that is what it takes to be successful in scientific endeavor. In (85f), *fen-xin*, which literally means "to divide the heart", refers to distraction. Their heart being "divided" on their study or work, people cannot learn or do it well. This, again, is remindful of Xunzi's argument for the "unity" and "oneness" of the heart when people get to know the world through their heart knowing the Way (see 2.2.2). Xunzi advocated for "emptiness", "oneness", and "stillness" of the heart, arguing that people should be receptive, attentive, and reflective when trying to understand the universe and its Way through their heart as the central faculty of cognition.

(86) a. 尽心 *jin-xin* (exhaust-heart) 'with all one's heart; put one's heart and soul into'
b. 呕心 *ou-xin* (vomit-heart) 'exert one's utmost effort (in creative work)'
c. 苦心 *ku-xin* (bitter-heart) 'trouble taken; pains'

d. 精心 *jing-xin* (meticulous-heart) 'meticulously; painstakingly; elaborately'

Supplied in (86) are more compounds for volitional efforts. When people put their heart and soul into something, they "exhaust their heart" (86a). In present-day Chinese *jin-xin* (exhaust-heart) means differently from when Mencius used it over two thousand years ago. According to Mencius, the heart, the thinking organ endowed by Heaven, is "preserved" only by "great men", who "exhaust" it so as to understand nature and Heaven (see 2.2.2). In (86b), people exerting their utmost effort in creative work "throw up their heart" for or into it. Here are two idioms that contain (86a) and (86b): 尽心竭力 *jinxin jieli* (exhaust-heart use up-strength) '(do something) with all one's heart and all one's might'; 呕心沥血 *ouxin lixue* (throw up-heart shed-blood) 'take infinite pains; work one's heart out'. Here, one refers to the utmost exertion of both mental and physical efforts whereas the other suggests the infinite pains taken in the work. Examples (86c) and (86d) describe people who are making painstaking or meticulous efforts in doing something: They do it with either a "bitter heart" or a "meticulous heart". In Chinese, the taste of "bitterness" is associated with hardships or pains, and "sweetness" with happiness. Thus, to bear, suffer, or endure hardships is to "eat bitterness" (吃苦 *chiku*). The idiom 苦尽甘来 *kujin ganlai* (bitterness-end sweetness-come) means "misery ends and happiness begins". In (87) are sentential examples illustrating the compounds in (86).

(87) a. 这些年青人干活可尽心呢。
Zhexie nianqing ren ganhuo ke ***jin-xin*** *ne.*
these young people work really exhaust-heart PRT
'These young people are really conscientious in their work (lit. really exhaust their heart when working).'

b. 这是他的呕心之作。
Zhe shi tade ***ou-xin*** *zhi zuo.*
this is his vomit-heart MOD work
'This is a work embodying his utmost effort (lit. a work for which he has thrown up his heart).'

c. 她煞费苦心教育她的子女。
Ta sha-fei ***ku-xin*** *jiaoyu tade zinü.*
she spend-a great deal bitter-heart educate her children
'She took great pains (lit. spent a great deal of bitter heart) in educating her children.'

d. 这是一个精心策划的阴谋。

Zhe shi	*yi-ge*	***jing-xin***	*cehua*	*de*	*yinmou.*
this is	a-CL	meticulous-heart	planned	MOD	conspiracy

'This is a carefully calculated plot / an elaborately planned conspiracy (lit. a conspiracy planned with a meticulous heart).'

If people "exhaust their heart" when working, they are indeed conscientious (87a). The sentence in (87b) refers to a creative work such as a novel. The writer has put so much painstaking effort into it and has toiled for so long on it that he has "worked his heart out". Related to the word *ou-xin* (throw up-heart), the compound 心血 *xin-xue* (heart-blood) is, other than taken literally as the heart qi and blood in Chinese medicine, generally used metaphorically to mean "painstaking effort", especially in an intellectual sense. Thus, 费尽心血 (exhaust the heart blood) means "expend all one's energies", and 毕生心血的结晶 (the crystallization of the heart blood of one's lifetime) means "the fruit of painstaking labor of one's lifetime". In (87c), a mother's love and affection for her children could taste "bitter" in her painstaking care and education of them. In (87d), *jing-xin* (meticulous-heart) usually refers to the elaborate care with which something is done. The care, based on one's volitional exertion, comes from the heart.

(88)
a. 决心 *jue-xin* (determined-heart) 'determination; resolution; be determined'
b. 横心 *heng-xin* (horizontal-heart) 'steel one's heart; become desperate'
c. 狠心 *hen-xin* (hardened-heart) 'harden one's heart'[82]
d. 铁心 *tie-xin* (ironed-heart) 'be unshakable in one's determination'
e. 死心 *si-xin* (dead-heart) 'drop the idea forever; have no more illusions about the matter; give up the idea forever; think no more of sth.'

The compounds in (88) represent a different type of volition, commonly known in English as determination or resolution, which suggests firm intention. Regardless of the words used for glosses in the parentheses, the first elements of these compounds actually have a verbal meaning. That is, they respectively mean, literally, to "make the heart determined", "make

82 The compound in (88c) is the same word as in (48e) in 4.3.3, but this word has different meanings. Here it is a verb meaning "harden one's heart" whereas in (48e) it is an adjective meaning "cruel; heartless; callous".

the heart horizontal", "harden the heart", "turn the heart into that of iron", and "deaden the heart" or "make the heart dead". In (88b), the image of the heart is such that its height is bigger than its breath. To "make the heart horizontal" is to place it horizontally or crosswise, which idiomatically means strong determination. For instance, 横下心来 *heng xia xin lai* (place the heart down horizontally) means "be dead determined to; harden the heart; steel oneself to (do something)". Example (88e) is a different case. While "deaden the heart" itself suggests desperation and hopelessness, an idiom containing it 死心塌地 *sixin tadi* (dead-heart collapsed-to-ground) means "be dead set; be hell-bent", i.e. with determination in desperation. The examples in (89) show how the compounds in (88a–d) are used in sentences.

(89) a. 他决心改正错误。

Ta	***jue-xin***	*gaizheng*	*cuowu.*
he	determine-heart	correct	mistake

'He is determined (lit. has his heart determined) to correct his mistake.'

b. 他横下一条心要学好英文。

Ta	***heng**-xia*	*yi-tiao*	***xin***	*yao*	*xue-hao*
he	place-down-horizontally	one-CL	heart	want	learn-well
Yingwen.					
English					

'He is dead determined (lit. places his heart crosswise) to learn English well.'

c. 我狠不下心去做这样的决定。

Wo	***hen**-bu-xia-**xin**-qu*	*zuo*	*zheyangde*	*jueding.*
I	harden-unable-heart	make	such-a	decision

'I can't make such a painful decision (lit. can't harden my heart to make such a decision).'

d. 他扎根农村可是铁了心啦。

Ta	*zhagen*	*nongcun*	*keshi*	***tie**-le-**xin***	*la.*
he	be-rooted-in	countryside	really	iron-PER-heart	PRT

'He was unshakable in his determination to settle in the countryside (lit. He had really become iron-hearted to be rooted in the countryside).'

In (89b), the classifier for the heart is *tiao*, which suggests something long and narrow (or thin). Originally, this long and narrow heart stands vertically. When the person becomes dead determined, he "places it horizontally or crosswise". The sentence in (89d) alludes to a period in Chinese history known as the "Cultural Revolution", when "educated youth" in cities were supposed to "be rooted in the countryside" for re-education, responding to the call of Mao Zedong.

(90) a. 逆心 *ni-xin* (go against-heart) 'not to one's liking; go against one's intention'
b. 违心 *wei-xin* (disobey/violate-heart) 'against one's will; contrary to one's convictions'
b. 降心 *jiang-xin* (lower-heart) 'against one's will'

The verb-object compounds in (90) are used to describe things that go against one's will or, literally, one's heart. One's thoughts that compose one's intention and will, like qi, move in a certain direction in circulation. Certain things go in the opposite direction, and they are not to one's liking or go against one's intention (90a). Things going against one's will or convictions are those that "disobey or violate one's heart" (90b). To do this kind of things one, sometimes, has to "lower one's heart", i.e. "go against one's will" (90c). Here are three sentential examples:

(91) a. 她遇着逆心的事，总要抹几滴眼泪的。
Ta yuzhe ***ni-xin*** *de shi, zongyao*
she come-across go against-heart MOD things always
mo ji-di yanlei de.
wipe a few-CL tears PRT
'Whenever she comes across things not to her liking (lit. going against her heart), she will shed a few drops of tears.'

b. 她绝不说违心的话，做违心的事。
Ta jue-bu shuo ***wei-xin*** *de hua, zuo*
she will-never utter violate-heart MOD words do
wei-xin *de shi.*
violate-heart MOD things
'She will never speak or act against her conscience (lit. utter words that violate her heart, or do things that violate her heart).'

c. 他只好降心相从。
Ta zhihao ***jiang-xin*** *xiang-cong.*
he cannot-but lower-heart follow/obey-others
'He cannot but obey others against his will (lit. lower his heart to follow/obey others).'

Both (91b) and (91c) have a moral implication. Remember that, as discussed in 4.3.3, one's conscience is associated with one's heart. Things that "go against one's heart" are perceived as bad or immoral. People who do them will have a guilty conscience, feeling "their heart violated" (91b). If they "lower their heart", i.e., lower their moral standard, to do things that "violate their heart", then they should feel guilty in doing so (91c).

(92) a. 雄心 *xiong-xin* (grand/mighty-heart) 'great ambitions; lofty aspirations'
b. 壮心 *zhuang-xin* (strong/robust/magnificent-heart) 'high aspirations; great aspiration; lofty or noble ideal'

As in (92), ambitions and aspirations are thoughts motivated by strong will in one's heart. Therefore, compounds meaning ambitions and aspirations contain *xin* 'heart'.

(93) a. 心胸 *xin-xiong* (heart-chest) 'breath of mind; aspiration; ambition'
b. 心怀 *xin-huai* (heart-bosom) 'intention; purpose; state of mind; mood'
c. 心襟 *xin-jin* (heart-bosom/front of a garment) 'aspiration; ambition'
d. 心气 *xin-qi* (heart-qi) 'motive; intention; aspiration; mood; frame of mind; tolerance'
e. 心度 *xin-du* (heart-extent/degree) 'mind; heart; tolerance; magnanimity'
f. 心量 *xin-liang* (heart-capacity) '(Buddhism) a cover term for all mental phenomena; mind; heart; breath of mind; aspiration; ambition'

The group of compounds in (93) concerns ambition, aspiration, intention, purpose, mood, motive, and tolerance, etc., and all these concepts are associated with the heart in Chinese. Since the heart is located in the chest or bosom, it combines with terms denoting the chest or bosom in (93a–c). In Chinese, one's "heart-chest" can be "broad" (心胸广阔 *xinxiong guangkuo*) or "narrow" (心胸狭窄 *xinxiong xiazhai*), which respectively mean "broad-minded" and "narrow-minded".[83] In (93c), *jin* originally refers to

[83] Sometimes, the "chest" or "bosom" (胸 *xiong*) can by itself also be the locus of the "mind", such as in 胸有成竹 *xiong you chengzhu* (chest has fully grown

the "front of a garment" in the area of the chest or bosom. By metonymic principle of contiguity, it also refers to the "bosom" or "chest" itself. In (93d), qi is the gaseous vital life force in the body. As discussed in the previous two chapters, how qi gathers and moves in the heart affects one's mental states. Both (93e) and (93f) suggest dimensions of the heart. It is understood that longer "extent" and larger "capacity" are better and imply more tolerance, greater ambition, and loftier aspiration.

(94) a. 耐心 *nai-xin* (endure-heart) 'patient; patience'
b. 恒心 *heng-xin* (constant-heart) 'perseverance; persistence'
c. 忍心 *ren-xin* (bear-heart) 'have the heart to; be hardhearted; endurance'

The three compounds in (94) respectively mean "patience", "perseverance", and "endurance", which manifest one's will too. As expressed in Chinese, they are also qualities of the heart. In (94b), to have a "constant heart" is a moral or personal virtue associated with perseverance and persistency (cf. relevant discussions on Mencius in 2.3.3). Persevering people all have a "constant heart", which will remain unchanged under various circumstances. Therefore, a "constant heart" is a key to success. The following examples illustrate these three compounds.

(95) a. 他正在失去耐心。
Ta zhengzai shiqu ***nai-xin***.
he IMP lose endure-heart
'He's losing his patience (lit. endure-heart).'
b. 你要是没有恒心可学不好。
Ni yaoshi mei-you ***heng-xin*** *ke xue-bu-hao*.
you if not-have constant-heart really can't-learn-well
'Unless you persevere with a subject you can't hope to master it (lit. If you don't have a constant heart, you can't learn anything well).'

c. 他不忍心拒绝他们的要求。
Ta bu ***ren-xin*** *jujue tamende yaoqiu*.
he not bear-heart turn-down their request

---

bamboo) 'have a well-thought-out plan', and 了然于胸 *liaoran yu xiong* (understand/be clear in chest) 'have a clear understanding of something; have a clear picture of something in the mind'. Apparently, the chest or bosom has gained this "cognitive function" through metonymic extension: The heart, being the locus of the "mind", is located inside the chest. In other words, the chest is the container of the heart, which in turn is the container of the "mind".

'He didn't have the heart (or couldn't bear) to turn down their request.'

In this subsection I have dealt with linguistic data concerning volitional efforts that demonstrate an individual person's will. Ample examples show that an individual person's will originates in, and stems from, the heart. When masses of people share a common will, then this combined will becomes the will of the people or popular will. That is what I will deal with in the next section.

4.4.5. The heart and popular will

People hold their thoughts and feelings in their heart. The thoughts and feelings shared by the people constitute a trend that moves in one direction with great forces, like a surging river. The trend of thinking and feeling in people's hearts is called "popular will". In Chinese, however, the will of the people is literally called "people's heart", as shown by the compounds in (96).

(96) a. 人心 *ren-xin* (people-heart) 'popular feeling; public feeling; the will of the people; human feelings'
b. 民心 *min-xin* (people-heart) 'popular feelings; popular sentiments; popular support; common aspiration of the people'

In present-day Chinese the word for "people" is 人民 *renmin*, a compound itself of which the two constituents *ren* and *min* respectively occur as the first morpheme of the two compounds in (96a) and (96b). That is, "the people's heart" metonymically represents popular feelings, popular support, or the will or common aspiration of the people. In Chinese there are also these idiomatic expressions: 人心所向 *renxin suoxiang* (people-heart PRT-direction) 'popular sentiment; the feelings of the people (lit. the direction or orientation of public feeling; the trend of public feeling)'; 民心所向 *minxin suoxiang* (people-heart PRT-direction) 'where the popular will inclines; the common aspiration of the people'; 人心向背 *renxin xiangbei* (people-heart turn to-turn back) 'whether the people are for or against (something)'. In the first two, "the people's heart" is oriented toward a particular direction in which it moves like a surging trend. In the third, "the people's heart" has a front and a back, whose orientation represents support or opposition. When it turns its front toward something, it supports that thing. When it turns its back against something, it opposes that thing. An ancient saying about the law of ruling goes, "Those who obtain people's hearts (i.e. gain popular support) will obtain all under Heaven, and those who lose people's hearts (i.e. lose popular support) will lose all under Heaven" (得民心者得天下，失民心者失天下). This is reminiscent of section 2.4, where it is argued that ancient Chinese thought holds "people's hearts" as the foundation of societal governance. For instance, Guanzi argued that success in government lies in following the hearts of the people whereas failure in government lies in opposing them. Mencius also advocated the "benevolent government" (仁政 *renzheng*) that rules by winning the heart of the people. In general, public opinion is fair and accurate: "There is a steelyard (a traditional weighing instrument in Chinese culture) in the hearts of a crowd of people" (众人心里有杆秤). That is, public opinion or judgment is usually right and unbiased.

Public feeling, which exists in the heart of the people, is an important social factor. Look at the following idioms:

(97) a. 人心安定 *ren-xin an-ding* (people-heart calm-settled) 'public feeling is calm and stable'
b. 人心浮动 *ren-xin fu-dong* (people-heart float-move) 'a public feeling of insecurity'
c. 人心涣散 *ren-xin huan-san* (people-heart lax-loose) 'widely divided in public opinion; people being not of one mind'
d. 人心惶惶 *ren-xin huang-huang* (people-heart fear-anxiety) 'popular anxiety'

When public feeling, or "people's heart", is calm and stable, the society is calm and stable. In general, public feeling is interrelated with political situation. Therefore, those who want to destabilize the political situation will try to destabilize or mislead public feeling or "people's heart", as the following idiomatic phrases or collocations show.

(98) a. 动摇人心 *dong-yao ren-xin* (move-shake people-heart) 'shake popular morale'
b. 惑乱人心 *huo-luan ren-xin* (confuse-mess people-heart) 'confuse and poison people's minds'
c. 收买人心 *shou-mai ren-xin* (gather-buy people-heart) 'buy popular support; curry favor with the public'

d. 笼络人心 *long-luo ren-xin* (rope-in people-heart) 'cultivate people's good will (by dispensing charity, favors, etc.); try to win people's support by hook or by crook'

The government should try to do everything it can to stabilize, satisfy, inspire, access, or gain "people's hearts", as expressed by the following idiomatic phrases or collocations.

(99) a. 安定人心 *an-ding ren-xin* (stabilize-settle people-heart) 'reassure the public; set people's minds at rest'
b. 大快人心 *da-kuai ren-xin* (great-happy people-heart) 'most gratifying to the people; to the great satisfaction of the people'
c. 振奋人心 *zhen-fen ren-xin* (shake-inspire people-heart) 'inspire people; fill people with enthusiasm; boost popular morale'
d. 深入人心 *shen-ru ren-xin* (deep-into people-heart) 'strike root in the hearts of the people'
e. 深得民心 *shen-de min-xin* (deeply-obtain people-heart) 'enjoy the ardent support of the people; win great popularity'

The same is true of the military. The "public feeling" of military troops, called the "army's heart", is their morale, as demonstrated by the following expressions.

(100) a. 军心 *jun-xin* (army-heart) 'soldiers' morale'
b. 惑乱军心 *huo-luan jun-xin* (confuse-mess army-heart) 'undermine the morale of an army'
c. 动摇军心 *dong-yao jun-xin* (move-shake army-heart) 'shake the army's morale'
d. 稳定军心 *wen-ding jun-xin* (stabilize-settle army-heart) 'stabilize the army's morale'

Different people usually have different thoughts and feelings. The differences in thoughts and feelings are often expressed metaphorically as the differences in physical traits of the hearts. The metaphor is, again, an extension of the metonymy CONTAINER FOR CONTAINED. "People's hearts are as different as their faces" (人心如面 *renxin rumian*). While people's faces look different, their hearts think and feel differently. Sometimes, however, it is important that people have the same thoughts and feelings. The uniformity in thoughts and feelings are often expressed as people having similar hearts, or even the same heart.

(101)	a.	齐心	*qi-xin* (even/uniform-heart) 'be of one mind/heart'
	b.	同心	*tong-xin* (same-heart) 'with one heart'
	c.	一心	*yi-xin* (one-heart) 'wholeheartedly; heart and soul; of one mind; at one'

Conventionally, the heart, or its "line of thoughts", is sometimes conceptualized as a long and narrow (or thin) object so that the classifier *tiao* (条) is used when the emphasis is on the function of heart for thinking and feeling (cf. 4.2.2). Thus, the differences in thinking and feeling of people are conceptualized as the differences in length of their hearts.[84] That is, people's hearts vary in length as much as they themselves vary in height. When people's thoughts or feelings are unified with a consensus about a certain matter, they are then conceptualized as having the hearts of the same lengths. That is the image evoked by (101a): People's hearts are even or uniform in length. "The people all working with their hearts even (in length) can move Mount Tai (a famous mountain in China)" (人心齐，泰山移). That is, people united with one heart/mind can move mountains. The compounds in (101b, c) express the meaning that people have "the same and one heart". An idiom in Chinese has the literal meaning of "ten-thousand-people crowd having one heart" (万众一心 *wanzhong yixin*), which is defined as "millions and millions of people having one (classifier: *tiao*) heart" (千千万万的人一条心 XDHYCD 1996: 1300). Here are some more idioms:

(102)	a.	齐心协力	*qi-xin xie-li* (even-heart joint-effort) 'make concerted efforts; be all of one mind; be of one heart; work together with one will'
	b.	同心同意	*tong-xin tong-yi* (same-heart same-intention) 'be of the same mind; with one heart and mind'
	c.	同心同德	*tong-xin tong-de* (same-heart same-mind) 'be of one heart and one mind; work with one mind'

---

84 The differences among people in terms of, say, thoughts and feelings, characters and personalities, are also idiomatically expressed as differences in length of the fingers of a person: "Even the ten fingers are different in length when stretched out" (十个手指头伸出来还不一般长呢).

d. 一心一德 *yi-xin yi-de* (one-heart one-mind) 'be of one heart and one mind; be dedicated to the same cause'

When the masses have "their hearts even" and make concerted efforts, things will be accomplished far more easily. In contrast, if "people's hearts" are "uneven" or "unlevel", there is a potential risk of social instability. For instance, it is said that China is faced with a social problem today, namely, the uneven distribution of social wealth and privilege among its people, as a result of negligence of societal harmony and fairness. This social problem has caused the "unlevelness of its people's hearts" (人心的不平) and has prompted the Chinese government to promote the construction of a "harmonious society" (和谐社会), as the following remark (Chinesenewsnet) points out:

> 我们相信：能够提出"和谐社会"原则，说明国家领导人心里面透亮着。
> We believe that the national leaders' promotion of the principle of a "harmonious society" shows that the interior of their heart is crystally bright.

In this comment, "the interior of their heart is crystally bright" refers to the wisdom and mental discernment of the leaders, and it is obviously a linguistic instantiation of the conceptual metaphor KNOWING or UNDERSTANDING IS SEEING. Remember that, in traditional Chinese culture, "the heart governs the spiritual light" (心主神明), where the "spiritual light" refers to the totality of one's mental power (see Chs. 2 and 3, and relevant discussions in 4.2). It is believed that the national leaders' promotion of the principle of a "harmonious society" should enhance the social stability in China today. A "harmonious society", after all, consists of people with "even and level hearts".

4.4.6. The heart and attention

Attention is another type of volition in which people are mindful of something. Since the "mind" is traditionally located in the heart in the Chinese cultural conceptualization, the heart is therefore the source of attention. Look at the following three compounds that all contain *xin* 'heart' as its second morphological component:

(103) a. 小心 *xiao-xin* (small-heart) 'take care; be careful; be cautious'
b. 轻心 *qing-xin* (light-heart) 'careless; totally inattentive'

c. 当心 *dang-xin* (bear/direct-heart) ‘take care; be careful; look out’

If people have a “small heart” or are “small-hearted”, they will act in a cautious manner or be very careful in doing things (103a). If they have a “light heart” or are “light-hearted”, that means they will be very careless or inattentive in handling things (103b). Note that in English to be “light-hearted” means to be happy. However, when in such an emotional state, especially with a feeling of complacency, people tend to be careless and inattentive, namely “taking things lightly”. That aspect of the frame of mind is what a “light-heart” in Chinese emphasizes. When people are careful and looking out, they “bear their heart” and “direct their heart” toward the things to which they need to pay attention (103c). That is, when people are mindful and vigilant, their heart is alert. As ancients already observed, when the heart is not attentive, one looks but does not see, listens but does not hear, eats but does not know the taste (cf. Ch. 2).

(104) a. 雨后路滑，她一不小心摔倒了。
Yu hou lu hua, ta yi bu ***xiao-xin***
rain after road slippery she one-moment not small-heart
shuaidao-le.
fall-PER
‘The road was slippery after the rain, and she fell for not being careful (lit. not being small-hearted) for a moment.’

b. 大敌当前，我们决不可以掉以轻心。
Da di dang qian, women jue-bu-keyi
large enemy be in-front we must-never
diao-yi ***qing-xin****.*
drop-with light-heart
‘Faced with a formidable enemy, we must not lower our guard (lit. deal with it with a light heart).’

c. 跟这种人打交道，你可千万当心。
Gen zhe-zhong ren dajiaodao, ni ke-qianwan ***dang-xin****.*
with this-kind people deal you must bear-heart
‘You must be careful (lit. bear the heart) when dealing with this kind of people.’

In (104a), the word *xiao-xin* (small-heart) ‘be careful’ indicates a one-occasion mental state. In (104b), the advice is not to “take the enemy lightly" or "underestimate the enemy" (轻敌 *qingdi*). Example (104c) is a piece of advice, too.

(105) a. 留心 *liu-xin* (keep-heart) 'be careful; take care'
b. 上心 *shang-xin* (go up to-heart) 'set one's heart on sth.'
c. 在心 *zai-xin* (exist-heart) 'feel concerned; mind; be attentive'
d. 搁心 *ge-xin* (place-heart) 'be careful; be mindful'
e. 铭心 *ming-xin* (engrave-heart) 'be engraved on one's heart – be remembered with gratitude'
f. 容心 *rong-xin* (contain/hold-heart) 'bear in mind; be concerned about'
g. 关心 *guan-xin* (enclose/involve-heart) 'be concerned about; show solicitude for; care for; be interested in'

The compounds in (105) represent different types of attention: carefulness, mindfulness, remembrance, and concern. The possible image for (105a) is that of a container, and whatever people pay attention to is "kept in the heart". That is, the thing having one's attention will "go up to the heart" (105b), and "stay in the heart" (105c), or "be placed in the heart" (105d). If people want to remember it forever, they will "engrave it in their heart" (105e), or "have it contained or held by the heart" (105f). When people are concerned about something, it is "enclosed or involved by their heart" (105g). Here are two idioms containing (105e) and (105f): 铭心刻骨 *mingxin kegu* (engrave-heart carve-bone) 'be imprinted on one's bones and in one's heart – bear in mind forever'; 无所容心 *wusuo rongxin* (nothing contained by heart) 'be concerned about nothing'. In the latter, if people are concerned about nothing, they "have nothing contained or held in their heart". Given below are sentential examples of the remaining compounds in (105).

(106) a. 他很留心股票的行情。

Ta	*hen*	***liu-xin***	*gupiao*	*de*	*hangqing.*
he	very	keep-heart	stock	MOD	market

'He watches the stock market very closely (lit. keeps in the heart much of the stock market / keeps much of his heart on stock market).'

b. 这孩子读书不上心。

Zhe haizi	*dushu*	*bu*	***shang-xin*.**
this child	study	not	go up to-heart

'This child doesn't set his heart on study (lit. This child studies without making what he learns go up to his heart).'

c. 别看他大大咧咧的，什么事他都很在心。
Bie-kan ta dadalielie de, shenme shi ta
although he look-unconcerned PRT whatever matter he
dou hen ***zai-xin.***
all very exist in-heart
'He appears unconcerned, but nothing escapes his attention (lit. but he has everything exist in his heart).'

d. 不论学什么技术都得搁心。
Bu-lun xue shenme jishu dou dei ***ge-xin.***
no-matter learn what technique/skill all should place-heart
'No matter what technique you learn, you should be mindful (lit. place it in your heart).'

e. 我们要关心国家大事。
Women yao ***guan-xin*** *guojia da-shi.*
we should involve-heart country/state/nation big-affairs
'We should concern ourselves with (lit. have our heart involve) state affairs.'

When people pay close attention to something, they "keep it in their heart" (106a). People have not learned anything unless what they study "goes up to their heart" (106b). Things studied will not turn into knowledge unless they are processed by the heart, the seat of intellect. Mindful people have everything in their heart even though they may look careless and inattentive (106c). Whatever people learn, they need to "place the thing they learn into their heart" (106d). People concerned about something "have their heart enclose or involve that thing" (106e). All these examples illustrate the heart as the seat of cognitive activities.

(107) a. 经心 *jing-xin* (pass through-heart) 'careful; mindful; conscientious'
b. 走心 *zou-xin* (walk/go through-heart) '*dial.* bear in mind; careful; mindful; conscientious'

The two compounds in (107) evoke a different image. This time, the thing that people pay attention to "goes through their heart". People are careless, casual, and negligent if things "spread out and do not go through their heart" (漫不经心 *man bu jingxin*).

(108) a. 她经心搜集各种资料。
Ta ***jing-xin*** *souji ge-zhong ziliao.*
she pass through-heart collect all-kinds data
'She takes great care (lit. pass through heart) to collect all kinds of data.'

b. 学习技术，不走心可学不好。
Xuexi jishu, *bu* ***zou-xin*** *ke xue-bu-hao.*
learn skills/techniques not go through-heart really learn-not-well
'To learn skills, you won't learn them well if you are not mindful/conscientious (lit. if you don't learn them going through your heart).'

If people do things "through their heart", they do them carefully or mindfully (108a). Again, whatever people learn, they cannot learn it well unless it "goes through their heart" (108b). This is because, according to the cultural conceptualization of the Chinese, the heart is the central faculty of cognition. That is why people have to "utilize their heart" when they are carrying out any cognitive activities. When the heart is not deployed or applied, whatever one is learning will not "go through the heart" (be processed by the heart) or "stay in the heart" (be saved in the heart).

4.5. The heart as the locus of emotional life

In the previous section I examined the linguistic evidence in Chinese demonstrating that the heart is the locus of mental life. I showed that various facultes of the "mind" such as intellect and volition, and mental activities in thought and intentions, are tied to the heart as conceptualized traditionally as the thinking organ of the person. In traditional Chinese culture, the heart is conceptualized as the feeling organ as well, as is the case in many other cultures. In this section I study the aspect of cognition involved in conceptualizing emotional experience through linguistic analysis. Specifically, I discuss various compounds of feelings and emotions that contain *xin* 'heart'.

In the Chinese cultural conceptualization, the heart is the seat of feelings and emotions. For instance, the following compound words have to do with feelings, emotions, and moods and their morphological components suggest that feelings, emotions, and moods constitute states of the "heart".

(109)
a. 心情 *xin-qing* (heart-feeling/situation) 'state/frame of mind; mood; feeling; emotion'
b. 心绪 *xin-xu* (heart-thread ends) 'state of mind; mind; feeling; emotion'[85]
c. 心气 *xin-qi* (heart-qi) 'mood; frame of mind'
d. 心境 *xin-jing* (heart-territory/area) 'state of mind; mental state; mood'

Remember that, according to traditional Chinese medicine, the heart is the "grand master of the five zang and six fu organs", presiding over all mental and emotional activities. Although the various mental and emotional activities are each categorized with particular zang organs in the five-element schema, they all originate in and arise from the heart, the "ruler of the body" and the "governor of the spiritual light" (see Ch. 3).

In what follows, I first discuss the relationship between the body and emotions in general. I will then discuss the relationship between the heart and emotions in particular.

4.5.1. The body and emotions

In the past decade, talk about feeling and emotion has received extensive linguistic attention, which has resulted in the publication of numerous monographs and edited volumes on the study of emotional expressions in various languages (e.g., Athanasiadou and Tabakowska 1998; Enfield and Wierzbicka 2002a; Harkins and Wierzbicka 2001; Kövecses 1986, 1988, 1990, 2000; Niemeier and Dirven 1997; Palmer and Occhi 1999; Wierzbicka 1999). Cross-linguistic studies show that although human beings may undergo similar bodily events or processes in their emotional experiences, their concepts of emotion, including their interpretations and descriptions of bodily responses to emotions, vary across languages and cultures. A question that emerges from these studies is "how the role of the body in emotion and the impact of emotion on the body is conceptualized in different cultures and manifested in different languages" (Yu 2002: 341). Enfield

85 In (109b) 绪 *xu* means "thread ends" in its physical sense. One's mental or emotional state consists of thoughts and feelings as "thread ends" that can get into a "mess". For instance, 心绪烦乱 *xin-xu fanluan*, 心绪缭乱 *xin-xu liaoluan*, 心绪不宁 *xin-xu bu-ning*, and 心绪沸腾 *xin-xu feiteng* all describe a disturbed or confused state of mind or an emotional turmoil.

and Wierzbicka (2002a) study the body in the description of emotions, focusing on the question of how speakers of the world's languages refer to the body in talking about emotions. As Enfield and Wierzbicka (2002b) point out in their introduction to their volume (2002a), while the experience and the description of emotions are "culture-situated" and "culture-specific", "it is universally true that when people talk about their emotions, they often talk about what is happening inside their bodies" (p. 5). "The role of the body in emotion has commonly been a subject of clinical research, but it has less often come into discussion of the semantics and pragmatics of how languages encode ideas about emotion" (p.2). Therefore, "data on how speakers refer to the body in their talk about emotions will be a valuable addition to the limited corpus of broad cross-linguistic data on the linguistics of emotion" (p. 3).

In my contribution (Yu 2002) to Enfield and Wierzbicka's (2002a) special issue, I presented a semantic analysis of how emotions and emotional experiences are described and conceptualized in Chinese, focusing on conventionalized expressions that contain body-part terms. The body-part terms are divided into two classes: those denoting external body parts and those denoting internal organs. It is found that, with a few exceptions, the expressions involving external body parts are originally metonymic, describing emotions in terms of their externally observable bodily events and processes. However, once conventionalized, these expressions are also used metaphorically regardless of emotional symptoms or gestures. The expressions involving internal organs evoke imaginary bodily images that are primarily metaphorical. I have found that the metaphors, although imaginary in nature, are not really all arbitrary. They seem to have a bodily or psychological basis, although they are inevitably shaped by cultural models. What follows in this subsection is a summary and discussion of my findings (adapted from Yu 2002: 355–362).

Chinese emotion expressions involving terms for external body parts are generally composed of body-part terms in collocation with other words that modify, predicate, or govern them. The words in collocation belong to a variety of semantic domains, as listed below:

(i) emotion (e.g., worried brows; angry hair)
(ii) color (e.g., red face [shyness, anger]; white eyes [contempt])
(iii) temperature (e.g., face hot [shame]; eyes hot [jealousy])
(iv) orientation/dimension (e.g., vertical eyes [anger]; neck thick [anger])
(v) bodily sensation (e.g., stiff tongue [fear, surprise]; flesh creepy [disgust])
(vi) bodily movement (e.g., gritting teeth [anger, hatred]; snorting nose [contempt])

As listed above, category (i) makes explicit use of emotion words, attributing them to the body parts that reveal the specified emotions metonymically. In category (ii), certain color terms are applied to certain body parts, both together metonymically signaling certain emotions. The choice of color words seems to reflect, to some extent, the physiological symptoms of certain emotions on certain body parts. The motivation behind the choice seems to be reinforced by the related category of temperature (iii). When viewed together, there seems to be some consistency between both categories, namely, "hot colors" tend to go with certain emotions while "cold colors" tend to go with a different set of emotions. For instance, "white eyes" (from the whites of eyes) goes with contempt, as do "cold brows", "cold eyes", and "teeth cold" (probably from a "cold grin"). The similar parallel is also found between "red face" and "red eyes" on the one hand, and "hot face" and "hot eyes" on the other. As noted earlier, however, there is a difference between Chinese and English in the color associated with jealousy: it is "red eyes" in Chinese and "green eyes" in English. It will be very interesting to make cross-linguistic and cross-cultural studies on what color and temperature words are used to conceptualize and describe what emotions.

Apparently, the choice of orientation words in category (iv) is less predictable. There, both "horizontal" and "vertical" brows denote anger, and so is the case with eyes. The effect here seems to be more cartoon-like, that is, to "catch" something real, physically or psychologically, in an artistically exaggerated manner. In category (v), the expressions describe emotions in terms of bodily sensations caused by the emotions. Thus, in Chinese, grief will cause a "tingling nose" and disgust will make the "flesh creep". Category (vi) is by far the largest category. It contains expressions that describe emotions by referring to the bodily movements in reaction to those emotions. As a broad category, bodily movements can be convulsive to varying degrees, from "eyes twitching" and "fine hair standing on end" with fear, to "stamping feet" and "pounding chest" with grief, for instance.

Viewed as a whole, the conventionalized expressions involving external body parts are metonymic in nature. They follow the metonymic principle THE PHYSIOLOGICAL EFFECTS OF AN EMOTION STAND FOR THE EMOTION (Lakoff and Kövecses 1987). They refer to emotions by describing their externally observable bodily events and processes. It seems that there are only a few exceptions, like "bosom opened (to release emotions)", which metaphorically implies a container.

In sharp contrast to the expressions with external body-part terms, those expressions containing terms of internal body parts are primarily metaphorical. They evoke internal bodily images that are imaginary in character (Wierzbicka 1999). As an overview, the following is a list of all seven internal organs and the emotions with which they are linked. Given in the parentheses are the images evoked in the expressions.

(i) spleen:	anger (gaseous energy of qi expanding)
(ii) liver:	anger (fire burning)
	sadness (split, ripped into pieces)
(iii) intestines:	anxiety (knotted, twisted, hanged)
	sadness (knotted, twisted, split, ripped into pieces)
(iv) stomach:	anxiety (hanged)
(v) lungs:	sadness (split)
(vi) gallbladder:	fear (void, frigid, hanged, dropped, lost, trembling, split)
(vii) heart:	anger (fire burning)
	anxiety (troubled, hanged, lifted, suspended, pinched, scorched, fried, burned by fire)
	sadness (pain, frigid, wounded, twisted, fragmented, pierced, torn apart, pounded)
	fear (shocked, throbbing, frigid, lifted, split)
	happiness (open, vast, bright, blooming)
	relief (laid down, settled down, calm down, broad)
	admiration (toppled, drunk)
	vexation (closed up, blocked, messed up, troubled, pain)
	disappointment (frigid, gray)
	disgust (vomiting)
	hatred (pain, rotten)
	guilt (void, lost)

Note that the list is based on my data consisting of conventionalized expressions found in dictionaries. In everyday Chinese, for instance, we can say something to the effect "Don't explode your lungs with gas (i.e. anger)" (see Yu 1995, 1998). While this saying is very idiomatic, it is not a compound or idiom listed in the dictionaries. Therefore, the link between lungs and anger is not listed here. As shown in the list and most relevant to the present study, the heart is linked to various emotions while the other internal organs are linked to one or two only. In my data, the heart is the most recurrent of all body parts in idiomatic emotion expressions. The linguistic evidence certainly reflects and reinforces the cultural conceptualization of the heart as the source and seat of all emotions. As discussed in Chapters 2 and 3, the heart is, after all, the "ruler of the body", the "governor of the spiritual light" and the "grand master of the five zang and six fu organs". As such, it is responsible for the operation and regulation of all bodily, mental, and emotional functions.

Obviously, the expressions involving internal body parts also contain words from such semantic domains as emotion (e.g. worried intestines, heart anxious), color (e.g. gray heart), temperature (e.g. gallbladder frigid), dimension (e.g. heart vast, broad heart), bodily sensation (e.g. heart aching, heart tingling), and bodily movement (e.g., heart throbbing, gallbladder trembling). However, there is a difference in quantity. For instance, bodily movement is the largest category with the external body parts, but it is a very small category with the internal body parts. The two examples given above are the only two, and only "heart throbbing" is the bodily movement we can really feel. In contrast, we cannot really tell how "gallbladder trembling" feels. The gallbladder example is certainly not on a par with "eyes twitching" or "flesh quivering" that has real physiological basis. Other examples that demonstrate the difference between the two categories of external and internal body parts include "worried brows" versus "worried intestines", "gray head" versus "gray heart", and "neck thick" versus "broad heart". In short, the difference under discussion is not just quantitative, but also qualitative. To summarize, the expressions involving external body parts are primarily metonymic, whereas those involving internal body parts are fundamentally metaphorical.

Now I turn to the major kinds of metaphorical images found in the expressions involving internal organs. The previous list has already provided an overview. Here I want to focus on the emotions that involve at least two internal organs. Notably, they are the four negative emotions listed below. In the list I use more general words where possible. For instance, "break" includes "split", "rip into pieces", "wound", "fragment", "pierce", and "tear apart".

(i) anger:	gas expanding spleen	Pain
	fire burning liver, heart	Damage
(ii) anxiety:	blocking (knot, twist) intestines	Pain
	lifting (pull, hang, suspend, lift) intestines, stomach, heart	Pain
	hurting (pinch) heart	Pain
	fire burning (scorch, fry, flame) heart	Damage
(iii) sadness:	blocking (knot, twist) intestines	Pain
	breaking (split, rip into pieces, wound, fragment, pierce, tear apart) liver, intestines, lungs, heart	Damage
	hurting (twist, pound) heart	Pain
	freezing (frigid) heart	Pain
(iv) fear:	lifting (hang, lift) gallbladder, heart	Pain

breaking (split) gallbladder, heart	Damage
freezing (frigid, trembling) gallbladder, heart	Pain
losing (void, dropped, lost) gallbladder	Damage

As this list shows, anger is linked to spleen, liver, and heart; anxiety to intestines, stomach, and heart; sadness to intestines, liver, lungs, and heart; fear to gallbladder and heart. The heart is the only organ linked to all emotions. Note that on the right column, I use "Pain" and "Damage" to characterize the physical impact of the negative emotions on the internal organs as dramatized by the metaphorical images. It should be pointed out that there is no cutting line between physical pain and physical damage. As the condition intensifies, pain can certainly change to damage. Thus, for instance, as the gas expands increasingly in the spleen, it will cause damage to the container (see Yu 1995). No matter what organs are involved, sustained hanging or a freezing temperature will convert pain to damage as well.

Although the negative emotions listed above inflict either pain or damage on the internal organs, we can see some interesting similarities and differences in how they do it. With anger, qi expands in the spleen and fire burns in the liver and heart. Both processes are related to heat, namely, heat causes qi to expand and fire produces heat. They both converge to the metaphor ANGER IS HEAT (see Lakoff and Kövecses 1987; Yu 1995). Another emotion that is heat-related is anxiety: it "scorches", "fries", and "flames" the heart. The similarity here seems to suggest that anxiety and anger overlap.

In contrast to anger and anxiety, which are heat-related to different degrees, fear and sadness are cold-related. Fear makes the gallbladder "frigid" and "trembling" and the heart "frigid" and "throbbing". Similarly, sadness, as well as (bitter) disappointment, causes the heart to be frigid. Fear and sadness also have another commonality, namely, as their intensity increases, they both "break" the internal organs involved. These organs are gallbladder and heart for fear, and liver, intestines, lungs, and heart for sadness. Moreover, fear also does some unique "damage" to the gallbladder. In "shaking" it, fear can "void" its content, or "snap its base" making it "drop off its stem" in a complete "loss".

Noticeably, both anxiety and sadness "block" the "pipes" of intestines by "knotting" and "twisting" them. They also "hurt" the heart, though in somewhat different ways. The former "pinches" it while the latter "twists" and "pounds" it. From the images here we can "feel" some similarities and differences between anxiety and grief. Moreover, there is another interesting point about anxiety and fear in Chinese. As pointed out earlier, these two emotions contrast with each other in the aspect of temperature. Anxiety is related to heat, and fear to cold. On the other hand, however, the two emotions also have a commonality: they both "lift into the air" the organs they affect. Thus, anxiety will "raise" the intestines, stomach, and heart and keep them "suspended in the air", while fear will "lift" the gallbladder and heart and "hang them up there". It is worth mentioning that the feeling of relief, linked to the heart in the overall list, poses an interesting contrast to anxiety and fear. While anxiety and fear "lift" the heart and "hang it up in the air", relief "lays it back down" and lets it "rest on solid ground".

The analysis presented above offers two implications. First, the similarities and differences between the four emotion concepts, namely anger, anxiety, sadness, and fear, suggest that they have more than one facade and they relate to one another in a complex network. Emotion concepts do not have clear-cut boundaries, and there may be overlaps between them. The multi-images cast in metaphorical mode mirror the multi-facades of the concepts and the multi-links in their relations. The finding here supports the script hypothesis that categories of emotions are fuzzy, with the borders between categories vague, the status of membership within a category varying, and different categories overlapping one another (Russell 1991).

Second, those metaphorical images, viewed as a whole, reflect the "Chinese way" of understanding emotions. In this particular way, for instance, anger is conceptualized as "hot gas" as well as "fire", the gallbladder as linked to courage, the heart as "governor" of all mental or psychological activities including emotions, and so forth. All these, and many more, seem to be modeled on the theory of internal organs of Chinese medicine. The underlying folk theories, or cultural models, have influenced how Chinese people talk about emotions in a specific way. On the other hand, viewed at a more abstract level, the metaphorical images seem to conform, in general, to a universal tendency expressed in the form of a conceptual metaphor EMOTION IS FORCE (Kövecses 2000). That is, they dramatize emotions as physical forces and emotional experiences as impact of those forces. The metaphor maps physical forces we experience around us onto cognitively based feelings we experience inside us. The mapping is imaginary, but not entirely arbitrary. Thus, at a more specific level, we see a division of labor among metaphorical images. For example, "heat" is linked to anger and anxiety, but "cold" to fear and sadness (as well as disappointment). "Lifting up" is linked to anxiety and fear, but "letting down" to relief. "Hurting" is linked to anxiety and sadness, and "breaking" to sadness and fear. The images of "blocking" and "closing up" are found with sadness and anxiety (and vexation), but that of "opening up" and "broadening" with happiness and relief. It seems that these metaphorical images in Chinese have a bodily or psychological basis, although they are inevitably affected by cultural models. It would be enlightening to know how other languages are different or similar regarding internal bodily images in their emotion expressions. That is why the study of emotion language should be a cross-linguistic enterprise.

4.5.2. Emotion metaphors

As the overview in the previous subsection shows, the heart features prominently in conceptualization and description of emotion in Chinese. The body-part term for "heart", *xin*, participates in talk about various emotions, since the heart organ is traditionally conceptualized as the source and seat of all feelings and emotions in Chinese culture. Before I discuss the relation between *xin* 'heart' and emotion, however, I would like first to touch upon the metaphorical conceptualization of emotion. As abstract as they are, emotions and feelings are generally understood metaphorically as various forms of substance – gaseous, fluid, and solid – which can produces forces (see Kövecses 2000: Ch. 5). Very often, the heart is conceptualized as receiving the impact of emotional forces. For instance, some emotions that are heat-related are understood as "fire":

(110) a. 他再也压不住心头的怒火。
Ta zai-ye ya-bu-zhu ***xin-tou*** *de* ***nu-huo****.*
he no-longer unable-to-contain heart-top MOD angry-fire
'He can no longer restrain his fury (lit. the angry fire on top of his heart).

b. 她的好奇心快烧着了。
Tade ***haoqi-xin*** *kuai* ***shaozhao*** *le.*
her curious-heart almost start-burning PRT
'Her curiosity (lit. curious heart) almost started burning.'

The sentence in (110a) is another instance of ANGER IS FIRE (see also Yu 1995, 1998). In (110b), the person's curiosity is so strong that she feels that "her curious heart almost starts burning". Curiosity is a kind of anxiety, which, as we saw in 4.5.1, is related to heat. Given below is another example that has to do with worry. When asked about his most difficult moment after he became the President of China, President Hu Jintao answered that it was the time when SARS burst out in China in 2003. Here is what he said according to a news report (Chinesenewsnet):

> 当数千国人处于萨斯威胁之中，数百人面临死亡之际，作为中国的领导人，我感觉自己的心都快着火了。
> When thousands of compatriots were amid the threat of SARS, and hundreds of them were faced with death, as the leader of China, I felt my heart was almost on fire.

He then added that he felt that he was responsible not only for 1.3 billion Chinese people, but also for the whole world. Worry, as well as anger and anxiety, is related to heat. Little wonder that Chinese has these words related to "worry" and "anxiety": 焦急 *jiaoji* (scorching-anxious/worried) 'anxious; worried', 焦虑 *jiaolü* (scorching-worry/concern) 'feel anxious; have worries and misgivings', 焦躁 *jiaozao* (scorching-impetuous/restless) 'restless with anxiety; impatient', and 焦心 *jiaoxin* (scorching-heart) 'feel terribly worried' (see also 116a and 117a, and 126a and 127a below). One thing in common is that they all contain the element that literally means "scorch; scorching; scorched".

(111) a. 他一股怒气涌上心头。
*Ta yi-gu **nu-qi** yong shang **xin-tou**.*
he one-CL angry-gas charge onto heart-top
'He was boiling with rage (lit. A puff/burst of angry gas charged or gushed onto the top of his heart).'

b. 她心里像打翻了五味瓶。
*Ta **xin-li** xiang dafan-le **wo-wei** **ping**.*
her heart-in like overturn-PER five-flavor bottle
'She had mixed feelings or emotions in her heart (lit. In her heart it seemed as if five-flavor bottles had been overturned).'

c. 他望着她娇美的身影，心里有酸酸的醋意。
*Ta wang-zhe ta jiaomei-de shenying, **xin-li** you **suansuan-de** **cu-yi**.*
he look-at-DUR her delicate-beautiful body-figure heart-in has sour vinegar-flavor
'He was looking at her delicate and charming figure, feeling a sour taste of jealousy in his heart (lit. having a sour taste of vinegar in his heart).'

In the three sentences in (111), emotions are understood differently. Other than “fire”, anger is also understood as hot “gas” or qi, as can be seen in (111a). As in (109c), “heart-qi” means “mood” and “frame of mind”, and “angry-qi” therefore refers to anger. In Yu (1995, 1998), I argue that the GAS metaphor for anger in Chinese contrasts with the FLUID metaphor for anger in English (see the English translation for 111a); furthermore, this contrast reflects some more fundamental difference in cultural models. Example (111b) contains an idiomatic way of saying that someone has mixed feelings or emotions. In Chinese culture, where cuisine is an important component, there are five basic flavors, which fall into the schematic pattern of the five elements: sweet, sour, bitter, pungent, and salty (see Table 4 in 3.1.1). The sensory image involved is that the seasoning bottles are all knocked down and overturned so that the five seasoning flavors inside all get spilt out and mixed together in one’s heart. Here one has mixed “tastes” (and smells) of emotions, not in the mouth (or nose), but in the heart. Example (111c) illustrates that the sour taste is associated with jealousy. Thus, feeling jealous, especially in love and sex, is “eating vinegar” (吃醋 *chicu*).

(112) a. 表面的平静一旦崩溃，汹涌的情绪又涌上心头。
Biaomian de pingjing yidan bengkui, ***xiongyong***
surface MOD tranquility once collapse rolling-surging
de qingxu *you yong shang* ***xin-tou****.*
MOD emotions again surge onto heart-top
‘Once the surface tranquility collapses, the rolling emotions will again surge onto the top of the heart.’

b. 你表面上装着没事，可心里早就乐得噼里啪啦直滴水了。
Ni biaomian-shang zhuang-zhe mei-shi, ke ***xin-li*** *zao-jiu*
you on-surface pretend-DUR no-thing but heart-in for-long
le de pilipala zhi di
be-happy COM crackling-and-spluttering keep dripping
shui *le.*
water PRT
‘You are pretending to be emotionless on the surface, but inside your heart has been brimming over with joy for long (lit. but inside you have for long been so happy that water has kept dripping, crackling and spluttering, from your heart).’

The two examples in (112) illustrate a different source domain for emotion metaphors. Here emotions are understood as fluid. In (112a) emotions with a strong impact are described in terms of rolling and surging tides (see, also, relevant examples in 4.2). In (112b), which is taken from a comedic TV drama series, there is an explicit reference to water, which is a metaphor for the feeling of joy or happiness. The heart is the container of emotion. When it is filled with an emotion, it is then "brimming over" with it. In this example, *pilipala*, rendered as "crackling and spluttering", is an onomatopoeic expression that, in this particular case, imitates the sound of water dripping onto a hard surface.

(113) a. 他长长吐了一口气，因为压在心头的一块大石头已经落地。

Ta	*changchang*	*tu-le*	*yi-kou*	*qi,*	*yinwei*	*ya*	*zai*
he	long-long	vent-PER	one-CL	breath	because	weigh	on
xin-tou	*de*	*yi-kuai*	*da*	***shitou***	*yijing*	*luo*	*di.*
heart-top	MOD	one-CL	big	rock	already	fall-to	ground

'He vented a long breath, for he had been relieved of his deep worry (lit. the huge rock weighing on the top of his heart had fallen to the ground).'

b. 你不道歉，他的心结就解不开，你俩就不能建立真正的友谊。

Ni	*bu*	*daoqian,*	*ta*	*de* ***xin-jie***	*jiu*	*jie-bu-kai,*
you	don't	apologize	his	heart-knot	then	cannot-be-untied
ni-lia		*jiu*	*bu-keneng*	*jianli*		*zhenzheng-de*
the-two-of-you		then	impossible	establish		real
youyi.						
friendship						

'If you don't apologize, his hard feeling won't melt (lit. his heart knot won't be untied), and the two of you will not be able to establish real friendship.'

In the two examples in (113) emotions or feelings are understood as solid. In (113a) the deep worry, or its cause, is "a huge rock weighing on the top of the heart", which is therefore both heavy and hard. One should have a very "heavy heart" when having such "a huge rock" weighing on its top. In (113b), the hard feeling is light and soft like, say, a string, but it has been tied into a tight knot that is very difficult to untie. We can also say that the hard feeling has "tied the heart itself into a knot", hence the "heart knot". Readers can also refer back to (19b) in 4.2.2 for another example of emotions or feelings as being solid. In that sentence, hatred, sorrow, and shame are "things" that can be "buried" deep in one's heart.

As shown by the above examples, human feelings and emotions are indeed conceptualized metaphorically in forms of substance – gaseous, fluid, and solid. Therefore they may be "flaming" or "glowing", "surging" or "trickling", "heavy" or "light", "hard" or "soft", "bitter" or "sweet", "tangled" or "straight", and so on. Also, as shown in these examples, the heart as the seat of feelings and emotions is often affected by them one way or another. In the next two subsections I will again focus on Chinese emotion compounds and idioms that contain *xin* 'heart' as one of their constituents, dealing with them separately as more negative or positive feelings, which however form a continuum with those in the middle more neutral than either negative or positive.

4.5.3. The heart and negative feelings

The first three compounds in (114) have a noun-noun construction with two possible semantic relations: subject-predicate (114a) and modifier-modified (114b, c).

(114) a. 心旌 *xin-jing* (heart-banner/flag) 'a fluttering heart – nervous excitement; flurry'
b. 心病 *xin-bing* (heart-disease) 'worry; anxiety; secret trouble'
c. 心火 *xin-huo* (heart-fire) 'hidden anger; pent-up fury'

Here (114a) has its two constituents forming the metaphorical formula A IS B, as discussed in 4.2.1, and in this case it is HEART IS A BANNER. Thus, a "fluttering heart" in the mental state of nervous excitement or flurry is a "banner flapping in the wind" (心旌飘荡 *xinjing piaodang*). In (114b), "heart-disease" refers to worry or anxiety that troubles one's heart. More often than not, it refers to mental problems, attributed to the heart, rather than to physiological conditions. In Chinese, cardiologic diseases are called 心脏病 *xinzang bing*, which literally means "heart-organ diseases". Here is a sentential illustration of (114b).

(115) 这事老悬着，一直是他的心病。
Zhe shi *lao* *xuan-zhe,* *yizhi* *shi* *tade*
this matter always hang-DUR-in-the-air always is his
***xin-bing*.**
heart-disease
'Not having this matter settled has always worried him (lit. This matter has been hanging in the air; it has always been his heart disease).'

Here, a thing that is not settled is a "heart disease", which is psychological rather than physiological and, therefore, 心病从来无药医 'No medicine can ever cure mental worries and/or pains (lit. heart diseases)'. The compound in (114c), which literally means "heart fire", refers to anger and fury (see 110a).

Now, I turn to a group of compounds that all have the subject-predicate structure and evoke various images focused on the heart.

(116) a. 心焦 *xin-jiao* (heart-scorched) 'anxious; worried'
b. 心急 *xin-ji* (heart-anxious) 'impatient; short-tempered'
c. 心切 *xin-qie* (heart-eager) 'eager; impatient; anxious'
d. 心重 *xin-zhong* (heart-heavy) 'care-laden; weighed with anxieties'
e. 心系 *xin-xi* (heart-tied to) 'worry about; miss; be anxious about; keep thinking of'
f. 心痒 *xin-yang* (heart-itch) 'have an itch for; be anxious to do sth.'
g. 心烦 *xin-fan* (heart-troubled) 'be vexed; be perturbed'

The compound in (116a), which characterizes the emotions of anxiety and worry, is heat-related. When extremely anxious and worried, one's heart will be "scorched" by the heat. Both (116b) and (116c), about impatience and anxiety, are also heat-related. Here are two idioms involving (116b): 心急火燎 *xinji huoliao* (heart-anxious fire-flaming) 'burning with impatience; in a nervous state'; 心急如焚 *xinji rufen* (heart-anxious like-being burned) 'burning with impatience'. According to XDHYCD (1996: 1400), "heart-heavy" in (116d) describes people who think and reflect too much. Their heart is full of thoughts and cares and therefore "weighs heavy" and they are "unable to lay down whatever is weighing in their heart" (遇事心里总放不下). That is why they tend to have a "heavy heart". The metaphorical image of (116e) is a string connecting two things. At one end it is the heart of the people who are worried about, or keep thinking of, an entity; at the other end it is the entity itself. Thus, a "physical tie" is established between the heart and the entity. When the entity moves one way or another, the heart is "pulled" by the string accordingly. Obviously, the mental connection between the heart and the entity is conceptualized metaphorically. In (116f), the sensational feeling in the heart, the itch, is related to the feeling of a desire to do something right away. The heart "troubled" by something (116g) often has a "mess" of thoughts in it, as in the idiom 心烦意乱 *xinfan yiluan* (heart-troubled thought-messed) 'be annoyed and perplexed;

be terribly upset; be in an emotional turmoil'. The examples in (117) respectively illustrate (116a, d, and f).

(117) a. 我们等得好心焦！
Women deng de hao ***xin-jiao****!*
we waited COM how heart-scorched
'How anxiously we waited! (lit. We waited so anxiously that our hearts were scorched.)'

b. 孩子心重，你不要过于责备。
Haizi ***xin-zhong****, ni buyao guoyu zebei.*
child heart-heavy you shouldn't too-much reproach
'The child tends to be care-laden (lit. heart-heavy). You shouldn't reproach her too much.'

c. 一见那清凉的水，个个都心痒，巴不得马上跳下去。
Yi jian na qing-liang de shui, gege
upon seeing that clear-cool MOD water everyone
dou ***xin-yang****, babude mashang tiao xiaqu.*
all heart-itch anxious at-once jump down-in
'Upon seeing the clear cool water, they all had an itch (lit. had an itching heart) to dive in at once.'

When people have their "hearts itching", as in (117c), they cannot scratch it because the itch in the heart is psychological rather than physical, as the saying goes, "It is difficult to scratch an itching heart" (心痒难搔 *xinyang nansao*). The compounds in (118) have similar meanings but a verb-object construction.

(118) a. 忧心 *you-xin* (worry-heart) 'a troubled heart; an anxious heart'
b. 烦心 *fan-xin* (trouble-heart) 'annoying; vexatious; troublesome'
c. 难心 *nan-xin* (put into a difficult position-heart) '*dial.* feel embarrassed; feel awkward; worry; be anxious'
d. 犯心 *fan-xin* (invade-heart) '*dial.* be on bad terms with sb. because of a difference of opinion; be at odds'
e. 闹心 *nao-xin* (stir up-heart) '*dial.* be vexed; be annoyed; feel sick'
f. 糟心 *zao-xin* (mess up-heart) 'vexed; annoyed; dejected'
g. 窝心 *wo-xin* (nest-heart) '*dial.* feel irritated; feel vexed'
h. 堵心 *du-xin* (block-heart) 'feel oppressed; having a load on one's mind'

In (118a and b), something causes the heart to be in the emotional state of *X*. In (118a), something "worries the heart" and it is therefore a "worried heart". Note that (118a) is also related to heat, as shown in the idioms 忧心如焚 *youxin rufen* (worried-heart like-being burned) 'burning with anxiety or worry' and 忧心如煎 *youxin rujian* (worried-heart like-being fried) 'one's heart burned with anxiety or worry'. That is, when people are worried or anxious, their heart feels like being burned or fried. In (118b), something "troubles the heart" and it is thus a "troubled heart". When people feel worried, troubled, or anxious, their "heart is put in a difficult position" (118c). In (118d–f), something with an external force "invades" (118d), "stirs up" (118e), and "messes up" (118f) the heart. People with an "invaded", "stirred-up" or "messed-up" heart feel vexed, annoyed, or troubled. In (118g), people feeling vexed have a heart-container closed up. In (118h), people feeling oppressed or having a load on their mind feel as if their "heart is blocked" by something that hampers the circulation of qi and blood.

(119) a. 你不要为这件事难心。
Ni buyao wei zhe-jian shi ***nan-xin****.*
you shouldn't for this-CL matter feel difficult-heart
'You shouldn't worry (lit. put your heart in a difficult position) about this matter.'

b. 前几天他和老张犯心怄气。
Qian-ji-tian ta he Lao Zhang ***fan-xin*** *ou-qi.*
a-few-days-ago he and Old Zhang invade-heart irritate-qi
'The other day he was vexed and sulky (lit. heart-offended and qi-irritated) with Lao Zhang.'

c. 你怎么这么闹心呀？
Ni zenme zheme ***nao-xin*** *ya?*
you how-come so stir up-heart PRT
'How come you are so annoying (lit. heart-stirring/annoying)?'

d. 他因失败而糟心。
Ta yin shibai er ***zao-xin****.*
he because-of failure so mess-heart
'He was vexed at (lit. messed up his heart because of) his failure.'

e. 他一口窝心气没出就归了天。
Ta yi-kou ***wo-xin*** *qi mei chu jiu*
he a-CL nest-heart anger wasn't vented then

gui-le-tian.
return-PRT-heaven
'He died with pent-up grievances (lit. He hadn't been able to vent the anger nested in his heart before he returned to heaven).'

People should try not to "put their heart in a difficult position" about anything (119a). When they are unhappy with each other, they feel their "heart is invaded" and their "qi is irritated" (119b). As in (119d), failures can "mess up people's heart". In (119e), which illustrates (118g), the person had qi or anger "nested in his heart", and he died before he had the chance to vent the qi or anger from his "heart-container".

In (120) below is another group of verb-object compounds that refer to feelings of anxiety, worry, and trouble.

(120) a. 操心 *cao-xin* (grasp-heart) 'worry; take trouble; take pains; be concerned over/with; rack one's brains'
b. 张心 *zhang-xin* (stretch-heart) '(*dial.*) be a tax on (one's mind); bother; trouble; worry; take trouble'
c. 揪心 *jiu-xin* (pitch-heart) 'anxious; worried; heartrending; agonizing; gnawing'
d. 费心 *fei-xin* (cost-heart) 'give a lot of care; take a lot of trouble'

In the first three, the heart undergoes physical manipulation by worry-related feelings. People's heart is "grasped" (120a), "stretched" (120b), or "pitched" (120c) when they are worried or concerned, or when they take pains to do something. The heart feels pressed when "grasped", tense when "stretched", and pain when "pitched". As in (120d), troubles can "cost the heart" (cf. 147d below), which can be used up if there are too many troubles.

(121) a. 多少父母为子女操碎了心。
Duoshao fu-mu wei zinü ***cao****-sui-le-****xin****.*
so-many father-mother for children grasp-fragment-PER-heart
'Many parents go to a lot of trouble for their children (lit. So many parents grasp their hearts into crumbs for their children).'

b. 只要我有个地方暂时住几天，您什么也不必张心了。
Zhiyao wo you ge difang zanshi zhu ji
as-long-as I have a place temporarily live a-few
tian, nin shenme ye bubi ***zhang-xin*** *le.*
days you anything else needn't stretch-heart PRT

'As long as I have a place to stay for a few days, you don't have to worry anything else (lit. stretch your heart for anything else).'

c. 她揪心事太多，人都显得老了。
Ta ***jiu-xin*** *shi tai duo, ren dou xiande*
she pitch-heart things too many person already look
lao le.
old PRT
'Too much worry had made her look an old woman (lit. She had too many heart-pitching things, and she already looked old).'

d. 您见到他时，费心把这封信交给他。
Nin jiandao ta shi, ***fei-xin*** *ba zhe-feng xin*
you see him time cost-heart PRT this-CL letter
jiao-gei ta.
give-to him
'Will you be so kind as to give him this letter when you see him? (lit. When you see him, please cost heart to give him this letter.)'

When worrying about their children, parents sometimes "grasp their heart" so hard that their heart "is crumbled into small pieces" (121a). The heart should not be further "stretched" when no more trouble needs to be taken (121b). Things that worry people actually "pitch their heart", and the "pitching" of the heart will not only cause pain but also cause aging (121c). A favor asked for can be done "at the cost of the heart" since the heart guides the action (121d).

(122) a. 担心 *dan-xin* (carry-heart) 'worry; feel anxious'
b. 提心 *ti-xin* (lift-heart) 'worry; feel anxious'
c. 悬心 *xuan-xin* (suspend-heart) 'be on tenterhooks; be filled with anxiety'
d. 牵心 *qian-xin* (pull-heart) 'worry; be concerned; be on one's mind'
e. 挂心 *gua-xin* (hang-heart) 'be on one's mind; keep in mind; be concerned about; be anxious for'

In (122) is another group of verb-object compounds regarding worry, anxiety, and concern. The first three suggest the semantic feature of "the heart going up". In (122a), the verb *dan* primarily means "carry", especially with a shoulder pole, a common tool for carrying things in traditional Chinese culture. The loads to be carried in this fashion are a burden weighing on the person's shoulder. The heart being carried in this manner is a "heavy burden" on the person. In XDHYCD (1996: 243), (122a) is defined as 放心不下 *fangxin buxia*, which literally means "unable to lay down one's heart", i.e., one carries one's heart weighing heavily on oneself and is unable to lay it down. By the same token, (122b and c) respectively evoke the metaphorical image of the heart being "lifted" or "suspended". Oftentimes, people very nervous, worried, anxious, or uptight are said to have their "heart hanging in the throat" (心吊在喉咙眼儿上), "leaping (i.e. beating wildly) in the throat" (心在嗓子眼里跳), or even "jumping into the mouth" (心跳到口里). The images here are very similar to that evoked by the English idiom *to have one's heart in one's mouth*, meaning "to feel very afraid or worried".

The heart in such situations "is not resting on the ground" and "is hanging in the air". The compounds in (122d and e) evoke similar images. In (122d), a string is tied to the heart at one end and is being "pulled" at the other end by the entity of worry and concern. Thus, when people are worried and concerned about something or somebody, they feel their "heart being pulled" by that thing or person (cf. 116e above). In (122e), the entity of worry and concern, tied to a loop of string, is being "hung on the heart". Thus, one's heart feels the load being "hung" from it and "pulling down". As XDHYCD (1996: 459) defines it, *gua-xin* means 牵挂在心上, literally "pulling and hanging on the heart". In all these cases, the heart can feel painful depending on the amount of weight or force being applied. The compounds in the following, which contain the same verbs as in (122d and e), evoke similar metaphorical images, although the term for "heart" is not directly involved: 牵念 *qiannian* (pull-think of/miss) 'worry about somebody or something; think constantly of'; 挂念 *guanian* (hang-think of/miss) 'worry about somebody who is absent; miss'; 牵挂 *qiangua* (pull-hang) 'worry; care'; 挂牵 *guaqian* (hang-pull) 'worry; care'. In the context of this study, no one would doubt that it is the heart that is doing the thinking or missing, or that is being "pulled" or "hung from" even though *xin* 'heart' is not explicitly used. The following sentence elaborates on the image evoked by (122d and e).

(123) 你的每一根头发都连着爸妈的心。
Nide *mei-yi-gen* *toufa* *dou lian-zhe* *ba-ma-de* ***xin***.
your every-one-CL hair all link-with-DUR dad-mom's hearts
'Every hair of yours is linked with your dad and mom's heart.'

In this sentence, the parents are so worried and concerned about their child that every hair on their child's head is linked with their hearts. Thus, every slightest "movement" of their child will make a pull on their hearts. The following are some idiomatic collocations that expanded on the compounds in (122).

(124) a. 牵动人心 *qian-dong ren-xin* (pull-move people-heart) 'affect people's feelings'
b. 牵心挂肠 *qian-xin gua-chang* (pull-heart hang-intenstine) 'be very worried'
c. 提心吊胆 *ti-xin diao-dan* (lift-heart hang-gallbladder) 'have one's heart in one's mouth; be on tenterhooks; be filled with anxiety or fear'
d. 悬心吊胆 *xuan-xin diao-dan* (suspend-heart hang-gallbladder) 'have one's heart in one's mouth; be on tenterhooks; be filled with anxiety or fear'

When something affects people's feelings, it literally "pulls and moves people's hearts" (124a). When people are very worried, their "heart is pulled" and their "intestine is hung" (124b). The heart and the small intestine are a pair of zang and fu organs that are closely related physiologically according to traditional Chinese medicine. Both (124c) and (124d) involve *dan* 'gallbladder', which is traditionally conceptualized as the container of courage (Yu 2003a). They express fear as well as anxiety. Notably, the heart and the gallbladder are both "up" from being "lifted", "suspended", and "hung". In the following are the sentential examples illustrating (122a) and (122e).

(125) a. 我真担心她的健康。
Wo zhen ***dan-xin*** *tade jiankang.*
I really carry-heart her health
'I do worry (lit. carry-heart) about her health.'

b. 他挂心家里，恨不得马上赶回去。
Ta ***gua-xin*** *jia-li, hen-bu-de mashang gan huiqu.*
he hang-heart family anxious at-once hurry home
'He was concerned about his family (lit. had his family hanging on his heart), and wished he could hurry home immediately.'

The three compounds in (126) below further show that worry and anxiety are related to heat as they all evoke the image of fire doing damage to the heart in different ways.

(126) a. 焦心 *jiao-xin* (scorch-heart) 'feel terribly worried'
b. 煎心 *jian-xin* (fry-heart) 'feel extremely anxious'
c. 熬心 *ao-xin* (cook-heart) '*dial.* pent-up in one's heart; worry'

Here, something "scorches" (126a), "fries" (126b), or "cooks" (126c) the heart. It is obvious that (126a) is related to (116a) above, with the two constituents of the latter reversed from a subject-predicate to a verb-object construction. That is, they provide a mirror image of each other: "(something) scorches the heart" and "the heart is scorched (by something)". Both (126b) and (126c) also highlight the suffering caused by anxiety and worry: The heart is either "being fried in boiling oil" or "being cooked in boiling water". Below are two sentences respectively exemplifying (126a) and (126c).

(127) a. 至今没有接到儿子来信，真叫人焦心。
Zhi-jin meiyou jiedao erzi-laixin, zhen jiao ren
to-date haven't received son's-letter really make people
jiao-xin.
scorch-heart
'I haven't received my son's letter to date. It really makes me feel terribly worried (lit. It really scorches my heart, or it's really heart-scorching).'

b. 提起这种熬心事儿，他又要诉苦了。
Ti-qi zhe-zhong ***ao-xin*** *shir, ta you yao*
speaking-of this-kind cook-heart things he again would
su-ku le.
talk-bitterness PRT
'Speaking of this kind of things pent-up inside his heart (lit. heart-cooking things), he would again pour out his woes (or vent his grievances).'

Now, I turn to the compounds concerning the feelings of fear, guilt, disappointment, or downheartedness that are cold-related. Look at (128) below.

(128) a. 心怯 *xin-qie* (heart-timid) 'be timid'
b. 心惊 *xin-jing* (heart-startled) 'be startled'

c. 心悸 *xin-ji* (heart-throbbing) 'be scared'
d. 心慌 *xin-huang* (heart-flustered) 'be flustered; be nervous; get alarmed'
e. 心虚 *xin-xu* (heart-void) 'afraid of being found out; with a guilty conscience; lacking in self-confidence; diffident'
f. 心疚 *xin-jiu* (heart-remorseful/guilty) 'feel agonized and guilty'
g. 心灰 *xin-hui* (heart-ashy/gray) 'be discouraged; be disheartened; be downhearted'
h. 心寒 *xin-han* (heart-frigid) 'be bitterly disappointed'

In (128e), the heart that is "void" cannot be strong, either because it feels guilty or because it lacks confidence. Here are two idioms that contain (128e): 心虚胆怯 *xinxu danqie* (heart-void gallbladder-timid) 'have a guilty conscience; apprehensive and cowardly'; 做贼心虚 *zuozei xinxu* (be-thief heart-void) 'have a guilty conscience like a thief'. In the first one, when people's "heart is void", their "gallbladder is timid". The heart is the container of thoughts whereas the gallbladder is the container of courage. In the second, a thief's heart should always be "void" because of a guilty conscience. Therefore, those who have a guilty conscience have their "heart void" like a thief. In (128g), *hui* originally refers to ashes, dust, or the color of gray that is associated with these substances. By metaphorical extension, it also means "discouraged", "disheartened", or "downhearted". A discouraged or disappointed heart is certainly more "ashy" or "gray" than "bright". Such a heart will make the thoughts, wishes, or intentions inside it "lazy" or "cold": 心灰意懒 *xinhui yilan* (heart-ashy/gray thought-lazy) 'be disheartened; be downhearted; be dispirited'; 心灰意冷 *xinhui yileng* (heart-ashy/gray thought-cold) 'be downhearted; be dispirited'. People in such "states of heart" do not want to think of anything, nor do they wish or intent to do anything. They are as "cold" as they are "lazy", because their heart has turned "ashy" or "gray". Note that a "scorched heart" may be burned into "ashes", which would soon become cold when anxiety turns into disappointment. In (128h), a bitterly disappointed heart can be so "cold" that it becomes "frigid". It is expected that such a "frozen" heart is more "dormant" than "active".

In the group below, (129a–d) present the "mirror images" of some compounds in (128) above.

(129) a. 惊心 *jing-xin* (startle-heart) 'startling'
b. 疚心 *jiu-xin* (remorseful/guilty-heart) 'feel remorseful'

c. 灰心 *hui-xin* (ashy/gray-heart) 'lose heart; be discouraged'
d. 寒心 *han-xin* (frigid-heart) 'be bitterly disappointed; be afraid; fear'
e. 亏心 *kui-xin* (lose-heart) 'have a guilty conscience; go against conscience'

In (129e), people with a guilty conscience have "lost their heart". It is unlikely that they have lost the heart itself. Instead, they may have lost the contents, such as confidence and conscience inside the container (i.e. CONTAINER FOR CONTAINED). Note that (129e) is related to (128e) above, which literally means "heart void". With a guilty conscience, people have "lost (the contents in) their heart" (129e) so that their "heart is void" (128e). A proverbial saying goes: 白天不做亏心事，夜里不怕鬼敲门 'A quiet conscience sleeps in thunder (lit. If one doesn't do heart-losing things during the day, one isn't afraid that the ghost will knock at the door, or isn't scared when the ghost knocks at the door, at night)'.[86] It is worth noting that both (128b) and (129a) are involved in a number of four-character set phrases, as listed in (130) below.

(130) a. 心惊胆怕 *xin-jing dan-pa* (heart-startled gallbladder-frightened) 'be filled with apprehension; feel alarmed; be in a state of anxiety'
b. 心惊胆战 *xin-jing dan-zhan* (heart-startled gallbladder-trembling) 'tremble with terror; shake with fright; quake with fear'
c. 心惊胆裂 *xin-jing dan-lie* (heart-startled gallbladder-split) 'be so frightened that one's gallbladder bursts; utterly demoralized with fear'
d. 心惊胆碎 *xin-jing dan-sui* (heart-startled gallbladder-fragmented) 'the gallbladder bursts with fright; utterly demoralized with fear'

86 The "mirror image" of 亏心 *kui-xin* (lose-heart) is 心亏 *xin-kui* (heart-lost), with more or less the same meaning. A proverb says, 心亏理短话不周 'When one has a guilty conscience, one is short of argument and will be unable to talk in a well-conceived and convincing manner (lit. When one's heart is lost, one's argument/reason is short and one's speech is not round)'. In the original, the word 周 *zhou* has a basic spatial sense of circle: "circumference; periphery; circuit". The circle itself suggests "fullness" and "perfection". If one's speech is "not round", it is not convincing, with many loopholes.

e. 心惊肉跳 *xin-jing rou-tiao* (heart-startled flesh-jumping) 'shudder with fear; be terribly frightened; feel nervous and creepy'

f. 心惊肉颤 *xin-jing rou-chan* (heart-startled flesh-quivering) 'be creepy and shivery; be filled with anxiety and fear; shudder with fear'

g. 惊心动魄 *jing-xin dong-po* (startle-heart move-corporeal soul) 'soul-stirring; be struck with fright; breath-taking; shake sb. to the core'

h. 惊心掉胆 *jing-xin diao-dan* (startle-heart drop-gallbladder) 'be frightened out of one's wits'

i. 惊心破胆 *jing-xin po-dan* (startle-heart break-gallbladder) 'heart startled and gallbladder broken – extremely frightened'

In addition to the heart, another element of the body is involved in each of these expressions: gallbladder, flesh, and corporeal soul. As discussed earlier, it is characteristic of Chinese culture where the gallbladder, a fu organ, is associated with the feeling of fear and the concept of courage (see Ch. 3). Below are the sentential illustrations of (129c and d).

(131) a. 他一遇上困难就灰心丧气。

Ta yi yushang kunnan jiu
he as-soon-as come-across difficulties then
hui-xin *sang-qi.*
ashy/gray-heart lost-qi
'He's easily disheartened by difficulties (lit. As soon as he comes across difficulties, his heart turns ashy and his qi is lost.'

b. 孩子这样不争气，真叫人寒心。

Haizi zheyang bu-zhengqi, zhen jiao
child so-much fail-to-live-up-to-expectations really make
ren ***han-xin.***
people frigid-heart
'Our child has failed to live up to our expectations, and that is so bitterly disappointing (lit. which really makes us frigid-hearted).'

Example (131a) contains an idiom that involves heart and qi. When people are disheartened, their heart is "ashen" and their qi is lost. Qi is the gaseous life force inside the body. A body that has "lost qi" is like a deflated ball that sags. In (131b), the failure of the child to live up to the expectations of the parents would turn their heart "frigid". When people are bitterly disappointed, they have a "cold" heart.

Next, I discuss the compounds denoting the feelings of sadness, grief, and sorrow.

(132) a. 心痛 *xin-tong* (heart-pain) 'pained; distressed; grieved'
b. 心疼 *xin-teng* (heart-ache) 'be distressed; feel sorry; love dearly'
c. 心酸 *xin-suan* (heart-tingle) 'be grieved; feel sad'
d. 心伤 *xin-shang* (heart-wounded) 'sad; grieved; broken-hearted'
e. 心碎 *xin-sui* (heart-fragmented) 'be heart-broken'

In (132a–c) *xin* 'heart' combines with a term for a sensational feeling, which is "pain" in (132a), "ache" in (132b), and "tingle" in (132c). These sensational feelings of the heart are related to emotions, such as distress, grief, sadness. With severe grief or sorrow, people have so much pain in their heart that they may think that their heart is "wounded" (132d) and is going to "break" (132e), as in the idiom 心痛欲碎 *xintong yusui*. Note that (132b) is also related to "love". People can love others so dearly that this feeling of love makes their "heart ache". The two different senses are illustrated by the two sentences below.

(133) a. 这么浪费，叫人看了心疼。
Zheme langfei, jiao ren kan-le ***xin-teng***.
being so wasteful make people see-PER heart-ache
'It makes one's heart ache to see such waste.'

b. 这样惯孩子不是心疼他。
Zhe yang guan haizi bushi ***xin-teng*** *ta.*
this way pampering child isn't heart-ache him
'Pampering a child like this is not loving (lit. heart-aching) him.'

In the group below, (134a–c) are obviously related to (132a, c, and d) as their "mirror images" respectively.

(134) a. 痛心 *tong-xin* (pain-heart) 'pained; distressed; grieved'
b. 酸心 *suan-xin* (tingle-heart) 'be grieved; feel sad'
c. 伤心 *shang-xin* (wound-heart) 'sad; grieved; broken-hearted'
d. 绞心 *jiao-xin* (twist-heart) 'sorrow-stricken; grief-stricken; need or exert great mental effort'

In (134c and d), emotions of sadness, sorrow, and grief "wound" and "twist" the heart. The heart being "twisted" will certainly be "broken", and it is great pain to have a heart like this. The examples in (135) show how the compounds in (134) are used in sentences.

(135) a. 这样浪费粮食令人痛心。
Zhe yang langfei liangshi ling ren ***tong-xin***.
this way waste food make people pain-heart
'It is distressing (lit. heart-paining) to see food being wasted like this.'

b. 这出戏看了叫人酸心。
Zhe-chu xi kan-le jiao ren ***suan-xin***.
this-CL play see-PER make people tingle-heart
'It was heartrending (lit. heart-tingling) to see the play.'

c. 别为这事伤心。
Bie wei zhe shi ***shang-xin***.
don't for this matter wound-heart
'Don't let it grieve you (lit. wound your heart).

d. 娘儿俩为失去了亲人而流着绞心的眼泪。
Niang er lia wei shiqu-le qin-ren er
mother son both for lose-PER loved-ones thus
liu-zhe ***jiao-xin*** *de yanlei*.
shed-DUR twist-heart MOD tears
'The mother and son were both shedding sad (lit. heart-twisting) tears for having lost their loved ones.'

The emotion of grief "hurts" people's heart, both figuratively and literally (135c). Note that in (135d) tears themselves are not "heart-twisting". Those are sad tears, and the emotion of sadness "twists the heart".

At this juncture, I would like to cite the following sentential examples, as relevant to the feelings of sorrow and grief. Although they do not illustrate any of the compounds under discussion, they apparently expand and elaborate on the images evoked by the compounds in (132) and (134).

(136) a. 他的心被戳了个血窟窿。
Tade ***xin*** *bei-chuo-le ge xue kulong*.
his heart was-jabbed a bloody hole
'His heart was jabbed so as to have a bloody hole in it (i.e. He felt so saddened or grieved).'

b. 我的心在流血。
Wode ***xin*** *zai-liu-xue*.
my heart is-bleeding

'My heart is bleeding (i.e. I'm extremely saddened).'

c. 自从那以后，我的心就彻底死了。
Zicong-na-yihou, wode ***xin*** *jiu chedi si-le.*
ever-since-then my heart then completely die-PER
'Ever since then, my heart has been completely dead.'

These sentences are all taken from the context of love or, to be more exact, loss of love. In (136a and b), the "heart" is badly "wounded" and "bleeding" resulting from the loss of love that one cherishes so much. No wonder people often say that true love is all their "life". After the loss of true love, their hearts would "die" and remain "dead" even though they or their bodies are still living (136c).

Finally, the following idioms also characterize some negative feelings in metonymic and metaphoric terms that are based on real or imaginary bodily processes and activities.

(137) a. 痛心疾首 *tong-xin ji-shou* (pain-heart ache-head) 'with bitter hatred'
b. 痛心切齿 *tong-xin qie-chi* (pain-heart gnash-teeth) 'gnash one's teeth with anger; make one burn with anger'
c. 腐心切齿 *fu-xin qie-chi* (rotten-heart gnashing teeth) 'with deep hatred'
d. 撕心裂肺 *si-xin lie-fei* (tear-heart split-lungs) 'be extremely grieved'
e. 椎心泣血 *chui-xin qi-xue* (pound-heart shed-blood) 'beat one's breast and shed tears of blood – be heartbroken'
f. 椎心痛哭 *chui-xin tong-ku* (pound-heart painful-cry) 'cry one's heart out'

The one in (137a) involves both "heart" and "head". Bitter hatred results in "heart pain" and "headache". Example (137b) characterizes the intensive feeling of anger in terms of bodily feeling and movement associated with the emotion: "heart pain" and "teeth gnashing". As shown in (137c), people with deep hatred have a "rotten heart" and keep "gnashing their teeth". The idiom in (137d) shows that the emotion of grief has the force to "tear the heart and split the lungs". Both (137e) and (137f) are about grief and sorrow. People keep "pounding their chest" while "crying in pain". In (137e), people are so grieved that they "shed tears of blood" rather than usual kind of tears.

4.5.4. The heart and positive feelings

Having dealt with the compounds that denote more negative feelings, I now look at those that describe more positive feelings. The first group consists of those characterizing happiness, joy, delight, and so on.

(138) a. 心花 *xin-hua* (heart-flower) 'happy mood'
b. 惬心 *qie-xin* (satisfy-heart) '*formal* be pleased; be satisfied'
c. 快心 *kuai-xin* (please-heart) 'find sth. satisfactory; be gratified'
d. 娱心 *yu-xin* (amuse-heart) 'pleasant; make happy'
e. 爽心 *shuang-xin* (brighten-heart) 'happy; feel good'
f. 开心 *kai-xin* (open-heart) 'happy; joyous; elated; feel happy; rejoice; be delighted; amuse oneself at sb.'s expense; make fun of sb.'
g. 舒心 *shu-xin* (smooth out-heart) '*dial.* comfortable; happy'

The compound in (138a) is a noun-noun one that refers to a happy mood and literally means "heart flower". An idiom describing people wild with joy is 心花怒放 *xinhua nufang*, i.e. the "heart flowers are blossoming wildly". The other examples in (138) have a verb-object structure. Semantically, however, they are stative or adjectival: something causes the heart to be *X* (process or event) and, as a result, the heart has the quality of *X* (result). For example, something "satisfies the heart" and it is thus a "satisfied heart" (138b). It is interesting to note that in Chinese the word *shuang* in (138e) means both "bright" and "feeling well". The relatedness in meaning may be based on experiential correlation. For instance, a bright day makes people feel well, and when people feel well, things appear "bright" to them. Conversely, a gloomy day makes people feel bad, and a bad feeling makes things appear "gloomy" to them. The compound in (138e) is often used in the idiom 爽心悦目 *shuangxin yuemu*, which describes something that "brightens the heart and pleases the eye". This idiom suggests a tie between the eye and the heart, and between the visual view and the mental view. In (138f), something "opens the heart" and it is thus an "opened heart". When the heart is "opened", it receives more "light" and therefore is "brighter" and happier. In (138g), something "smoothes out the heart" and it is thus a "smoothed heart". What is "smoothed out" usually feels more comfortable and makes one happy. The sentences below exemplify (138c and f).

(139) a. 老战友在一起畅叙往事是一件快心的事。
Lao zhanyou *zai-yiqi* *chang-xu* *wang-shi*
old comrade-in-arms together cheerfully-chat bygone-things

shi *yi-jian* ***kuai-xin*** *de* *shi.*
is a-CL please-heart MOD thing
'It is a gratifying (lit. a heart-pleasing) thing for old comrade-in-arms to get together and chat cheerfully about bygones.'

b. 孩子们开心地围着他跳舞。
Haizi-men ***kai-xin*** *de* *wei-zhe* *ta* *tiaowu.*
children open-heart MOD surround-DUR him dance
'The children danced around him in delight (lit. with open hearts).'

In (139a), the compound word that literally means "please-heart" functions as an adjectival modifier. In (139b), the compound functions as an adverbial modifier that modifies the verb: the children were dancing happily (lit. open-heartedly).

The compounds in the next group denote the feelings of love, admiration, fascination, etc. It is the heart that is experiencing these feelings or is in these emotional states.

(140) a. 心爱 *xin-ai* (heart-love) 'loved; treasured; dear to one's heart'
b. 心羡 *xin-xian* (heart-admire/envy) 'admire; envy'
c. 心仪 *xin-yi* (heart-yearn for) 'admire; respect'
d. 心醉 *xin-zui* (heart-be drunk) 'be charmed; be enchanted; be fascinated; be overcome with admiration'
e. 心折 *xin-zhe* (heart-snap) 'be filled with admiration'

As shown in (140a), when people love someone or something, their love comes from the heart (cf. 4.3.4). In present-day Chinese, those loving and caring people are said to have a "loving heart" (爱心 *aixin*), and those who demonstrate their affection for others are said to "donate their loving heart" (献爱心 *xian aixin*). In (140d), when people are charmed, enchanted, fascinated, or overcome with admiration, their heart is "drunk", not because of alcohol, but because of admiration and related feelings. Admiration or any of the related feelings can be so intensive that it makes people who experience it lose senses. The compound in (140e) is somewhat related to (140d). In (140d), the feeling of admiration is like alcohol that fills the heart so that it gets "drunk". Here, the force of the feeling takes effect from within the heart. In (140e), however, the force of admiration comes from outside the heart. It "hits" the heart with such an impact that the "heart snaps" into two halves, like a twig of a tree. Given below are two sentences exemplifying (140d and e) respectively.

(141) a. 无边的春色令我心醉不已。
Wubian *de* *chun-se* *ling* *wo* ***xin-zui***
boundless MOD spring-colors make me heart-drunk
buyi.
incessantly
'The boundless spring scenery makes me irresistibly enchanted (lit. heart-drunk a great deal).'

b. 他的一席话使人心折。
Tade *yi-xi* *hua* *shi* *ren* ***xin-zhe***.
his one-CL words made people heart-snapped
'His words made people filled with admiration (lit. made people's hearts snapped).'

When enchanted or charmed, people have their hearts "drunk", which is an irresistible feeling that completely "overpowers" them (141a). In (141b), the words spoken are so powerful that they inflict "physical damage" upon other people's hearts. The "snapping" of the heart by admiration suggests psychological "conquering" or "overwhelming".

The three compounds in (142) are related to those in (140) as they denote similar kinds of feelings, but they have a verb-object construction.

(142) a. 动心 *dong-xin* (move-heart) 'one's mind is perturbed; one's desire, enthusiasm or interest is aroused'
b. 倾心 *qing-xin* (topple/overturn and pour out-heart) 'be overcome with admiration; fall in love with; lose one's heart to; admire; adore'
c. 醉心 *zui-xin* (intoxicate/drunk-heart) 'be bent on; be wrapped up in'

The moment people's desire, enthusiasm, or interest is aroused, their "heart is moved" (142a). That is why Mencius suggested that gentlemen should have "unmoved heart" (不动心 *budong xin*) so that they will not be swung by desires (see 2.3.3). In (142b), *qing-xin* has two literal senses: "topple the heart" and "overturn and pour out the heart". In the first sense, one's heart "falls" in admiration for or in love with another person. That is, some people are so attractive that their force of attraction, or "magnetic force", makes the heart of other people "topple" in their direction. When the heart "collapses" with such intense feeling of admiration or love, it no longer "stands" in good balance of senses. For the second sense of the word, the image can be either of the two versions. First, people "overturn and empty their heart" so that other people can "see the thoughts and feelings poured out of their heart-container". Second, people "overturn their body and pour out their heart" so that other people can "see their heart". The second one can be seen as a metonymic version of the first (i.e. CONTAINER FOR CONTAINED). Sometimes, (142b) also has the meaning of "going all out". Here are four idiomatic collocations that contain it.

(143) a. 一见倾心 *yi-jian qing-xin* (first-sight topple-heart) 'fall in love at first sight; lose one's heart to sb. at first sight'

b. 倾心交谈 *qing-xin jiaotan* (pour out-heart hold-conversation) 'have a heart-to-heart talk'

c. 倾心吐胆 *qing-xin tu-dan* (pour out-heart throw up-gallbladder) 'pour out one's heart; unbosom oneself; lay bare one's heart'

d. 倾心竭力 *qing-xin jie-li* (pour out-heart use up-strength) 'exhaust every effort to; exert oneself to the utmost'

Example (143a) literally means that one's heart "topples" at the first sight of another person, i.e. this person has fallen in love with another at the first sight. In (143b), people are having a heart-to-heart talk when they "pour their thoughts and feelings out of their heart". In (143c), people can "pour out their heart and throw up their gallbladder" in an effort to unbosom themselves. The idiom in (143d) describes people who spare no effort to accomplish something when they "pour out their heart and exhaust their strength".

The compound in (142c) may have a slightly different meaning from its mirror-image version in (140d), as the following two sentences illustrate.

(144) a. 他醉心于数学的研究。

Ta	***zui-xin***	*yu*	*shuxue*	*de*	*yanjiu.*
he	drunk-heart	in	math	MOD	research

'He's deeply engrossed (lit. drunk-hearted) in mathematical research.'

b. 这美妙的音乐使我心醉。

Zhe meimiao	*de*	*yinyue*	*shi*	*wo*	***xin-zui.***
this beautiful	MOD	music	made	me	heart-drunk

'I was enchanted with the sweet music (lit. The beautiful music made my heart drunk).'

In (144a), *zui-xin* may suggest initial self-control, that is, when people "bury themselves in something" or "throw themselves into something", they indeed choose to do it although they may lose that self-control once they are actually "in" it. On the other hand, *xin-zui*, as in (144b), suggests that people cannot help it when they "slip into something". It is the same as "falling in love"; people cannot keep themselves from doing it.

In the next group there are four subject-predicate compounds characterizing positive mental states.

(145) a. 心安 *xin-an* (heart-peaceful) 'with one's mind at ease'
b. 心静 *xin-jing* (heart-still/quiet) 'calm'
c. 心宽 *xin-kuan* (heart-broad) 'not lend oneself to worry and anxiety; broad-minded'
d. 心顺 *xin-shun* (heart-smooth) 'be in a good mood'

As we can see in (145a and b), the absence of emotions means that the heart is "peaceful", "quiet", and "still". In traditional Chinese thought, such "states of heart" are seen as virtuous (cf. Ch. 2). In (145c), when people's heart is "broad", it means that they do not lend themselves to worry and anxiety.[87] Here is a literal translation of the definition in XDHYCD (1996: 1398): "the heart and chest being open and wide (i.e. be broad-minded), able to think open things that do not turn out as one wishes (i.e. able to look at the bright side of things)" (心胸开阔，对不如意的事情想得开). People "able to think things open" (想得开 *xiang de kai*) will not be "trapped" by bad things that may otherwise "enclose" them psychologically. In (145d), when people are in a good mood, their heart is "smooth". A "smooth heart" actually refers to the circulation of qi in the heart. A good mood is embodied in the smooth circulation of qi in the heart whereas the disturbed circulation of qi in the heart is the physiological symptom of a bad psychological state (cf. 149g below). The compound in (145d) is used in the following sentence:

(146) 趁他心顺的时候去跟他说。

Chen	*ta*	***xin-shun***	*de*	*shihou*	*qu*	*gen*	*ta*	*shuo.*
while	he	heart-smooth	MOD	time	go	with	him	talk

'Go and talk to him while he is in a good mood (lit. while his heart is smooth with its circulation of qi).'

---

[87] Note that the same example is also used in 4.3.2, under the heading of "Heart and personal disposition" (cf. 45a above and 147a and 148a below). Obviously, there is a close relationship between emotional states and personalities. A repeated or sustained emotional state is part of the character of a person.

When people are in a good mood, that is, when the circulation of qi is smooth in their heart, they are more agreeable. That is why the timing of talking to "him" is important.

The next group of examples consists of verb-object compounds that express more relaxed states of mind, having to do with relief from worry and anxiety.

(147) a. 宽心 *kuan-xin* (broaden-heart) 'feel relieved; be relaxed; be at ease; feel at rest; set one's mind at ease; feel free from anxiety'
b. 松心 *song-xin* (loosen-heart) 'feel relieved; have ease of mind; feel carefree and happy'
c. 散心 *san-xin* (disperse-heart) 'drive away one's cares; relieve boredom; ease up; enjoy a diversion; be carefree'
d. 省心 *sheng-xin* (save-heart) 'save worry'

When people are angry, worried, anxious, etc., their heart is "packed" with such negative feelings. A heart like this is "nested", "blocked", or "stretched". That is why they have a "heavy" and "tense" heart. The relief from those negative feelings is then to "broaden" (147a), "loosen" (147b), and "disperse " (147c) the heart. Example (147c) is metonymic: What is dispersed is not the heart itself, but the negative emotions inside it. The heart relieved from negative feelings has more room in it, and therefore is more relaxed. The compound in (147d) is an antonym of (120d) in 4.5.3. When people are saved from worries, they "save their heart" from being "consumed" by those worries. What follows are sentential examples.

(148) a. 他对我说了几句宽心话。
Ta dui wo shuo-le ji-ju ***kuan-xin*** *hua.*
he to me say-PER a-few-sentences broad-heart speech
'He said a few reassuring words (lit. heart-broadening words) to me.'

b. 有了个帮忙的，老太太松心多了。
You-le ge bangmang-de, lao taitai ***song-xin***
have-PER a help old lady loosen-heart
duo le.
a-lot PER
'The old lady feels much relieved (lit. has a much looser or loosened heart) now that she's got a help.'

c. 她建议举行一个茶会来散散心。
Ta jianyi juxing yi-ge cha-hui lai ***san-san-xin****.*
she suggest hold a-CL tea-party to disperse-disperse-heart

'She suggested holding a tea party for relaxation (lit. to disperse [cares or worries in] the hearts).'

d. 孩子进了托儿所，我省心多了。
Haizi jin-le tuo'ersuo, wo ***sheng-xin*** *duo le.*
child enter-PER nursery I save-heart a-lot PER
'Having the child in kindergarten saves me a lot of worry (lit. heart).'

In (148c), a tea party can help "disperse" the cares or worries in people's hearts. With fewer or no worries or cares in their hearts, people have "broadened" or "loosened" hearts (148a, b). The hearts that have been rid of their negative contents should feel "lighter" too. In (148d), since the parent does not have to take care of, or worry about, the child, who is now in the kindergarten, it "saves this parent a lot of heart".

In the following list, the compounds, which all have a verb-object construction too, have to do with satisfaction, gratification, etc.

(149) a. 称心 *chen-xin* (fit-heart) 'find sth. satisfactory; be gratified'
b. 可心 *ke-xin* (fit/suit-heart) 'satisfying; to the satisfaction/liking of'
c. 遂心 *sui-xin* (satisfy/fulfill-heart) 'after one's own heart; to one's liking; fulfill one's desire'
d. 如心 *ru-xin* (in compliance with/according to-heart) 'after one's own heart; to one's liking'
e. 趁心 *chen-xin* (go with-heart) 'find sth. satisfactory; be gratified'
f. 随心 *sui-xin* (follow-heart) 'follow one's inclinations; find sth. satisfactory; be gratified'
g. 顺心 *shun-xin* ([go] in the same direction-heart) 'be satisfactory'

As can be seen, the concepts related to satisfaction are also expressed in terms of the heart. The overall image is that satisfaction is something fitting or following the heart. More specifically, things that are satisfactory "fit", "suit", "fulfill", "satisfy", "accord with", "follow", or "go with" the heart. Of course, the heart here may be interpreted simply as a metonymy for thoughts, wishes, and intentions inside it (CONTAINER FOR CONTAINED). Here are some sentential examples.

(150) a. 你想要什么尽管说，我包你称心如意。
Ni xiang-yao shenme jinguan shuo, wo bao ni
you want what just say I guarantee you
chen-xin *ru-yi.*
fit-heart accord with-wishes/thoughts

'Just tell me what you want, and I'll see that your wishes are met (lit. it fits your heart and accords with your wishes).'

b. 他是我们的可心人。
Ta shi womende ***ke-xin*** *ren.*
he is our suit-heart person
'He is the person we really like (lit. who suits our hearts).'

c. 这几件事办得太不遂他的心了。
Zhe-ji-jian shi ban de tai bu ***sui****-tade-****xin*** *le.*
these-few-CL things handle COM too not satisfy-his-heart PER
'He was far from being satisfied with the way the things were done (lit. These few things were done in a way that really did not satisfy or fulfill his heart).'

d. 他父亲晚年过得挺顺心。
Ta fuqin wan-nian guo de ting ***shun-xin****.*
his father late-years pass MOD rather go with-heart
'His father spent the evening of his life in happiness (lit. life that went in the same direction as his heart).'

In (150a), *chen-xin ru-yi* is an idiom, which is one of many that suggest the connection between *xin* 'heart' and *yi* 'thoughts; wishes; intentions'. The heart is the container whereas thoughts, wishes, and intentions are contents inside the container. The heart as a container has its own size and shape. It can only hold things that fit its size and shape. The thoughts, wishes, and intentions inside the heart "move" in specific directions. Things "following" the same direction will "go with the flow" whereas those "going" in the opposite direction will "go against the flow". Thus, things that are satisfactory "fit the heart and accord with the wishes inside the heart". In (150d), a happy life is the life that "goes in the same direction as the heart". Again, the heart itself does not move around, but thoughts, wishes, and intentions inside the heart "move" in specific directions (i.e. THINKING IS MOVING), as much as the qi and blood in the heart circulate following specific routes. Things "going with" thoughts, wishes, and intentions are satisfactory, and vice versa.

In (122) in 4.5.3, the compounds that indicate worry and anxiety express the concepts in terms of the heart going up from the normal position. In the following group, the compounds that indicate relief from worry and anxiety all express the concept in terms of the heart going down, back to its normal position.

(151) a. 放心 *fang-xin* (lay down-heart) 'set one's mind at rest; be at ease; rest assured; feel relieved; have confidence in sb.; trust sb.'
b. 落心 *luo-xin* (fall-heart) '*dial.* feel relieved; be relaxed; to one's liking/taste'
c. 歇心 *xie-xin* (rest-heart) 'in a relaxed mood; free from worries; peaceful and carefree'
d. 息心 *xi-xin* (rest-heart) '*dial.* be at ease; rest assured; feel relieved'
e. 定心 *ding-xin* (settle-heart) 'feel relieved; feel at ease'

When people are relieved or assured, they "lay down their heart" (151a). The heart that "rests on the ground" is more at ease than the heart that "hangs in the air". The heart "hanging in the air" has to "fall" down before it can become relieved or relaxed (151b). A related image is not to have the heart itself "fall", but to "have a rock in the heart fall to the ground" (心里落下一块石头), as also illustrated by (113a) in 4.5.2. After the "rock" (i.e. worry, anxiety, etc.) has been removed from the top of one's heart, one now has a "light heart". As in (151c and d), people who are in a relaxed mood or rest assured are those who are able to "rest their heart" or "make their heart rest". In (151e), people who feel relieved or at ease are those who are able to "settle their heart" or "have their heart settled". In Chinese, idiomatically, things that are capable of setting people's mind at ease are called "heart-settling pills" (定心丸 *ding-xin wan*), and those who are reassured or feel relieved are said to "have taken heart-settling pills" (吃了定心丸).

(152) a. 看到这样的前景，他们放心了。
Kandao zhe yang de qian-jing, tamen ***fang-xin*** *le.*
seeing this kind MOD front-view they lay down-heart PER
'They felt relieved (lit. laid down their heart) at this prospect (lit. front-view).'

b. 你就把心放在肚皮里，在家耐心等待吧。
Ni jiu ba ***xin*** *fang zai-dupi-li, zai jia*
you just PRT heart lay-down in the belly at home
nai-xin *dengdai ba.*
endure-heart wait PRT
'You just rest assured (lit. lay down your heart in your belly) and wait patiently (lit. with an endure-heart) at home.'

The sentences in (152) illustrate (151a). "Feeling relieved" is literally "laying down one's heart". Also in (152a), the compound for "prospect" is literally "front-view", i.e. "the view that lies ahead". The example in (152b), cited from a TV drama series, contains an "extended" usage of (151a), where the object (i.e. "heart") and the verb (i.e. "lay down") are reversed in order in a *ba*-sentence. Note that, normally, the heart is in the chest. In this idiomatic way of asking someone to relax and rest assured, however, the "heart" is to be "laid down in the belly", namely below its normal position. We know that in worry, anxiety, fear, etc., people's "heart goes up" from its normal position in the chest (see 122 and 124 above). Now that the "heart" is placed even below its normal position, "in the belly", the person addressed should be more relaxed, relieved, and assured than normal. Again, as in (152b), people doing something patiently have an "enduring heart" (see 94a in 4.4.4).

(153) a. 任务完成了，他总算可以睡个落心觉了。
Renwu wancheng-le, ta zongsuan keyi shui ge
task be-accomplished-PER he finally can have a
luo-xin *jiao le.*
fall-heart sleep PER
'The task has been accomplished, and he can finally have a reassured sleep (lit. a fallen-heart sleep).'

b. 他仔细地听着，句句入耳，字字落心。
Ta zixi-de ting-zhe, ju-ju ru-er, zi-zi
he carefullylisten-DUR sentences-all enter-ears words-all
***luo-xin*.**
fall-into-heart
'He was listening carefully, all sentences appealing (lit. entering his ears), and all words pleasing (lit. falling into his heart).'

Both sentences in (153) illustrate (151b). After people have accomplished the mission that has for long kept them from sleeping well, they can finally have "a fallen-heart sleep", i.e. a sound sleep that one can have with a reassured and relieved mood. Sentence (153b) exemplifies another meaning of (151b). In this sentence, the words that "fall into the heart" of the listener are those that find "echoing" in his heart.

(154) a. 听说孩子的伤势很轻，家里人都息心了。
Ting shuo haizi-de shangshi hen qing,
hear say child's injury very light

jia-li-ren *dou* ***xi-xin*** *le.*
family-members all rest-heart PER
'After they heard that the child's injury was not serious at all, the family members all felt relieved (lit. rested their heart).'

b. 那笔钱找到了，这一下她可定心了。
Na bi *qian* *zhaodao-le,* *zhe-yi-xia*
that amount money was-found-PER under-such-circunstances
ta ke ***ding-xin*** le.
she could settle-heart PER
'Now that the money was found, she could feel relieved (lit. settle her heart).'

The two sentences in (154) exemplify (151d and e). In (154a), when the family members felt relieved at the news that the child had not been seriously injured, they "rested their heart". In (154b), after she recovered the lost money, she "settled her heart", namely, she felt relieved. The heart that is "settled" is peaceful, quiescent, and calm. Since in traditional Chinese culture, the heart is conceptualized as the seat of both emotional and intellectual faculties, one's emotion and intellect are closely related to, and incessantly interactive with, each other, as illustrated by the following sentence:

(155) 心定了，他就有了慧心、慧眼，才能听到心音。
Xin ***ding**-le,* *ta jiu* *you-le* *hui-xin,*
heart settle-PER he then have-PER intelligent-heart
hui-yan, *cai* *neng* *tingdao xin-yin.*
intelligent-eye then can hear heart-voice
'Once the heart has settled down, he gains wisdom (lit. intelligent-heart) and mental discernment (lit. intelligent-eye), and then one can hear the heart-voice (i.e. heartfelt wishes or thinking) of others.'

This sentence, short as it is, involves three occurrences of *xin* 'heart' and one occurrence of *yan* 'eye'. The first occurrence of "heart" is the "mirror image" of (151e). Only after one is emotionally calm, i.e. one's "heart has settled down", can one has an "intelligent heart" (i.e. "wisdom"; see 73a in 4.4.2) and an "intelligent eye" (i.e. "mental discernment; mental perception; insight"; see 22c in 4.2.2) and, as a result, "hear other people's heart voice" (i.e. gain insights into other's minds; see 12c in 4.2.1). The "intelligent eye", meaning "mental discernment", is a linguistic instantiation of the conceptual metaphor THINKING, KNOWING, or UNDERSTANDING IS SEEING (Yu 2004), as much as the English word *insight*, which refers to a "mental sight *in* something". In Buddhism, for instance, the "intelligent eye" refers to "a mind which perceives both past and future" (H-YCD 1995: 433).

4.6. Summary and discussion

In this chapter, I have analyzed the conventionalized expressions revolving around *xin* 'heart' as a key word in the Chinese language that provides an important key to the understanding of human experience and cognition in the context of Chinese culture. The linguistic evidence shows that the Chinese *xin* 'heart' is culturally conceptualized as the central faculty of cognition, which is the agent of thinking, feeling, understanding, knowing, reasoning, and judging; as the seat of both mental and emotional lives of a human being, where cognitive and affective activities and processes are housed, and where feelings and thoughts are stored; and as the locus of human nature and true self, where personal character and moral sense are located. In sum, as manifested in the conventionalized expressions, the Chinese heart is conceptualized as embodying and permeating all aspects of human experience and cognition.

Related to the above finding is the large number of conventionalized expressions, studied in this chapter, all containing *xin* 'heart' as their central constituent. My analysis covers over 300 compound words plus over 200 idiomatic phrases and proverbial sayings (Appendix 1 lists over 50 compound words and over 250 idiomatic phrases and proverbial sayings, which I have not used in this chapter), excluding the many sentential examples cited to illustrate the usage of the lexical items. My coverage is not exhaustive at all. Due to space restrictions, I had to leave out many other expressions I had collected for my research. The participation of *xin* 'heart' in the large number of conventionalized expressions in the Chinese language reflects the central importance of the concept of "heart" in human cognition and human experience as conceptualized in Chinese culture. The Chinese "heart" is simultaneously mental, spiritual, moral, intellectual, rational, volitional, temperamental, and emotional. As we have seen in Chapters 2 and 3, this conceptualization has a long history, rooted deeply in Chinese philosophy and medicine for at least two thousand and five hundred years.

As I have shown in this chapter, the conventionalized expressions of compounds, idioms and proverbs all have *xin* 'heart' as their central element and, for that reason, evoke culturally constructed images centered on the heart as an internal organ of the body. As discussed in 4.2.1, the heart itself is understood metaphorically in terms of a number of source concepts (e.g. ruler, lamp, mirror, plant, instrument, house, nest, field, land, water source). At a more abstract and general level, however, are the following conceptual metaphors:

(i)	THE HEART IS A PERSON
(ii)	THE HEART IS AN OBJECT
(iii)	THE HEART IS A CONTAINER
(iv)	THE HEART IS A LOCATION

Here (i) is a special case of metaphor known as personification, by which the heart is conceptualized as the "ruler" of the body; and (iii) is a special case of (ii) since a container is a kind of object too.

Semantically, various abstract aspects of human cognition and experience are embodied in terms of the heart as the qualities it possesses, functions it plays, and activities it performs or undergoes. Therefore, the "heart" can be a Theme, a Location, an Agent, or a Patient. As a Theme, the "heart" has a variety of qualities of physical objects, such as found in the following:

(i)	Color:	red, black, gray, bright, dark
(ii)	Dimension:	thick, thin, broad, narrow, high, low, big, small
(iii)	Sound:	quiet, noisy
(iv)	Temperature:	hot, warm, cool, cold
(v)	Weight:	heavy, light
(vi)	Feel:	hard, soft, loose, tense
(vii)	Flavor:	sweet, bitter, sour
(viii)	Others:	solid, void, floating, pure, clear, clean, messy, even, uneven, open, close, poisonous

Among these qualities, (i) and (ii) belong to the sense of sight, (iii) to hearing, (iv–vi) to touch, (vii) to taste, and (viii) contains qualities that are mixed in character and that can belong to more than one category. As can be seen, these qualities are attributed to the heart metaphorically. As a Theme, the heart also has a variety of human qualities and feelings, such as the following:

(i)	Mental:	arrogant, modest, sincere, loyal, filial, pious
(ii)	Moral:	good, fine, kind, ruthless, bad, crooked, thievish
(iii)	Intellectual:	intelligent, clever, smart
(iv)	Sensational:	painful, aching, tingling, hurting, itching, drunk

This is because the heart as the central organ of a person can function as a metonymy or synecdoche for the person. In a similar vein, the heart, being the central faculty of cognition, performs various mental activities in the role of an Agent: thinking, understanding, knowing, wishing, expecting, suspecting, appreciating, designing, calculating, etc. As a Location, the heart is the place that stores thoughts and feelings or houses mental activities and processes. Thus, for instance, something can be "put", "kept", "contained", "engraved" in the heart, "placed" or "hanged" on it, or something can "grow out of" or "go through" it. In the role of a Patient, the heart is manipulated in a wide variety of ways by sorts of external forces. Thus, it can be "scorched", "fried", "cooked", "pitched", "twisted", "pulled", "lifted", "suspended", "hanged", "laid down", "settled down", "moved", "snapped", "fragmented", and so on.

As discussed in this chapter, the compounds and idiomatic phrases are part of the daily vocabulary that actually stays at the "heart" of Chinese lexicon. It is obvious that metaphor and metonymy play crucial roles in their construction. Various images are stretched out, via metaphor (e.g. HEART IS A CONTAINER, HEART IS AN OBJECT) and metonymy (e.g. CONTAINER FOR CONTAINED, OBJECT FOR ITS QUALITY), around and from the basic image of "heart", to structure various abstract concepts for aspects of human cognition and experience. In this way, "language evokes imagery and requires imagination for its interpretation" (Palmer 1996: 3). That is why for Cognitive Linguistics "language analysis should begin with conventional imagery" (p. 27).

At this point, it is necessary to emphasize that the images evoked by the compounds and idiomatic phrases discussed in this chapter are culturally constructed rather than universally existent. They all stem from a proposition that is a literal cultural belief by tradition: THE HEART IS THE CENTRAL FACULTY OF COGNITION. That is, in traditional Chinese culture, the heart is believed to be the home of inner self, the residence of personal disposition, the abode of moral character, the center of thought, the seat of emotions, and so forth. The heart is, therefore, the organ holding or possessing all these cognitive and affective faculties. It is from this cultural belief that metaphors (e.g. HEART IS A CONTAINER, HEART IS AN OBJECT) and metonymies (e.g. CONTAINER FOR CONTAINED, OBJECT FOR ITS QUALITY) have arisen. This observation should shed light on a linguistic difference between Chinese and English, not explicitly discussed in this chapter. That is, the Chinese expressions containing *xin* 'heart' mostly do not involve *heart* in their respective English translations. We can, for instance, make the following list of equivalents:

English	Chinese
sincerity	*cheng-xin* (sincere-heart)
conscience	*liang-xin* (good-heart)
intimate friend	*zhi-xin pengyou* (knowing-heart friend)
careless person	*cu-xin de ren* (a thick-heart person)
think to oneself	*xin-xiang* (heart-think)
be genuinely convinced	*xin-fu* (be heart-convinced)
be willing	*xin-gan* (be heart-willing)
good intention	*hao-xin* (good-heart)
on purpose	*cheng-xin* (establish-heart)
with concentrated attention	*yong-xin* (use-heart)
determination; be determined	*jue-xin* (determined-heart)
against one's will	*wei-xin* (disobey/violate-heart)
perseverance; persistence	*heng-xin* (constant-heart)
be careful; be cautious	*xiao-xin* (small-heart)
feel terribly worried	*jiao-xin* (scorch-heart)
feel happy	*kai-xin* (open heart)
be charmed; be enchanted	*xin-zui* (be heart-drunk)

The list can go on and on. The difference in phraseology may suggest differing ethno-philosophical and ethno-medical views in the interpretation of the workings of the body and its heart organ in particular and how they are related to the "mind" in the conceptualization of the person (see Ch. 6). The Chinese phraseology points to an embodied view of "mind", but this embodiment is situated in the context of Chinese culture that traditionally holds the proposition THE HEART IS THE CENTRAL FACULTY OF COGNITION.

Certainly the Chinese word *xin* is polysemous. While its most prototypical meaning refers to that "internal organ of blood and flesh", it has also come to refer to the "seat" of the innermost being, the locus of moral character and personal disposition, the "container" of feelings and thoughts, and to various feeling-related and thought-related concepts. Of course the Chinese word *xin* 'heart' cannot be an "online polysemy" (Enfield and Wierzbicka 2002b; Enfield 2002) by which people will have the "physical organ" in mind when speaking or hearing the word *xin*. However, various meanings of the word are indeed connected in a spiderweb fashion with its central sense of "internal bodily organ", and such a connection can be established whenever and wherever the circumstances are appropriate, as illustrated by the following example taken from a TV drama series:

(156) A: 我的心已经破了一个大洞。
A: My heart is already broken with a big hole.
B: 你的心要是已经破了一个大洞你不是早就死了吗？

B: If your heart is already broken with a big hole, shouldn't you have died a long time ago?

Here A, a girl, is saddened by a serious misunderstanding between her and the young man she truly loves. B is a close friend of A. It so happens that he loves A very much in his heart, but has never expressed his feeling openly to her. In this instance, he is just trying to console her. It is interesting to see that, while A is referring to her "mental heart", B is referring to her "physical heart" instead. The connection between the two is established for a pragmatic purpose.

It has become clear that the Chinese *xin* 'heart' is the combination of "heart" and "mind" in the English sense. It is where both emotions and thoughts are stored, processed, and manipulated in its traditional conceptualization. As I pointed out elsewhere (Yu 2003d), there exists a conceptual difference between Chinese and English that reflects a significant difference between the corresponding cultures. That is, Western cultures' binary contrast between the heart and the mind does not exist in traditional Chinese culture. "It is a case in which different cultural models interpret the functioning of the mind and the body differently" (p. 141). In light of the surveys in ancient Chinese philosophy and traditional Chinese medicine presented in Chapters 2 and 3, it is clear that the linguistic evidence analyzed in this chapter is actually embedded in its cultural context. The language is but a part of the cultural system (Palmer 1996). Manifested linguistically, the conceptualization of the Chinese "heart" is indeed a phenomenon at the cultural level of cognition (Sharifian 2003).

As I have also observed (Yu 2003d), however, in present-day Chinese, 头脑 *tou-nao* 'head and brain' can also mean "mind" as understood in English. It is also where one's thoughts and ideas are stored and one's thinking takes place, as illustrated by the examples in (157), of which the first three are taken from Yu (2003d: 159):

(157) a. 我们要有冷静的头脑。
Women yao you lengjing de ***tou-nao****.*
we should have cool-quiet MOD head-brain
'We should have a cool head (or, be sober-minded; lit. have cool-quiet head-brain).'

b. 我们应该把头脑里的错误思想清除出去。
Women yinggai ba ***tou-nao*** *li de cuowu sixiang*
we should PRT head-brain in MOD wrong ideas
qingchu chuqu.
clear out

'We should rid our minds (lit. head-brain) of erroneous ideas.'

c. 僵化思想束缚着一些人的头脑。
Jianghua sixiang shufu-zhe yixie ren-de ***tou-nao***.
stiffened ideas bind-DUR some people's head-brain
'An ossified way of thinking shackles some people's minds. (lit. Stiffened ideas are binding some people's head-brain.)'

d. 这个硬头脑不能正确认识问题。
Zhe-ge ying ***tou-nao*** *bu-neng zhengque renshi wenti.*
this-CL hard head-brain cannot correctly understand problem
'This stiffened brain (lit. hard head-brain) cannot understand problems correctly.'

In (157a), to be "sober-minded" is to have a "cool and quiet head and brain". In (157b), thought and ideas exist in people's "head and brain", from which erroneous ones should be removed so that they do not have bad thoughts and ideas in their minds. As in (157c), the "head-brain" is the part that fulfills the function of thinking. When it is "bound" by stiffened ideas that restrict its "movement", the "head-brain" can no longer "take the action of active thinking". In Chinese, to use one's mind is literally to "move one's brain" (动脑 *dongnao* or 动脑筋 *dongnaojin*). When the brain is "tied up", it of course cannot "move" any more. The example in (157d) contains the metonymy BRAIN FOR PERSON. When the brain is "stiffened" or "fossilized" and as "hard" as a "rock", it of course has lost the function of thinking and understanding.

(158) a. 脑子 *nao-zi* (brain-PRT) 'brain; brains; mind; head'
b. 脑袋 *nao-dai* (brain-bag) 'head; brains; mind'
c. 脑汁 *nao-zhi* (brain-liquid/juice) 'brains'
d. 脑海 *nao-hai* (brain-sea) 'brain; mind'
e. 脑际 *nao-ji* (brain-boundary/inside) 'mind; memory'
f. 脑筋 *nao-jin* (brain-muscle/vein) 'brains; mind; head; way of thinking; ideas'
g. 脑力 *nao-li* (brain-strength) 'mental power; intelligence'

The compounds in (158) all contain as their first morpheme 脑 *nao* 'brain', and they are in one way or another associated with "mind", "memory", "thinking", "idea", "mental power", and "intelligence". As shown here, the "brain" (158a) is a container of "bag" (158b) that contains "liquid" (158c) in it. This "pool of liquid" is so big that it is as vast as a "sea" (158d) with a remote "boundary" (158e). Also, this "brain" has its "muscle" (158f) and "strength" (158g). Given below are sentential examples.

(159) a. 问题是复杂的，我们的脑子也要复杂一点。
Wenti shi fuza de, womende ***nao-zi*** *ye*
problems are complicated PRT our brain also
yao fuza yi-dian.
must-be complicated a-bit
'The problems are complicated, and our brains must be a little complicated, too.'

b. 他的脑袋瓜子好使。
Tade ***nao-dai****-gua-zi hao shi.*
his brain-bag-mellon-SUF good use
'He's got a clever mind (lit. His brain-bag is good to use).'

c. 我绞尽脑汁设法离间她们。
Wo jiao-jin ***nao-zhi*** *she-fa*
I wring-all brain-liquid think-of-a-way
lijian tamen.
drive-a-wedge-betweem them
'I rack my brains (lit. wring out all my brain liquid) to think of a way to drive a wedge between them.'

d. 多年前的旧事又重现在他的脑海里。
Duo-nian qian de jiu shi you chong-xian
many-years ago MOD old things again re-appear
zai tade ***nao-hai*** *li.*
at his brain-sea in
'Memories of things long past flashed across his mind (lit. brain-sea).'

e. 突然一个念头浮上脑际。
Turan yi-ge niantou fu shang ***nao-ji****.*
suddenly one-CL idea float onto brain-boundary
'An idea flashed across my mind (lit. Suddently an idea emerged within the boundary of the brain).'

f. 你问老杨去，他脑筋好，记得清。
Ni wen Lao Yang qu, ta ***nao-jin*** *hao, ji*
you ask Lao Yang go his brain-muscle good remember

de *qing.*
COM clearly
'Ask Lao Yang; he has a good memory (lit. You go and ask Lao Yang; his brain-muscle is good, and can remember it clearly).'

g. 我们要逐步消灭脑力和体力劳动的差别。
Women *yao* *zhubu* *xiaomie* ***nao-li*** *he*
we should gradually wipe-out brain-strength and
ti-li *laodong de* *chabie.*
body-strength labor MOD difference
'We should gradually eliminate the distinction between mental and manual labor (lit. the difference between the brain-strength and body-strength labor).'

The example in (159a) shows that it is the brain that copes with problems. In (159b), those who have "a clever mind" have a "brain-bag" that is "good for use". In (159c), when people are trying very hard to think of a way to do something, they "wring out all the liquid inside their brain". The "brain sea" in (159d) has to do with memory. When "he" recalls the things many years ago, these things "emerge again on the surface of the brain sea". In a similar vein, when an idea occurs to people, it "floats up inside their brain" (159e). Those people who have "a good memory" are said to have "good brain muscle" (159f), i.e. their brains are more "powerful" than others. In (159g), the difference between mental and manual labor is that between "brain strength" and "body strength".

All the examples above show, beyond any doubt, that the brain, an organ in the head, is the seat of thought, memory, and intellect. In short, it is the locus of the "mind", too. That is, it seems, we are faced with a contradiction between the brain versus the heart as the locus of the "mind" in present-day Chinese. Now the questions are how this conflict can be resolved or and how the brain and the heart stand in relation to each other.

Of course, it could be argued that the heart being the locus of the "mind", as outlined in this chapter, is but a "linguistic relic" of the past that does not have its conceptual counterpart in the current "minds" of Chinese people. In the following I will argue, however, that the Chinese still hold the cultural conceptualization that the heart is the cognitive center of a person even though they know, scientifically, that the brain should take over that status. In other words, we should distinguish between the "cultural mind" and the "scientific mind", or a "scientific level" and a "cultural level" within a single mind, which are not necessarily identical and may operate separately and alternatively under different circumstances, resulting in views of a seemingly paradoxical nature (see 3.5). This argument is similar in spirit to Pritzker's (2007) view that people can hold multiple and contradictory cultural models of the thinking and feeling self.

First of all, it needs to be pointed out that the usage involving the "brain" as the locus of the "mind", as presented above, is limited to present-day Chinese with a relatively small number of conventionalized expressions, despite the fact that it is consistent with the findings of modern science. In fact, the compounds in (158), only seven of them, are all that I could find in the dictionaries. On the other hand, the bulk of conventionalized expressions, hundreds of them, presented in this chapter (see more in Appendix 1), including compounds, idioms, and sayings, demonstrate that the heart, rather than the brain, is the locus of the "mind" in Chinese. In other words, while both "brain" and "heart" are supposed to be the locus of the "mind", they are distinguished from each other in two important dimensions. Diachronically, the "brain" is quite "young" in taking up this role as compared with the "heart", which has a history of at least two thousand five hundred years playing the same function. Synchronically speaking, there exists a significant disparity between the two in terms of quantity of conventionalized expressions that they each involve. The "heart" is involved in a great number (hundreds) of "mind-related" expressions while this number is very small (not a lot more than the seven found) for the "brain". Their huge quantitative difference in Chinese phraseology itself is very significant evidence for their qualitative difference even though they both are now conceptualized as having certain identical functions.[88]

Secondly, it should be stressed that scientific knowledge and cultural conceptualization are not the same thing and they are not always in agreement with each other. People may have a certain level of scientific knowledge but still cling to a certain cultural conceptualization that contradicts the scientific knowledge that they possess. As an illustration I will cite from two newspaper articles (Feng 2003; Gu 2005). The translations provided below of the Chinese originals are my own.

---

88 Readers are referred to Pritzker (2007), where the researcher reports her quantitative findings of her analysis of some spontaneously generated speeches obtained from her interviews of 49 Chinese patients suffering fromn depressions. Her findings show that while 45 out of 49 (92%) patients referred to the heart to express thinking and feeling, 18 of the 45 (37%) also referred to the brain to express thinking and feeling, and 4 out of 49 referred to neither the heart nor the brain. I will come back to this study in 7.3.

The first quotation is from an article titled "Good health depends on regular use of the brain (健身在于勤动脑)" (Feng 2003), which appeared in the "Health" section on the *People's Daily* (Overseas Edition) on October 27, 2003:

> 大脑是人的指挥部，不但人的一言一行均由脑来指挥，而且人的所有器官的健康状况也与脑的健康直接相关。……人体的大脑功能是不用则废，勤用则健。现代医学的研究发现，脑子动得越多，人的思维越敏捷，人也不容易衰老。那些未老先衰者，往往是思想懒惰的人。
> 冯活源《健身在于勤动脑》载《人民日报 (海外版)》2003 年 10 月 27 日第 10 页(“健康”版)。
> The brain is the command post of the human being. Not only is people's every word or action commanded by their brain, but also the health of their organs is directly related to the health of their brain. … The human brain is such that the lack of its use will lead to the loss of its function and its frequent use will make it sharper and keener. Modern medical research has discovered that the more people use the brain, the sharper and quicker their thinking will become, and they are also less likely prone to aging. Those who have aged prematurely are usually those who are too lazy to think.
> Feng Huoyuan, "Good health depends on regular use of the brain", *People's Daily* (Overseas Edition), October 27, 2003, p. 10 ("Health" section).

Note that, as already mentioned, the article from which the above quotation is cited appears in the "Health" section of the newspaper. It addresses the relations between people's mental and physical health. The point, as is made clear by its title, is that people's good physical health (健身 *jianshen,* literally "healthy body") depends on the frequent and regular use of their brain. This point is made based on scientific knowledge discovered by "modern medical research". Thus, the brain is regarded as the "command post" of the human body. It "commands" people's linguistic competence and physical action, and is directly responsible for the soundness of their other organs. Unlike other things that are worn out with regular and frequent use, the more people's brain is used, the more sharp-minded and physically sound they will become. Obviously, the knowledge of "scientific" nature promoted here departs from the cultural belief traditionally held in Chinese philosophy and medicine that the heart is "the ruler of the body" and "the governor of the spiritual light" discussed in Chapters 2 and 3. It is interesting to note that the point made here about the brain is quite parallel to that made about the heart by Mencius over two thousand years ago: i.e., "The organ of heart is for thinking. If you think, you will get it; if you do not, then you will not get it" (see 2.2.1).

The point most relevant to my discussion here is that the Chinese in general, especially those with some education, will accept the above quotation as it is and will not challenge its validity since it "fits" well with their schema of scientific knowledge, or their "scientific mind", as I would call it. Nevertheless, scientific knowledge is not all there is in the conceptual system of human beings. They also have other knowledge than the scientific one, for example, cultural knowledge that may very well be in conflict with their scientific knowledge and that constitutes their "cultural mind". Now, let us turn to the quotation from the second newspaper article (Gu 2005), titled "The spirit of the Chinese" (中国人的精神), which appeared in *China Tribune* on June 3, 2005 as a reprint of an essay by Gu Hongming (1857–1928), a well known scholar of Chinese and Western studies and once a professor at Peking University. Gu studied in a number of European countries such as Britain, Italy, Austria, Germany, and France and learned more than ten foreign languages including Greek and Latin. The Chinese name of the newspaper *China Tribune* is 《文化与生活》, which, if translated literally, means "Culture and Life". It is a biweekly published by some Chinese-Americans living in the greater Chicago metropolitan area. In this article, the author discusses what he thinks is a distinct cultural characteristic of the Chinese as being "gentle and kindhearted" (温良 *wenliang*). He believes that this cultural characteristic stems from Chinese people's "sense (lit. heart) of compassion" (同情心 *tongqing xin*). The reason why the Chinese have this sense of compassion is, he argues, that they lead a "life of heart" (心灵的生活).[89] He makes this answer his hypothesis: namely, that "the Chinese, entirely or almost entirely, lead a life of heart", and that their "entire life is a life of emotion" (Gu 2005: 27). By "emotion" (情感 *qinggan*) he refers to the "kind of feeling that arises from the depth of our humanity – in the sense of heart's passion (心灵的激情) or human love" (p. 27). He then goes on to support his hypothesis with what he be-

---

[89] As shown in (73b) in 4.4.2, the compound word 心灵 *xin-ling* (heart-soul/spirit) can mean "mind; heart; soul; spirit; psyche". What is relevant and important is the fact that in Chinese "mind", "soul", and "spirit" are all located in, and associated with, the heart. Therefore, 心灵的生活 *xinling de shenghuo* here is translated into "life of heart". See, also, the relevant discussions in Chapters 2 and 3.

lieves are four pieces of evidence. Such discussion leads to the following passage, where the first two pieces of his evidence are given:

> 下面让我们看看中国人是否过着一种心灵的生活。对此，我们可以用中国人实际生活中表现出来的一般特征，来加以说明。
>
> 首先，我们来谈谈中国的语言。中国的语言也是一种心灵的语言。一个很明显的事实就是：那些生活在中国的外国人，其儿童和未受教育者学习中文比成年人和受过教育者要容易得多。原因在于儿童和未受教育者是用心灵来思考和使用语言的。相反，受过教育者，特别是受过理性教育的现代欧洲人，他们是用大脑和智慧来思考和使用语言的。有一种关于极乐世界的说法也同样适用于对中国语言的学习：除非你变成一个孩子，否则你就难以学会它。
>
> 其次，我们再来指出一个众所周知的中国人日常生活的事实。中国人具有惊人的记忆力，其秘密何在？就在于中国人是用心而非脑去记忆。用具同情力量的心灵记事，比用头脑或智力要好得多，后者是枯燥乏味的。举例来说，我们当中的绝大多数儿童时代的记忆力要强过成年后的记忆力。因为儿童就象中国人一样，是用心而非脑去记忆。
>
> 辜鸿铭《中国人的精神》载《文化与生活》2005 年 6 月 3 日第 27 页。
>
> In the following let us see whether or not the Chinese lead a life of heart. To that end, we can use, for illustration, the general traits displayed by the Chinese in their actual life.
>
> First, let us talk about the Chinese language. The Chinese language is also a language of heart. An obvious fact is that, among those foreigners living in China, children and uneducated people can learn Chinese much more easily than adults and educated people. This is because children and uneducated people think and use language via their heart. On the contrary, the educated, especially those modern Europeans who have received a rational education, think and use language via their brain and intelligence. A saying about the Land of Ultimate Bliss applies to the learning of the Chinese language too: You will not be able to learn it well unless you become a child.
>
> Next, let me point out a well-known fact in the Chinese people's daily life, that is, the Chinese have an amazingly good memory. What is the reason for that? The reason is that the Chinese utilize their heart rather than brain for memorization. It is much better to use the heart with compassion to memorize things than to use the brain or intellect, which is dry and dull. For instance, most of us have a better memory in childhood than in adulthood, because children, like the Chinese people, use their heart rather than brain for memorization.
>
> Gu Hongming, "The spirit of the Chinese", *China Tribune / Culture and Life*, June 3, 2005, p. 27.

The last two pieces of evidence, according to the author, lie in Chinese politeness, which "arises from the inner heart", and the Chinese habitual lack of accuracy or precision, which is so typical of the flexible heart, but not of the precise brain. To illustrate the difference between the flexibility of the heart versus the precision of the brain, the author cites the example of the Chinese brush pen, in contrast with the Western fountain pen, as symbolic of the spirit of the Chinese. The brush pen is difficult to handle in writing and painting; it also lacks the precision of the Western hard pen. However, once it is mastered, the author argues, it can create wonderful and graceful arts of calligraphy and painting. The author argues that it is because the Chinese lead a life of heart, a life like that of children, they appear to be quite naïve in many respects. Apparently, they lag behind in sciences, especially more abstract sciences. "Leading a life of heart, like children, the Chinese show no interest in abstract sciences, about which the heart and emotion can do noting". In short, the author concludes, "real Chinese people have the heart of a child and the wisdom of an adult" (Gu 2005: 27).

In the above I cited Gu's (2005) argument at length, not because I believe how much of it is truth or fallacy, but because I want to show a "view", if not a "worldview", which is established, obviously, not on modern scientific knowledge, but on culturally constructed knowledge or belief rooted deeply in the cultural conceptualization or, more generally, the cultural model of the Chinese formulated and renegotiated over the past several thousand years. In this view, therefore, the Chinese think and use language "with their heart" instead of their brain, and they "use their heart" rather than brain for memorization. Obviously, this view, or cultural belief, conflicts head on with the view presented in the first newspaper article cited earlier. My point is that those who accept the view of the first article may as well accept the view of the second article, regardless of the fact that they are indeed in contradiction with each other. However, the two views can co-exist in two separate "minds" of a person: the "scientific mind" and the "cultural mind", which occupy different domains of one's conceptual system and make sense in different contexts. In other words, we may say that people can hold multiple, and sometimes contradictory, cultural models (Pritzker 2007). I hope that the citation of the passages from these two articles accounts for the seemingly contradictory fact that in Chinese both heart and brain are manifested linguistically as the locus of the "mind", but the former holds a much more high-profiled status than the latter within the Chinese cultural models for the "mind" and "person".

For further illustration, I now provide some more examples from popular culture in China today – TV commercials. Thus, as a key word of Chinese culture, *xin* 'heart', but not *nao* 'brain' or *tou* 'head', represents a recurring theme in TV commercials in China, both for business and for educational purposes. The following are just a few recent examples of commercial scripts on China Central Television (CCTV) and Phoenix TV (Hong Kong):

(160) a. 每个人心中都有一个大舞台，心有多大舞台就有多大。
In everyone's heart there is a big stage; however big one's heart is, that is how big the stage is. (CCTV)

b. 发于点滴，行于心田， 融于交流，盛于久远。
Originating in drips and drops, functioning in the heart, fusing in communication, and flourishing in eternity. (CCTV)

c. 人与自然彼此共存，人与社会协调发展，人与人友好互助；从我心做起。
Humans and nature coexist, humans and society harmoniously develop, and humans are friendly and helpful to each other. Let it all start from my heart. (CCTV)

d. 关爱老人，用心开始；将爱心传递下去。
Care for and love the elderly, starting with the heart; pass the loving heart down. (CCTV)

e. 文明在身边，心心相传。
Civility is beside us; pass it on from heart to heart. (CCTV)

f. 让心畅通，我能。
Let the heart be unimpeded, I can. (Phoenix TV)

g. 心动，梦想的起点。
The heart moving, the starting point of dreams. (Phoenix TV)

h. 云动，心动，行动。
The clouds move, the heart moves, and the action moves. (Phoenix TV)

i. 心静，思远，志在千里。
The heart is quiescent, thinking afar, and determined to reach a thousand *li* (or Chinese miles). (CCTV)

The English translations are quite literal to provide a better flavor of the originals. The examples from (a) to (e) are from the so-called "commercials for public good" (公益广告) on CCTV, which are educational in nature, designed to influence people's way of thinking and understanding for the purpose of promoting public welfare. In (a), which is based on the Chinese cultural conceptualization of the heart as the organ for thinking and understanding, as well as feeling, and more generally as the central faculty of cognition, the verbal message is an instantiation of the popular conceptual metaphor LIFE IS A STAGE. On the "stage" of life, people play various roles, some being more important and successful than others. One's degree of success in the external life (the size of the stage) is attributed and related to the mental capacity of one's internal world, the "heart" (the size of the "heart"), in a metaphorical fashion. That is, only when one can "think big" (i.e., with "a big heart") can one "act big" on the "big stage" of life (see Yu 2007c). Example (b) is from an educational TV commercial that promotes Chinese virtues by means of a conceptual metaphor, VIRTUE IS WATER, manifested multimodally. Thus, virtues originate in "drips and drops" and "flow" in the heart, the locus of one's moral sense. Only when virtues "flow" in individual hearts can they "merge" harmoniously into a "long river" before pouring into the eternity of "seas and oceans". In (c), which is from a commercial promoting the construction of a "harmonious society", all the effort to that end "starts from one's own heart", the cognitive, affective, and moral center of a person. Without the heart "moving" in that direction, one will not move to take actions. As in (d), filial piety is a traditional moral value which originates in one's heart. Therefore, if one really wants to take good care of the elderly, in a loving manner, one needs to "start with one's heart". The commercial advocates that parents pass down the traditional value of filial piety (or more generally a "loving heart") by setting good examples for their children. Example (e) promotes good manners of courtesy, decorum, and so on, in everyday life. The daily practice of good manners is something so close to us that it is right "beside us". As part of good moral values, they should be passed on "from heart to heart". Example (f) is the script from a commercial promoting the GoTone Mobile Communications. When people can talk, to their heart's content, on their cellular phone to their loved ones, they feel good about it. The good feeling in this case is having their "heart unimpeded", which is a "conduit metaphor" for communication as having the "traffic" of thoughts and feelings traveling back and forth between two persons' hearts (see Reddy 1993). The interrupted communication will result in one's heart "being impeded", and it is a bad feeling both physiologically and psychologically. In (g), which is from a commercial for a company called "Sinotech", the heart is believed to be the source and origin of having one's dreams come true. One's "heart moving" refers to one being excited with cognitive and affective activities in one's heart, the site of those activities. Example (h) is from a commercial for a wine producer, the "Red Clouds" Group. When one sees the "clouds moving" (the "Red Clouds" products), one's heart, the ruler of one's body, will "move", and when one's "heart moves", one will "move into actions". Again, the "heart moving" means that one is active in both thinking and feeling. The last one, example (i), is from a commercial for Buick automobiles produced by GM based in Shanghai. The superior quality of the car is expressed in term of the "heart". When the heart is quiescent – quiescence of the heart being a virtue advocated by Xunzi (see section 2.2.2) – its thinking extends far, and it is determined to reach a thousand *li*.[90] After all, a quiescent heart has great potential to "reach a long goal".

In Chinese, thinking and feeling are not so clearly distinguished from each other, as residing separately in the head and the heart as in the West. As in the scripts of the commercials discussed above, thinking and feeling are mixed and both attributed to the heart, but not to the head or brain. There are many more TV commercials involving the concept of "heart" that I have noticed, too many to discuss them here one by one. That is why I would say again, based on the large number of such examples, that *xin* 'heart' is a key word of Chinese culture, but neither *tou* 'head' nor *nao* 'brain' is. The only example that I noticed involving the latter is one in a commercial on Phoenix TV that promotes its own serial programs hosted by five of their analysts and commentators of international and domestic

---

90 One *li*, or one Chinese mile, is half a kilometer. A thousand *li* is therefore five hundred kilometers, which, though not a long distance by today's criteria applied to automobiles, suggests both a high speed and a long distance in ancient times when the horse was the main means of transportation. Thus, there are, e.g., following idiomatic expressions in Chinese: (a) 千里 *qianli* (a thousand *li*) 'a long distance or a vast expanse'; (b) 千里马 *qianlima* (thousand-*li* horse) 'a horse that covers a thousand *li* a day; a winged steed'; (c) 千里驹 *qianliju* (thousand-*li* colt) 'a son who is showing great promise'; (d) 千里眼 *qianliyan* (thousand-*li* eye) 'farsighted person'; (e) 千里迢迢 *qianli tiaotiao* 'from a thousand *li* away; from afar'; (f) 千里之堤溃于蚁穴 *qianli zhi di kui yu yixue* 'one ant hole may cause the collapse of a thousand-*li* dyke – slight negligence may lead to great disaster'; (g) 千里之行始于足下 *qianli zhi xing shi yu zu xia* 'a thousand-*li* journey is started by taking the first step'.

political affairs (including cross-straight political situations) on five weekdays. These analysts and commentators are called "five brilliant heads-and-brains" (五个精彩的头脑), i.e., "five brilliant minds", which is an instance of metonymy. In this case, understandably, the analysts and commentators are supposed to detach themselves from any emotions, feelings, or ethical and cultural values, which could cause bias or prejudice. Whether this is possible or not is another matter, but they are supposed to keep their analyses and comments at an intellectual and rational level, as much as they can. In any event, this represents a case in conflict with the more general and traditional conception of the heart as the organ for thinking. It demonstrates that people can hold multiple and contradictory cultural models of the thinking and feeling self (Pritzker 2007). In general, the differences between two conflicting models may be such that one is huge and heavy whereas the other is small and light, or one is much older and stronger while the other is much younger and weaker. Going back to the COMPUTER metaphor, we can say that the five political analysts' way of thinking is "data processing".

To conclude my account for the seemingly conflicting facts about the heart and the brain, I would like to cite two more examples, which I hope would add the finishing touch. These examples were found in two news articles posted on DWNEWS.COM (多维新闻网). The first example is from the report that a leader of the Chinese government attended the Eighth National Congress of the Chinese Association of Literature and Arts late in 2006. In his talk he said the following (of which the English translation is rather literal):

(161) 我一直要求自己用心思考，用心讲话，用心做事，用心写文章。对于文学艺术家来讲，可能还要求你们用心创作，用心演出。
I have always required myself to think with my heart, to speak with my heart, to work with my heart, and to write with my heart. Of the writers and artists I would probably require that you compose with your heart, and perform with your heart.

In these two sentences, as can be seen, the recurring element is 用心 *yongxin*, which literally means "to use the heart (to do something)" or "(to do something) with the heart". This example indeed reveals a traditional Chinese value, which is manifested here linguistically in quite an emphatic fashion, namely, it is a virtue to do things (thinking, speaking, working, writing, etc.) "with one's heart". Only things out of one's heart represent one's "true self".

The second example is the title of a news article about the new strategy of the government of mainland China in dealing with the cross-straight relationship. The title goes as follows:

(162) 大陆提出对台工作策略：“入岛、入脑、入心”。
Mainland put forward the working strategy in dealing with Taiwan: “Into the island, into the brain, and into the heart”.

The mainland proposed this new strategy in order to attain the ultimate goal of peaceful unification with Taiwan. This is the “reaching-out” strategy, namely, they need to reach out “into the island” so as to “touch” the people in Taiwan. Just reaching out to “touch” the people there is not sufficient. They also need to reach “into the brain” of the people so as to influence their thinking and thought. But that is still not enough. They need to reach further and deeper “into the heart” of the people because, as discussed earlier, the heart is the innermost being where one’s secret feelings and thoughts are stored and is therefore the seat for the inner and true self. The ultimate success in peaceful unification with Taiwan depends on “winning the hearts” of Taiwanese people. Any effort short of reaching “into their hearts” is doomed to be unsuccessful. The word order of the three short phrases reflects the sequence of critical importance and the relationship between the brain and the heart as perceived in Chinese.

Chapter 5
The HEART in present-day Chinese discourse

5.1. Introduction: Textual analysis

The study to be presented in this chapter methodologically complements and supplements my study in the previous chapter by adding a perspective from textual analysis on the cultural conceptualization of the heart as manifested in the present-day Chinese language and discourse. Instead of focusing on conventionalized linguistic expressions in isolation, I will examine a few authentic texts that are chosen for my study because they all pertain to the Chinese concept of *xin* 'heart'. I hope that the contextualized analyses at the textual level will add another dimension to my research into the Chinese conceptualization of the heart and its underlying cultural models.

As Holland and Quinn (1987) suggest and show, cultural knowledge organized in cultural models can be propositional, metaphorical, and metonymic, enabling the performance of different kinds of cognitive tasks (see Quinn 1987; Quinn and Holland 1987). In this chapter, I will limit my goal to the discovery of the propositions, metonymies, and metaphors that underlie the discourse of the texts and play their roles in the construction of the Chinese conceptualization of the heart shaped in its cultural models.[91] My primary question is: Is the conceptualization of the *xin* 'heart' as manifested by the propositions, metonymies and metaphors in these authentic texts consistent, in one way or another, with the one delineated in Chapter 4 in particular, or in Chapters 2–4 as a whole? To answer this question, I will analyze the authentic texts that belong to two different kinds of discourse: prosaic and poetic. The prosaic text is an essay on the supreme importance and significance of the concept of "heart" in Chinese thought and culture,

---

[91] I use the term *proposition* in the sense of Quinn (1987) and Quinn and Holland (1987), where it refers to nonfigurative, cultural assumptions, in contrast with metaphors and metonymies, which are figurative in nature. In this sense, propositions represent what Lakoff and Johnson (1999) refer to as cultural beliefs, which can serve as components of complex metaphors. In other words, cultural beliefs and assumptions refer to "nonfigurative propositions" whereas metaphors and metonymies are "figurative propositions", now generally known as conceptual metaphors and metonymies (Dirven, personal communication).

written by a renowned contemporary scholar of Chinese philosophy and history. The essay was found in a newspaper that carried it as a reprint. The sample from the poetic discourse consists of eight poems about the inner life and self of the people living in a modern environment. The inner life and self, as we know, are localized in the "heart" in Chinese culture. These poems are composed by a "nameless" (only the pen name is known) poet who prefers to share his or her verbal artifacts on the Internet. With my sample texts from two different genres, my secondary question is: What are the similarities and differences, if any, in terms of the propositions, metonymies and metaphors as they are manifested in the two kinds of discourse, i.e. between the essay and the poems?

My selection of these sample texts was actually quite random and accidental: In my leisure reading I came across them and spotted the key word *xin* 'heart' in their titles, so I saved them for my future study. My sample texts, the essay and poems, are all in Chinese, but my analysis will be based on my English translations of them so that it can be accessed and appreciated by a wider audience. Since my study delves into the underlying conceptual level, rather than focuses on the linguistic surface, to grasp the propositional, metonymic, and metaphoric concepts that stay on an abstract plane, I hope that the use of the English translations, instead of their Chinese originals, for my analysis and discussion can be justified.

Methodologically, the study in this chapter is inspired and informed by Cognitive Stylistics, or Cognitive Poetics, which is a field "at the interface between linguistics, literary studies and cognitive science" (Semino and Culpeper 2002b: ix). Focused on textual analysis of language and cognition, Cognitive Stylistics may be seen either as part of the Cognitive Linguistics (CL) paradigm or as being fed into by the cognitive theories or paradigms including CL (Semino and Culpeper 2002a, 2002b). In contrast with formal linguistics that is interested only in a theoretical account of linguistic competence, CL adopts an encyclopedic view of language and attempts a scientific account of natural language in use, showing "increasing awareness of how literary texts might provide a productive source of data for investigation" (Freeman 2006: 404). Freeman (2006) believes that Cognitive Poetics as part of CL serves as a bridge between literary studies and linguistics. "Whereas literary critics focus on illuminating the language of the text, cognitive linguists focus on illuminating the language of the embodied mind. This is where cognitive poetics comes in" (pp. 404–405).

Having laid out the rationale, goal, and methodological issues of my study in this chapter, I now proceed to the analysis itself. In section 5.2, I will look into the essay on the supreme importance and significance of the concept of "heart" in Chinese thought and culture. In section 5.3, I will examine the poems on the concept of "heart" as the inner life and self of the people living in a modern environment. Section 5.4 concludes with a summary and some discussion.

5.2. The heart in an essay on the "heart"

The Chinese essay, titled "On the 'Heart' for the New Year" (新年话"心"), is written by Ying-shih Yu (Yu 2005), a historian and philosopher and professor emeritus of Chinese studies at Princeton University. In 2006, Ying-shih Yu was "the co-winner of the third John W. Kluge Prize for lifetime achievement in the study of humanity", states News@Princeton (December 3, 2006). According to the same online source, "The prize rewards accomplishment in the wide range of disciplines not covered by the Nobel prizes, including history, philosophy, politics, anthropology, sociology, religion, criticism in the arts and humanities, and linguistics".

Provided below is my own translation of the essay, with every fifth line numbered for convenient reference. The Chinese original can be found in Appendix 2. In the translation, the italic font face is added for emphasis. This very literal translation may appear somewhat unnatural in English, but it enables the reader to perceive the metaphorical imagery and structure of the original Chinese.

On "Heart" for the New Year

> The heart is the *most important thing to the Chinese*, and therefore you should *cultivate your heart*. The heart should be *cultivated* so that it is *clean*. Only if the heart is *clean* can a *pure* society emerge; if the heart has become *dirty* and gone *bad*, then the whole society will go *bad*. This is not idealism;[92] this is to talk about the *importance* of the heart. Instead of being completely determined by material conditions and social identity, the *human spirits* exert a strong influence on material conditions as well. If you want everyone to lead a good life, then, as the Chinese saying goes, "Do not impose on others what you do not desire yourself". The reason why Confucius and Confucian classics said this is that people should *compare their own hearts with others' hearts*.[93] "Other people

[92] Idealism in Chinese is 唯心论 *wei-xin lun*, literally it is the "only-heart theory".

[93] That is, to put oneself in somebody's shoes, or be empathic.

have the heart, and we should *conjecture it*".[94] If I think about *how others' heart would be* and *compare it with my own heart*, I would not do certain things. That is why the Chinese believe the heart is *extremely important*.

Why should Chinese culture talk emphatically about the heart? This is because, according to the Chinese, the heart is *equivalent to a kind of god*, which is very *changeable* and *all-inclusive*. Therefore, some philosophers, such as Lu Xiangshan and Wang Yangming, said: *My heart is the universe; the universe is my heart*. This is not idealism. Instead, it argues that if we want to build up a *human* society, in which everyone leads a happy life, we need to *expand our heart*, rather than employ a *selfish heart*. The selfish heart should have its *limit*. This limit is not to interfere with the *public heart*.

---

[94] It is worth noting that the Chinese original for the English translation *conjecture* is the compound word 忖度 *cunduo* 'speculate; conjecture; surmise', which is represented by two characters that have a spatial connotation. The first character is composed of the "heart" radical on its left and the character for "inch" on the right; the second character, with a change in pronunciation (*du*) and tone (from the second to the fourth), means "linear measure". Thus, by "face value", to "conjecture someone's heart" is to "measure it for its dimensions". That is, SPECULATING, CONJECTURING, or SURMISING IS MEASURING. Interestingly, in a related compound 忖量 *cunliang* 'think over; turn over in one's mind; conjecture; guess', the second character can mean "measure" when used as a verb (and "capacity", "volume", etc. when used as a noun); when its tone is changed (from the fourth to the second), it becomes a verb that again means "measure". In another related word 忖摸 *cunmo* 'reckon; estimate; conjecture', the second character means to "feel", "stroke" or "touch" with one's hand. The metaphorical mapping from bodily onto mental experience is very obvious. It is again interesting to note that, while the first character 忖 *cun* 'think over; ponder; speculate' contains the "heart" radical on its left, the second character of the compound 摸 *mo* 'feel; stroke; touch' contains the "hand" radical on its left side. Applying the metaphorical formula A IS B, we can say that the first character represents the target concept whereas the second represents the source concept. The metaphor so derived is THINKING OVER, PONDERING, or SPECULATING (IN ONE'S HEART) IS FEELING, STROKING, or TOUCHING (WITH ONE'S HANDS). That is, at the generic level, it is MENTAL FUNCTION IS MANUAL ACTION, or MIND IS BODY.

[95] The Chinese original for this saying is 人心不同，各有其面, that is, "People's hearts all differ, each (heart) having a unique face". This one is synonymous to another idiomatic saying 人心不同，各如其面'People's hearts differ just as their faces do'. In the former, however, the heart is said to have its own face, whereas in the latter people have their faces.

Zi Chan in the Spring and Autumn period said: *Human hearts differ with their unique faces*.[95] That is, the Chinese also affirm the *individual heart*. However, there also exists a *big collective heart* operating at the same time. This way, we will not be subject to the so-called absolute collectivism, nor will we be subject to absolute individualism. We should try to find a point of balance between the individual and the collective. *The function of finding this point of balance comes from the heart*. Zhang Zai in the eleventh-century Song dynasty wrote an essay titled "Enlarging the Heart", that is, one should try to *enlarge one's heart*. For instance, Zhuangzi in the Warring States period said: *Heaven and Earth and the ten thousand things are all one with me*. The Chinese often talk about *heaven and man being one*, and this also means that the *heart should be expanded*.

On the one hand, one should not *give up one's own unique heart*, and on the other hand, one should *enlarge one's heart so as to think of others*. Only in this way can we lead a *better*, and *more orderly*, life. This is because the Chinese do not very much believe that there is an after-life heaven and especially they, influenced by Confucianism, believe that this world is a true and real one. We should treasure and value it. If we treasure and value it, our heaven lies in this world, so does our hell. This is one view of the Chinese.

Mencius wrote the essay titled *Cleaning the Heart*, which argues, as we all know, that if we know *our own nature*, we know Heaven. Zhuangzi said, the *heart should be empty*; only after the heart is *empty* can the *Dao 'Way' enter into it*. As Mencius said, "Everyone has the *heart of compassion*". In "Benevolence, Righteousness, Propriety, and wisdom", *"Benevolence" refers to the heart that is most critical to humans*. Here, "Benevolence" means "*love people*", love other people; not only love yourself, but also love others. That is why, when Mencius talked about "heart", he would always talk about "*push*": people should *push their own heart*, and *the more they push it, the bigger it will become*, and *the further it will reach*, so that *it will include the whole society*. People like Hui Shi and Zhuang Zhou would *push it even further*; *their heart would become so big* that they would *love Heaven and Earth and the ten thousand things*.

This is the reason why *the Chinese's heart is so important*. It has *become* the *heart* that *everyone possesses*. It is *a special tradition in Chinese thought*. Under this tradition in China, there is no organized religion, and there is no tradition of church as organized and centralized as in the West. Something akin to the supreme commanding by the Roman Pope during the Middle Ages has never happened in China. Among the Chinese, *everyone is a heart*, and *everyone's heart is connectable with Heaven*. But you have to *cultivate your heart*. *If you do not cultivate it, your heart will become smaller and smaller, and more and more selfish*.

> Then, the society will be in turmoil.
>
> For this reason, I believe, *when we talk about the issue of values, the issue of spiritual values, in China, we must trace it to the heart*. It is almost *as important as the concept of God* in the West; it is *indispensable. Once it is lost, humans are not different from animals*. Therefore, in China, it has always been asserted that one should *clean one's heart*. In the past one hundred years in China, I think, *the heart has become a big problem* because we no longer believe ancient Chinese thought, *having lost the Chinese heritage*, whereas we cannot believe in the Western God either. Thus, our *heart has lost its locus*. Everyone's *heart has almost been seduced by material profits*. … Under such circumstances, *the Heart of China has been lost*. The *loss of the Heart is one of the biggest keys to the crises of Chinese culture* in the past one hundred years.
>
> I raise the issue of the heart to you all so that you can think it over. This is what I want to address for the New Year.

As is obvious, the author of the essay is trying to expound and promote a valuable moral heritage from ancient Chinese thought, which he thinks has been lost in modern and contemporary China. He argues for the restoration of this moral heritage from traditional Chinese culture (cf. Ch. 2). What is of special interest is the fact that this ethical heritage from ancient Chinese thought and traditional Chinese culture, which is abstract in nature, is understood in terms of *xin*, a term that originally denotes the heart organ, the most critical part of the body. According to the embodiment hypothesis, human cognition, including human language and thought, is embodied. That is, abstract values and concepts and subjective experiences and judgments are, at least partially, conceptualized, in one way or another, in terms of our body and grounded in our bodily experience in the physical and cultural world (see Gibbs 1994, 2006; Johnson 1987, 2007; Lakoff 1987a, 1993; Lakoff and Johnson 1980, 1999). In this particular case, the moral values and ethical codes that guide Chinese people's thought and action are conceptualized as originating in their heart and, for that matter, are talked about in terms of their heart. This is when cognitive mechanisms and structures such as metaphor and metonymy play a crucial role in the conceptualization of higher mental functions in terms of lower bodily experiences or, vice versa, in the projection of lower bodily experiences onto higher mental functions. It has been convincingly demonstrated in Cognitive Stylistics, and CL at large, that conceptual metonymy and metaphor, which involve mappings within one or across two domains, and conceptual blending based on the interaction between two or more domains, play important roles in the construction of both meaning and form in literary and nonliterary discourse (e.g. Barcelona 2005; Freeman 2002, 2006; Hamilton 2002; Nerlich 2005; Oakley 1998; Panther 2005; Popova 2002; Semino 2002; Steen 2002, 2004, 2007).[96] After all, the dichotomy between literary and everyday language is false since basic mental processes for language production and perception are not context-specific (Hamilton 2002).

In what follows, I analyze the Chinese cultural models for morality in terms of the heart, which in turn is understood as the central faculty of cognition and the organ of moral judgment. The Chinese cultural models for morality consist of propositions (i.e. cultural beliefs), metonymies, and metaphors involving the "heart" and demonstrating how the "heart" is understood in Chinese culture. Here is a list of relevant propositions, metonymies and metaphors involving "heart" that I formulated through close reading of the text:

(1) Propositions:
- a. HEART IS THE CENTRAL FACULTY OF COGNITION
- b. HEART IS THE LOCUS OF MORAL SENSES AND VALUES
- c. HEART IS THE SEAT OF THE INNER SELF
- d. HEART IS A MICROCOSM OF THE UNIVERSE
- e. HEART IS SACRED AND HOLY

(2) Metonymies:
- a. HEART STANDS FOR MORALITY (CONTAINER FOR CONTAINED)
- b. HEART STANDS FOR HUMAN NATURE (CONTAINER FOR CONTAINED)
- c. HEART STANDS FOR PERSON (PART FOR WHOLE)[97]

---

96 Both metaphor and metonymy can serve as inputs to conceptual blends. See e.g. Coulson and Oakley (2003), Fauconnier and Turner (1999), Grady (2005) for detailed discussions.

97 I must point out that there are different views on metonymy in CL. During the past decade, CL research on metonymy has virtually flourished (see, e.g., many of the contributions in Barcelona 2000a; Dirven and Pörings 2002; Otal, Navarro I Rerrando, and Bellés Fortuño 2005; Panther and Radden 1999; Panther and Thornburg 2003; Panther et al. in press; Radden and Panther 2004; Ruiz de Mendoza Ibáñez and Otal Campo 2002; Ruiz de Mendoza Ibáñez and Peña Cerval 2005a), although some of the basic issues involved are still under discussion and debate (see e.g. Ruiz de Mendoza Ibáñez and Otal Campo 2002; Panther 2006). The lack of consensus is reflected in the title of a recent theme session organized by Antonio Barcelona and Francisco Ruiz de Mendoza Ibáñez at the 10th International Cognitive Linguistics Conference held in Krakow, Poland, in July 2007: "What do we want to call a metonymy? An at-

(3) Metaphors:
- a. HEART IS AN OBJECT
  - HEART IS AN ORGANISM
  - HEART IS A CONTAINER
- b. BEING MORAL IS HAVING A CLEAN HEART
  - MORAL IS CLEAN (MORAL IS GOOD + GOOD IS CLEAN)
  - HEART FOR MORALITY IS AN OBJECT
- c. BEING IMMORAL IS HAVING A DIRTY HEART
  - IMMORAL IS DIRTY (IMMORAL IS BAD + BAD IS DIRTY)
  - HEART FOR MORALITY IS AN OBJECT
- d. BEING MORAL IS HAVING A BIG HEART
  - MORAL IS BIG (MORAL IS GOOD + GOOD IS BIG)
  - HEART FOR MORALITY IS AN OBJECT
- e. BEING IMMORAL IS HAVING A SMALL HEART
  - IMMORAL IS SMALL (IMMORAL IS BAD + BAD IS SMALL)
  - HEART FOR MORALITY IS AN OBJECT

In (3), indention denotes either subversions, as under (3a), or constituents, as under (3b–e). In proposition (1a), traditional Chinese culture believes that the heart is the central faculty of cognition (see Chs. 2 and 3). What this cultural belief, expressed in (1a) as a proposition, means is that the heart plays all-inclusive mental functions: feeling, thinking, knowing, understanding, reasoning, judging, etc. That is, the heart is the faculty of thought, knowledge, reason, and judgment, as well as emotion. Thus, for instance, it is believed that the heart is the locus of the human "spirits" (see Chs. 2 and 3), the totality of all spiritual and mental aspects of a person (line 7), including thinking, reasoning and judging (lines 29–31), and feeling and love (lines 49–54). The heart therefore guides one's actions (lines 12–14). Like one's "god", the heart is "all-inclusive", capable of comprehending the universe (lines 17–20). It is where one stores one's share of the Dao 'Way' (lines 48–49), with which one can relate to the whole society and connect with "Heaven and Earth and the ten thousand things" (lines 34–35, 57–59, 65–67). That is "the reason why the Chinese heart is so important" (line 60 and a number of other places).

---

tempt at building a consensus view on the limits of metonymy in Cognitive Linguistics". The theme session consists of 12 paper presentations, plus three discussions engaged in by the invited discussants Klaus-Uwe Panther, Zoltán Kövecses, and Günter Radden. As Radden indicated in his discussion, the views expressed at the theme session remained diversified and no consensus had been reached yet.

What is especially relevant to the essay under discussion is that the heart is culturally constructed as the locus of moral senses and values, as the proposition in (1b) states, since moral senses and values all originate and exist in the heart. This is why when the Chinese "talk about the issue of values, the issue of spiritual values", they "must trace it to the heart" (lines 70–71). This is also why the "function of finding the point of balance" between "the individual and the collective" comes from the heart (lines 29–31). While each heart exists as an "individual heart", it should also contribute to a "big collective heart", thus striking an ideal balance within itself between a "selfish heart" and a "public heart", or between an "individual heart" and a "collective heart" (lines 26–30). The so-called "individual heart" (lines 26–27) and "unique heart" (line 33) represent one's inner or true self, i.e. HEART IS THE SEAT OF THE INNER SELF, which is the proposition in (1c). That is also why it is said that "Human hearts differ with their unique faces" (lines 25–26).

As discussed earlier in Chapters 2 and 3, the human is believed to be a microcosm of the universe in ancient Chinese philosophy. However, since the heart, the critical organ of the body, is generally held as a metonymy or synecdoche for the person (see 2c; i.e. PART FOR WHOLE), it is then microcosmic of the whole universe, as the proposition (1d) states. Thus, as cited in this essay, as well as in Chapter 1, "My heart is the universe; the universe is my heart" (lines 19–20; cf. relevant discussions of Lu and Wang's theories of "heart" in 2.3.4). Notably, the heart is also a microcosm of the universe when it is able to "reflect" or "contain" Heaven and Earth and the ten thousand things (lines 58–59, 66–67). This is what Zhuangzi suggested when he said that "Heaven and Earth and the ten thousand things are all one with me" (lines 34–35): "the heart should be expanded" so as to "reflect" or "contain" the whole universe (line 35–37; see also lines 54–59).

In traditional Chinese culture, since the heart is believed to be the central faculty of cognition and the microcosm of the universe, it is therefore associated with special values to the extent of being sacred. This is what proposition (1e) says. Thus, it is regarded as "equivalent to a kind of god" (lines 17–18), comparable with "the concept of God in the West" (lines 71–72) when equated to the whole universe. After all, the heart performs the crucial guiding function: It guides people's thought and action (e.g. lines 12–14). That is why the whole society and culture would fall into crises and turmoil when the heart has "gone bad" and "lost its locus" (lines 4, 67–68, 76–78). Good moral values and right moral senses are not only the contents inside the heart, but also the prop beneath it. Without its support, the heart will "fall".

The essay under discussion displays a strong "current" of metonymies and metaphors in its "flow" of discourse. Two obvious cases of metonymies are HEART STANDS FOR MORALITY in (2a) and HEART STANDS FOR HUMAN NATURE in (2b), both of them being instances of the more general metonymy CONTAINER STANDS FOR CONTAINED. This is because the heart is believed to be the organ of moral judgment and human nature. Thus, morality, compassion, benevolence, and so forth, all originate and exist in the heart. The heart is therefore conceived of as the "container" of moral values and dispositions of human nature (see the relevant discussions in Ch. 2). By the prototypical metonymy CONTAINER FOR CONTAINED, the "heart" is used referentially in the place of "morality" and "human nature".[98] For instance, when the author speaks of "the Heart of China" being lost and the "loss of the Heart" being "one of the biggest keys to the crises of Chinese culture" (lines 79–81), he is talking about the loss of moral values and sense of morality in the minds of the Chinese. Also, when saying that having lost their heart "humans are not different from animals" (line 73), the author is referring to the loss of human nature. Besides, the HEART FOR PERSON metonymy in (2c), which is an instantiation of the more general PART FOR WHOLE metonymy, is also manifested in the essay. For example, the statement that in China "everyone is a heart" (line 66) is based on the metonymic conceptualization that the heart, which is the central and critical organ of the body, can stand for the whole person.[99] Similarly, we can say

---

98 However, I do not want to exclude the possibility of "heart" being interpreted as a metaphor of morality and human nature, especially considering the fact that the metonymy is embedded within the target domain of the metaphor HEART IS AN OBJECT (i.e. HEART FOR MORALITY IS AN OBJECT, as listed under 3b–e above). After all, "the distinction between metaphor and metonymy is scalar, rather than discrete: they seem to be points on a continuum of mapping processes" (Barcelona 2000b: 16). As I suggest elsewhere (Yu 2008a), metonymy is often the link between bodily experience and metaphor in the mapping process from concrete experience to abstract concepts: bodily experience → metonymy → metaphor → abstract concepts. In the past ten years or so, cognitive linguists have substantially demonstrated that metonymy is a more fundamental cognitive phenomenon than metaphor (Panther and Radden 1999b) and, very often, metaphor is motivated by metonymy (Barcelona 2000c; Panther 2006; Radden 2000; see also another view in Ruiz de Mendoza Ibáñez and Otal Campo 2002: 66–80).

99 Obviously, only certain parts of the body have the privilege of standing metonymically for the whole person (PART FOR WHOLE), and they carry different emphases and highlight different aspects in serving this function, e.g., in Chinese, the heart carries the emphasis on cognition and the inner self (Yu 2007a,

that the heart is a metonymy or synecdoche for the whole person when it is said that people's heart is "seduced by material profits" (lines 78–79). Furthermore, when the heart is said to be "the universe" (lines 19–20), it stands for the person who is the microcosm of the universe.

While moral values and human nature are conceptualized metonymically in terms of the "heart", the "heart" itself is also understood metaphorically as an object, i.e. HEART IS AN OBJECT (3a), which can get "lost" (lines 79–80). This metaphor has two different forms: HEART IS AN ORGANISM and HEART IS A CONTAINER. As the HEART AS ORGANISM metaphor entails, the heart needs to be "cultivated" (lines 2, 67). When the heart is cultivated, it will grow bigger and bigger. When one's heart is "big", one will "think of others" (lines 57–59). That is why it is always desirable to "expand" and "enlarge" the heart (lines 32–37). The heart may be so "expanded" and "enlarged" that it can include "other people", the "whole society", and even "Heaven and Earth and the ten thousand things" in it (lines 34–37, 39, 55–59). When that happens, the heart becomes a microcosm of the universe. If not cultivated, the heart will "become smaller and smaller, and more and more selfish" (lines 67–68). As an object, one heart can be "compared with" another heart so that the difference between the two can be "seen" in comparison (lines 12–15). The heart can also be "pushed", and the act of pushing causes it to be "expanded" and "enlarged" (lines 54–59). As is obvious, the heart as an "object" is a "container" too. Thus, it is "empty" inside so that the "Dao" or "Way" can "enter into it" (lines 48–49). The HEART AS CONTAINER metaphor is also at work when the heart is said to include the "whole society" or "Heaven and Earth and the ten thousand things" in it (lines 31–37, 57).

In addition, two metaphorical entailments of the heart-object are very obvious throughout the essay: its degree of cleanness and its size, both of them being directly related to the values of morality. These two aspects are expressed by two pairs of "complex metaphors", which are combinations of "primary metaphors" and other components (Grady 1997a, 1997b, 2005; Lakoff and Johnson 1999, 2003; see also section 1.5). According to Lakoff and Johnson (1999: 46), primary metaphors pair subjective experience and

---

2007b, 2008c), the face on social identity and outer self (Yu 2001), the hand on skills and capability of doing things (Yu 2003c), and the mouth and/or tongue on characteristics of talking or the function of the speaker (Yu 2007d). In the essay under discussion, when the author says that "Among the Chinese, everyone is a heart", he is emphasizing the fact that the heart as the central faculty of cognition is considered as the microcosm of the person.

judgment with sensorimotor experience, and each of them "has a minimal structure and arises naturally, automatically, and unconsciously through everyday experience by means of conflation, during which cross-domain associations are formed". So defined, a primary metaphor is an atomic component of the molecular structure of complex metaphors. In the essay under discussion, the first pair of complex metaphors is BEING MORAL IS HAVING A CLEAN HEART in (3b) and BEING IMMORAL IS HAVING A DIRTY HEART in (3c). They are respectively composed of the metaphors MORAL IS CLEAN and IMMORAL IS DIRTY in combination with HEART FOR MORALITY IS AN OBJECT (to be discussed in detail below). Parallel to the CLEANNESS metaphor is the SIZE metaphor. Again, there is a pair of complex metaphors: BEING MORAL IS HAVING A BIG HEART in (3d) and BEING IMMORAL IS HAVING A SMALL HEART in (3e). These two complex metaphors contain MORAL IS BIG and IMMORAL IS SMALL respectively in combination again with HEART FOR MORALITY IS AN OBJECT. That is why it is said in the essay that one needs to "cultivate" and "clean" one's heart. With a "clean" heart, one is morally good; if one has a "dirty" heart instead, one is morally bad (lines 1–4). In the same vein, the size of one's heart, which is variable, is also related to one's morality. A "big" heart is metaphorical of moral goodness, whereas a "small" heart suggests metaphorically the lack of morality (lines 31–37, 54–59, 67–68).[100] Therefore, it is morally good to "expand" and "enlarge" one's heart, and one is immoral when letting one's heart shrink to a smaller size. People with a "small heart" are mean and selfish, and necessarily narrow-minded; people with a "big heart" are caring and loving, and especially broad-minded, even having the whole universe "reflected" or "contained" in their heart. In sum, one's morality is distinguished, metaphorically, by two parameters of one's heart: its degree of cleanness and its size.

100 It is worth clarifying that metaphorical values are not absolute, and are affected by, and dependent on, context. For instance, in English, a person who is "big-hearted" is generous and kindly, but someone with a "big head" thinks too highly of one's own importance. It is also worth mentioning that 小心 *xiaoxin*, which literally means "small heart", has evolved into a neutral or more positive word in contemporary Chinese, meaning "take care; be careful; be cautious", whereas 小心眼 *xiaoxinyan* (lit. small heart-eye) is definitely derogatory, meaning "narrow-minded; petty" (see Ch. 4). Incidentally, 小人 *xiaoren* (lit. "small man" or "petty man") in Chinese means "base person; vile character; villain" (see also 2.3.3).

As mentioned above, complex metaphors are combinations of primary metaphors and other complex metaphors and of cultural beliefs. In the following I attempt to show in detail how they may be combined at different levels, taking (3b) and (3c) as examples.[101] The complex metaphors in (3b) and (3c) can be decomposed into its components at different levels of combination, as shown in (4) and (5) below, where indention denotes lower-level components:

(4) Complex metaphor BEING MORAL IS HAVING A CLEAN HEART

a.	MORAL IS CLEAN	(a complex metaphor)
b.	MORAL IS GOOD	(a proposition)
c.	GOOD IS CLEAN	(a primary metaphor)
d.	HEART FOR MORALITY IS AN OBJECT	(a complex metaphor)
e.	HEART IS THE SEAT OF MORALITY	(a proposition)
f.	HEART STANDS FOR MORALITY	(a metonymy)
g.	MORALITY IS A QUALITY	(a proposition)
h.	A QUALITY IS AN OBJECT	(a primary metaphor)

(5) Complex metaphor BEING IMMORAL IS HAVING A DIRTY HEART

a.	IMMORAL IS DIRTY	(a complex metaphor)
b.	IMMORAL IS BAD	(a proposition)
c.	BAD IS DIRTY	(a primary metaphor)
d.	HEART FOR MORALITY IS AN OBJECT	(a complex metaphor)
e.	HEART IS THE SEAT OF MORALITY	(a proposition)
f.	HEART STANDS FOR MORALITY	(a metonymy)
g.	MORALITY IS A QUALITY	(a proposition)
h.	A QUALITY IS AN OBJECT	(a primary metaphor)

The decomposition of (4), the complex metaphor BEING MORAL IS HAVING A CLEAN HEART, is interpreted as follows. This metaphor arises from the combination of two lower-level complex metaphors: (4a) and (4d). Of these two (4a), MORAL IS CLEAN, is composed of two lowest-level constituents: a proposition MORAL IS GOOD (4b) and a primary metaphor GOOD IS CLEAN (4c) that has arisen from pairing our subjective experience and judgment

---

[101] The analysis provided reflects my own thought developed along the line of a "decomposition account" of conceptual metaphors in terms of "primary metaphor" and "complex metaphor" (Grady 1997a, 1997b, 2005; Lakoff and Johnson 1999, 2003). I first applied such a decompositional analysis of conceptual metaphors to practice in Yu (2008b). I think such an approach is a good analytical tool for understanding how conceptual metaphors work and why some of them are widespread or even universal while others are culture-specific.

(GOOD and BAD) with our sensorimotor experience (CLEAN and DIRTY). As a primary metaphor, (4c) has a minimal structure that cannot be further decomposed, having arisen naturally from everyday experiential correlation in which cross-domain association (GOOD and CLEAN) is formed.[102] The complex metaphor HEART FOR MORALITY IS AN OBJECT in (4d) is also subject to further decomposition into four lowest-level constituents in (4e–h). Thus, (4d) is interpreted as follows. As a complex metaphor, its target itself contains a metonymy HEART STANDS FOR MORALITY (4f), which is based on (4e) HEART IS THE SEAT OF MORALITY. As a proposition, (4e) is a cultural belief that grounds (4f). That is, because the heart is the seat of morality, it can metonymically stand for morality (i.e. CONTAINER FOR CONTAINED). While MORALITY IS A QUALITY in (4g) is a proposition, A QUALITY IS AN OBJECT in (4h) is a primary metaphor that pairs subjective experience (QUALITY) with sensorimotor experience (OBJECT). So interpreted, the complex metaphor BEING MORAL IS HAVING A CLEAN HEART in (4) has two important bases: the proposition HEART IS THE SEAT OF MORALITY in (4e) is its cultural basis whereas the metonymy HEART STANDS FOR MORALITY is its metonymic basis. The complex metaphor in (4), combined from (4a) and (4d), involves metaphor-metonymy interaction, which can be diagramed as in Figure 7. As shown in this figure, the target of a metaphor contains a metonymy (i.e. HEART FOR MORALITY or CONTAINER FOR CONTAINED), which involves a target-in-source mapping (see Ruiz de Mendoza Ibáñez and Otal Campo 2002).

---

[102] The primary metaphors GOOD IS CLEAN and BAD IS DIRTY are manifested in our everyday language and thought. For instance, a *clean* copy of a document is one free of errors that are considered bad; a *clean* piece of work is a "good" job "well" done; a person who keeps a *clean* tongue is one that does not use "bad" language, or "dirty" words; a ship with *clean* lines is one with a "good" shape. What is related is the verb *cleanse* when it means "to remove something bad". Thus, e.g., to *cleanse* one's mind means to remove "bad" thoughts from one's mind. Similar metaphorical thought is reflected in such phrases as *ethnic cleansing*, where those who do the cleansing believe that people from other ethnic groups are not as "good" or, rather, "bad". During the so-called Cultural Revolution of China (1966–1976), a political movement is called *purification campaign*, where those who were considered as "bad" elements were "cleared" out of their units in order to "purify the class ranks". In a similar vein, the primary metaphors GOOD IS BIG and BAD IS SMALL are manifested in various expressions, e.g., *great* in "That's great!" can mean "very good" or "excellent" whereas *belittle* and *slight* can mean, at least in one sense, to cause to appear "worse" or "not as good".

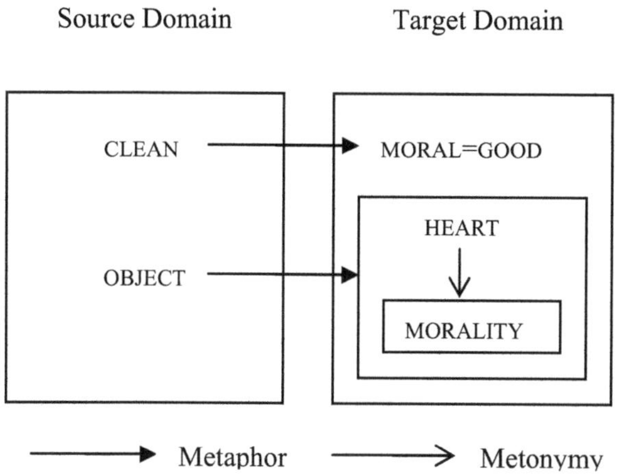

Figure 7. Metaphor-metonymy interaction in BEING MORAL IS HAVING A CLEAN HEART

The complex metaphor, BEING IMMORAL IS HAVING A DIRTY HEART, in (5) can be decomposed in exactly the same fashion. The only change consists in the complex metaphor in (5a), IMMORAL IS DIRTY, which is composed of a proposition IMMORAL IS BAD (5b) and a primary metaphor BAD IS DIRTY. In a similar vein, the complex metaphors in (3d) and (3e) can be analyzed by the same decompositional account.

As we can see, the text of the essay on the "heart" is structured by a group of metaphors and metonymies that form a scaffold of conceptual relations. The network of the metaphoric and metonymic mappings and entailments can be illustrated by Figure 8. As shown in this figure, the heart, which is culturally believed to be the central faculty of cognition in general and the organ of moral judgment and human nature in particular, stands metonymically for morality and human nature (CONTAINER FOR CONTAINED) and for the person (PART FOR WHOLE), represented by thick lines with open-headed arrows. That is, the heart as the container stands for the sense of morality and moral values stored inside it. Similarly, ever since the time of Mencius, human nature has been seen as the disposition of the heart, which is then supposed to be its container. Therefore, when the heart is "lost", human nature is gone, and humans are reduced to animals. Besides, the heart can stand for the whole person because it is the central faculty of cognition and the locus of the inner self.

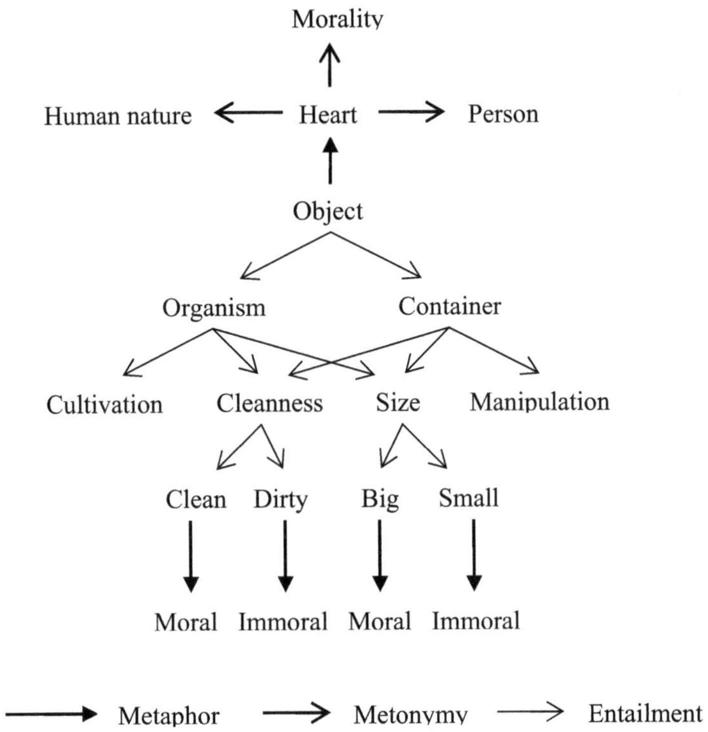

Figure 8. The network of metaphoric and metonymic mappings and entailments in the essay

It needs to be stressed that the "heart" in the essay under analysis is itself understood metaphorically in terms of "object". For one, it is an "object as organism" (i.e. a living being) and, for the other, it is an "object as container", although in effect these two cannot be completely separated from each other. Both versions of the OBJECT metaphor are bodily and metonymically based. In reality, the heart organ is indeed an "object", both as an organism and as a container. However, it is obvious that the author of the essay is not talking about our physical or biological heart. This heart-object can be "cultivated" as many organisms can, but our heart cannot. This heart-object can be "manipulated" (e.g. "compared", "pushed", "expanded", "given up", "lost", and it would "fall" when its "locus" of support is removed) as our heart cannot. Moreover, this heart-object can get "dirty" and be "cleaned" as our heart cannot. Finally, this heart-object can change its size drastically (e.g. "expanded" or "enlarged", or "becoming smaller and smaller") as our heart cannot. Both "organism" and "container" as metaphors of the heart have some entailments. Shown in the figure are highlighted ones in the essay. Thus, "Cultivation" is an entailment of "organism", and "Manipulation" is one of "container", whereas "Cleanness" and "Size" are shared by both. That is, both organism and container have physical dimensions, big or small, and they both can get dirty and be cleaned. It needs to be clarified that, although "Cultivation" and "Manipulation" are not listed as shared by "Organism" and "Container", these two entailments are tied to each other and can be possibly shared by both "Organism" and "Container". In reality, an organism can be a container and a container can be organic, as is our heart organ. Thus, for instance, when the author of the essay cites Mencius as saying that people should "push their heart" so that it will "become bigger" and "reach further", even to "include the whole society" in it, the heart here is simultaneously an "organism" being "cultivated" (i.e. it is capable of growth and change) and a "container" being "manipulated" (i.e. it seems to be "pushed" from within and able to "contain" more). After all, both "Cultivation" and "Manipulation" are entailments of "Object", the superordinate of "Organism" and "Container" in the figure.

In conclusion, the cultural models, consisting of those propositions, metonymies, and metaphors listed in (1–3), actually frame and structure the text of the essay like the skeleton of the body. It gives the essay its unity. More specifically, the scaffold of metaphoric and metonymic mappings and their entailments, as shown in Figure 8, provides the text with its coherence when the underlying conceptual metaphors and metonymies and their entailments are manifested at the surface level by linguistic expressions such as words, phrases, and sentences. These linguistics expressions, emphasized by the italic font type, also provide the text with its cohesion. In short, this essay is a good example of how underlying conceptual metaphors and metonymies help create coherence of a text through their conceptual governance of surface linguistic expressions (see, e.g., Barcelona 2005; Feng 2004: 150–238).

5.3. The heart in some poems on the "heart"

In this section I switch from prosaic discourse to poetic discourse in the hope that a study of poetic language will further flesh out the Chinese cultural conceptualization of the heart as the central faculty of cognition. Poetic language is characterized by its novel and original use of metaphors for aesthetic, artistic, and sometimes didactic purposes. The cognitive linguistic theory of conceptual metaphor claims that poetic metaphor basically uses the same cognitive mechanisms as everyday metaphor; what makes poetic metaphor special are its extension, elaboration, and combination of those mechanisms in unusual ways (Lakoff and Turner 1989). Since literary language shares much with ordinary language, and artistic usage with everyday usage, discoveries about one usually bear on the other (Lakoff 1987b). Sweetser (1992: 722) sees "strong arguments in favor of approaching artistic metaphor together with everyday metaphor, even via everyday metaphor" (see also Yu 2003b).

Taking the approach of Cognitive Poetics, Freeman (2000) argues that metaphors are not just strategies for enlivening otherwise prosaic language, but also markers of poets' ways of thinking about the world, and signs of their conceptual universe. "In linking the processes of language in literary text construction and interpretation to the processes of language in the workings of the human mind, cognitive poetics provides a bridge between the two fields" (Freeman 2006: 405). More broadly, Cognitive Poetics entails the following assumptions (p. 406):

> 1) the embodiment of the mind-brain constrains what humans can do; 2) human works, including works of art, are attempts to push the boundaries of what can be controlled, known, understood; 3) any study of cognitive issues in a specific work of art must be historically grounded. Thus, cognitive poetics includes not just interpretation from the reader's perspective, but creativity and cultural-historical knowledge of the writer too.
>
> At its best, cognitive poetics is Janus-faced: looking both toward the text and toward the mind. In so doing, it offers the possibilities of developing both a true theory of literature and contributing to a theory of mind.

In what follows, I will analyze a series of eight poems, with the series title *Depiction of the Heart* (心的描述).[103] The series was posted on Yahoo

[103] I now realize that there exist different versions of this series, posted on different websites, varying somewhat with its number of poems and the number of lines or the wordings within some individual poems. This is a characteristic of

China in 2005 by the poet with the pen name Ming Hushui, literally meaning "Clear Lake-water" (Ming 2005). Each of the poems has the key word *xin* 'heart' in its title. I cite them below with the Chinese originals each followed by my English translation. Once again I need to make it clear that the translations are rather literal and are not meant to reproduce the aesthetic and artistic effects of the originals. Instead, they are meant to preserve the Chinese metaphorical imagery and structure.

The goal of my analysis is limited to answering two questions: First, what is conceptualized in terms of the heart? Secondly, in what terms is the heart conceptualized? Both questions involve metaphor. In the first, the heart is the source domain concept that is mapped onto a target domain concept. In the second, the heart is the target concept onto which a source concept is mapped. As usual, however, what at first appears to be metaphorical may turn out to have derived from, or motivated by, a metonymy or a once literally accepted cultural belief. This analysis ignores the difference between metaphor and simile while concentrating on their similarity as mechanisms of conceptual connection and projection. I examine the poems one by one, in the order in which they were originally posted online.

《心事》

心事放在心里最温柔的地方，
虽然从未提起，但是永远不会忘记。
沧海桑田，事过境迁，心事仍然。
好象流浪的人，无论再怎样飘泊，
总是一心想着要回家。
人的家在你出生的地方，而心的家在哪里？

生活在繁华城市，居住在高楼大厦。
人不寂寞心孤独，白天人忙碌，夜晚心迷失。
物质越丰富，好象内心越痛苦。
最终，心事成了灵魂不敢去探望的角落。

Heart Matters

"Heart matters" are stored in the most gentle and softest place in the heart,

---

online publications: Authors can repost new versions of their works after changing, adding or cutting, a flexibility that is not readily available to print publications.

Although they have never been touched, they will never be forgotten either.
Time brings great changes to the world, but the heart matters remain unchanged.
A vagrant, no matter where he is wandering and drifting,
Will always think about returning home.
People's home is wherever they are born, but where is the heart's home?

Living in a busy city, and residing in a high-rising building.
One is not lonesome but one's heart feels lonely.
One is busy by day and one's heart is lost at night.
The richer one is materially, the more pain one seems to feel inside the heart.
Eventually, the heart matters become the corner that the soul dares not to visit.

Here, "heart matters" is the literal rendering of the Chinese compound word *xinshi* 心事, which usually refers to "things weighing on one's mind". "Heart matters" can be one's inmost thoughts and secret feelings that represent one's true self, as is the case in this poem. Obviously, they are kept somewhere inside the heart, and that "most gentle and softest place" is the seat of the inner self. The metaphors are HEART IS THE CONTAINER OF THOUGHTS AND FEELINGS and HEART IS THE CONTAINER OF THE SELF. This container, nevertheless, is also an organism inside of which one finds "the most gentle and softest place" (i.e. HEART IS AN ORGANISM). It also needs a "home" of its own, which of course is spiritual rather than physical in nature, and it has its own senses, subject to feeling "lonely" and "lost". That is, the heart as the seat of the inner self needs some kind of spiritual sustenance or locus to support itself. Otherwise, it will "fall" and "get lost" (cf. lines 75–81 of the "heart" essay above). The second stanza suggests the solitude of the heart of the modern man, who is materially rich but spiritually barren when living in a big city and leading a busy life. When one is making a lot of money, one has lost one's self, i.e. the heart, which is now compared to a "homeless vagrant". The inner self, where the "heart matters" are stored, is simply deserted by the soul. The contrast between day and night and between the outer and inner self highlights the "torn nature" or "split self" of modern man.[104] The outer self is above all the surface; it is the inner self or the "heart" that "matters". In short, what we see in this poem is consistent with the cultural conceptualization of the heart as the central faculty of cognition and in terms of an object, either a container or an organism.

---

[104] See Emmot (2002) for a detailed cognitive stylistic analysis of "split selves" in fiction and in medical "life stories".

《让心飞翔》

心象只大鸟，欲望是鸟食。
因为吃得太饱，而无法飞翔。
因为大家都在地上扑腾，
而忘记飞翔。
因为天长地久的生活在地上，
而不会飞翔。
我们都渴望自由，
但又不断地用欲望将自己束缚。
不断膨涨的欲望，
使我们的心越来越笨重。
飞翔的要求是越来越轻巧。
得到使我们的心不能飞翔，
得到有什么好呢？
失去使我们的心能够飞翔，
失去又有什么不好呢？
不会飞翔，就不会知道鸟的乐趣。
知道鸟的乐趣后，
才明白地上是多么的苦恼。
望着天上的鸟，减少自己的欲望。
试一试，让心飞翔！

Let the Heart Fly

The heart is a big bird while desires are bird food.
Because it has overeaten, it cannot fly.
Because all are hustling and bustling on the ground,
They forget to fly.
Because their everlasting and unchanging life is on the ground,
They are unable to fly.
We all long for freedom,
But also continuously bind ourselves with desires.
The forever swelling desires
Make our heart clumsier and heavier.
Flying needs being light and slim.
When gaining makes our heart unable to fly,
What is so good about gaining?
When losing makes our heart able to fly,
What is so bad about losing?
Unable to fly, one would not know the joy of a bird.

Only after one experienced the joy of a bird,
Would one know how vexing it is to be on the ground.
Looking at the birds in the sky, one should reduce one's desires.
Have a try, and let the heart fly!

This poem criticizes the immoral situation in modern life where people, according to the poet, are too much filled with desires for both material and immaterial gains (e.g. money, power, sex, and wealth). This is also a main theme of Yu's (2005) essay "On the 'Heart' for the New Year" that I analyzed in section 5.2. The obvious central metaphor in this poem is HEART IS A BIRD, which may appear to be quite novel and unique, although the metaphorical and symbolic image of "bird" for freedom has been around for a long time. A bird is after all an "organism" and a "container", especially in the sense of eating its food. The related metaphors are DESIRES ARE BIRD FOOD and DESIRES ARE FETTERS. Desires have long been associated with the heart in Chinese culture, ever since the time of the earliest Daoism and Confucianism (see Ch. 2). When it is argued that one should "empty" and "cultivate" one's heart, it is to remove or reduce desires in the heart. That is why, according to Zhuangzi, the "fasting of the heart" is necessary. As Guanzi argued, when one's heart is filled with desires, one will lose one's senses; thus, "things passing across the eyes will not be seen, and sounds coming to the ears will not be heard" (see 2.3.1). Mencius also asserted that for the nurturing of the heart there is nothing better than to reduce the number of desires in it (see 2.3.3).

As in this poem, when the bird has eaten too much food (i.e. desires), it is getting more fat, i.e. HAVING MORE DESIRES IS HAVING MORE WEIGHT. As a result, the folk theory assumes, the bird will become too heavy to fly, thus imposing restriction on its own freedom. In addition, therefore, the poem under analysis involves some more conceptual metaphors and their entailments, such as POSSESSION IS BODY WEIGHT, GAINING POSSESSION IS GAINING WEIGHT, LOSING POSSESSION IS LOSING WEIGHT, FREEDOM FROM WORRIES OF POSSESSION IS ABILITY TO FLY, RESTRICTION BY WORRIES OF POSSESSION IS INABILITY TO FLY, MENTAL FUNCTION IS PHYSICAL ACTION AND SPATIAL MOVEMENT. As we know, according to the cultural beliefs and assumptions of the Chinese, the heart is the central faculty of cognition, which is supposed to perform all mental functions. As Mencius' famous saying goes, the organ of heart is for thinking. Thinking is the salient mental function that the heart performs, as much as flying is the bird's salient physical function. From the metaphor MENTAL FUNCTION IS PHYSICAL ACTION AND SPATIAL MOVEMENT, we can infer that the "freedom" longed for in this poem, the "freedom to fly" that our heart tends to lose because it is getting too heavy and too clumsy, is not physical freedom, but freedom to think and understand and to make moral judgments. According to the embodiment hypothesis, abstract mental functions can be conceptualized as physical actions or spatial movements. In this particular case, it is the heart-bird being able to fly. Finally, it must be pointed out that the heart in this poem is also metonymic for the person as a whole, i.e. HEART STANDS FOR PERSON. For example, while the heart-bird has overeaten and is therefore unable to fly, people are "hustling and bustling on the ground" and "forget to fly". They are also "unable to fly" because "their everlasting and unchanging life is on the ground". While "We all long for freedom", we "also continuously bind ourselves with desires". Here, the borderline between "us" and "our heart" is blurred. We are our heart, and our heart is us. The conceptual mechanism in play is the metonymy HEART FOR PERSON. As the essay discussed above says, "Among the Chinese, everyone is a heart, and everyone's heart is connectable with Heaven".

《人心》

心坏了，人只是一堆肉。
虽然还能行动，但是已经不是在生活。
道德润滑着心，失去道德人心必废。
道德好象心与心之间做人工呼吸的那口气，
帮助别人救活自己。
每一颗心象一口井，
道德就是使之连成一体的地下水源。
水源一断，井必枯干。
文明是人行为的准则，
道德是心交流的法则。
如果心枯干了，就向心灵深处挖掘，
直达道德之源吧！
生活中的人心，好象行驶中汽车的发动机。
只要汽车能正常行驶，就不论发动机的优劣。
只要人能道德生活，就不论心的贵贱。

The Human Heart

If the heart has gone bad, the human is just a pile of flesh.
Although one can still move around, one is no longer leading a life.
Morality lubricates the heart; having lost morality the human heart will become waste.

Morality is like that breath of artificial respiration between two hearts,
Helping someone else also saves oneself.
Every heart is like a well.
Morality is the underground water source that connects them.
Once the water source runs out, the wells must run dry.
Civilization is the code of conduct for humans,
Whereas morality is the law of communication between the hearts.
If the heart runs dry, dig deep into the heart
Till reaching the source of morality!
The human heart in life is like the engine of a running automobile.
As long as automobiles can run well, we should not talk about how good or bad their engines are.
As long as one can lead a moral life, we should not talk about how noble or base this person's heart is.

This piece again focuses on morality metonymically associated with the heart as its container, i.e. HEART FOR MORALITY or, more generally, CONTAINER FOR CONTAINED. When the heart, or the organ of moral values and moral judgment, "has gone bad", the human being is reduced to "a pile of flesh" or a walking corpse. This also highlights the critical functions of the heart as the locus of human nature and the central faculty of cognition. Metaphorically, morality is understood as an essential element or force, i.e. MORALITY IS AN ESSENTIAL ELEMENT or MORALITY IS AN ESSENTIAL FORCE, with a variety of source concepts or images including lubricant, breath/air, water, binding force (of the law), and motive force (of the engine). For instance, a salient pair of metaphors is HEART IS A WELL and MORALITY IS WATER. Here the metaphors fall again into the convention where the heart, now the target concept, is conceptualized as a source of water (see Ch. 4) and morality as water from that source (see also Feng 2004: 154–168). If the morality-water runs out, the heart-well will run dry. Whereas the HEART AS WELL metaphor is conventional, the metaphor HEART IS AN ENGINE (OF AN AUTOMOBILE) at the end of the poem seems to be quite novel. Nonetheless, an engine is still a kind of source, a source of force or power, or horsepower to be more exact. Once the engine breaks down, the whole automobile becomes a heavy piece of junk (cf. "a pile of flesh"). Note that the MECHANICS metaphor is consistent with the earlier line: "Morality lubricates the heart; having lost morality the human heart will become waste". In the case of "morality is the law of communication between hearts", MORALITY IS A BINDING FORCE that regulates the interaction between human hearts or between human beings as a whole if we see "hearts" as metonymically standing for humans (i.e. HEART FOR PERSON or

PART FOR WHOLE). Moreover, this poem also deploys another metaphor for morality, MORALITY IS BREATH. The source concept, BREATH, is a kind of air, which is an essential element of life, as much as water.

《洗心》

衣服脏了，可以用水洗净。
心污染了，用什么清洗？
是什么污染了我们的心呢？
道德高尚的人，心一定纯洁。
一切不道德的行为，会把我们的心污染。
被污染的心，就是我们痛苦的根源。
能把心洗净，就找到了幸福的源泉。
怎么样把心洗净呢？
心是被人不道德的行为所污染，
做个有道德的人，就能把心洗净。
现在追求的是自由啊，人性解放啊。
什么是道德呢？
树木连根拔起，大地离它远去，
树会手舞足蹈欢呼自由解放吗？
人扎根在道德。

Wash the Heart

When our clothes are dirty, we can wash them with water.
When our hearts are polluted, what can we wash them with?
What has polluted our hearts?
Morally noble people must have pure hearts.
All immoral conduct can pollute our hearts.
The polluted hearts are the sources of our pain.
If we can wash and clean our hearts, we have then found the fountainhead of happiness.
How can we wash and clean our hearts?
Our hearts are polluted by immoral conduct.
Be a moral person and we can wash and clean our hearts.
Nowadays people seek for freedom, for emancipation of humanity.
What is morality then?
When trees are uprooted, away from the earth,
Will they dance for joy and cheer for their freedom and liberation?
Humans are rooted in morality.

This is another poem focused on the heart and morality. The metaphors in this poem overlap to some extent those found in the essay on "heart" discussed in section 5.2. These are conceptual metaphors of morality in terms of cleanness, i.e. MORAL IS CLEAN and IMMORAL IS DIRTY, which are also complex metaphors composed respectively as follows: MORAL IS GOOD + GOOD IS CLEAN and IMMORAL IS BAD + BAD IS DIRTY (see 5.2). As analyzed in the preceding section, being moral and immoral is culturally conceived of as a trait of the heart and the heart is culturally viewed as the seat of morality and moral values (hence, the metonymy HEART STANDS FOR MORALITY). Furthermore, the heart itself is also understood metaphorically as an "object", i.e. HEART IS AN OBJECT, which can get "dirty" and be "cleaned" by washing. Therefore, we have here the related complex metaphors at a higher level: BEING MORAL IS HAVING A CLEAN HEART and BEING IMMORAL IS HAVING A DIRTY HEART.

Besides, the heart is also a "source of water", i.e. HEART IS A SOURCE OF WATER, where water refers metaphorically to morality and emotion or feeling, i.e. MORALITY IS WATER, and EMOTION/FEELING IS WATER. Thus, a moral person can get the heart "washed clean", and that being done, one will find one's heart a "fountainhead of happiness". In terms of emotions and feelings, the metaphor HEART IS A SOURCE OF WATER is equivalent to the more propositional formula HEART IS THE SEAT OF EMOTIONS AND FEELINGS. Because the heart as a source of water can be "polluted" by immorality or immoral conduct, we have the following pair of metaphors that connect morality with the heart and its feeling or emotion: A POLLUTED HEART IS THE SOURCE OF PAIN and A CLEANED HEART IS THE SOURCE OF HAPPINESS. The poet here is referring to the "pain" and "happiness" at one's core of inner self, at a higher spiritual, rather than a simple physical, level. That is, one can go through much physical hardship and pain while being moral, but one feels happy "deep in the heart" where one's inner self is. Conversely, one can have much sensual fun and pleasure being immoral, but one feels guilty and troubled by one's conscience, which would be one's "good heart" in Chinese (see 4.3.3).

Finally, morality is also understood as another essential element, earth, in which humans as trees should be rooted: i.e. MORALITY IS EARTH, HUMANS ARE TREES (or A HUMAN IS A PLANT), and HEART IS THE ROOT (OF A PLANT) (see 4.3). When trees are uprooted from the earth, they will wither and die. That is to say, humans (trees) will "die" when their hearts (roots) are void of (uprooted from) morality (earth). Note that the poet, apparently speaking against people nowadays seeking after "freedom" and "emancipation of humanity", is actually criticizing them for their loss of morality in so doing. Seeking after "freedom" and "emancipation of humanity" without the "binding force" of morality is of course negative to human society as a whole.

《善心》

如果胸怀善心，不用人人如近敌。
人无善心，时刻小心，
惊醒得象睁着眼睛睡觉的鱼一样。
人无善心，日夜提防，
惊慌得象过街的小鼠一样。
人无善心，生活就象冬天睡觉裹铺盖。
折腾了一夜，也只为保暖。
对于名利，我们总是争在人先。
对于善心，我们往往落在人后。
如果胸怀善心，万物之灵的人类，
就不用再去符合动物的生存规律。
动物永远不能象人一样文明生活，
人也不应该象动物一样野蛮生存。
人类有多少善心，世界就有多么美好。
如果胸怀善心，
人生收获的就不再只是过眼烟云。
善心源于人类本性，善行符合自然规律。
持之以恒，终将获得最好的回赠。
对胸怀的善心，从未置疑。
虽然磨难不断，但是也有机会经常亲近真理。
这是人生最大的安慰。

The Kind Heart

If one harbors a kind heart in one's chest, one doesn't have to feel as if everyone else is an enemy at hand.
Without a kind heart, one will have to be small-hearted (i.e. suspicious, small-minded) all the time,
And be as alert as a fish sleeping with its eyes open.
Without a kind heart, one will have to be on high guard day and night,
And be as alarmed as a mouse running across the street.
Without a kind heart, one is leading one's life as if sleeping in the cold,
Turning and tossing the whole night just to keep oneself warm.
For fame and gain, we usually strive to be the first.
For a kind heart, we usually lag behind.

Harboring a kind heart in the chest, humans, as the soul of ten thousand things,
No longer have to abide by the laws of existence for animals.
Animals can never lead a civilized life as humans,
Nor should humans live for a barbarous existence of animals.
How much kind heart humans have, that's how much beauty the world will have.
If we harbor a kind heart in our chest,
What we harvest in our life will no longer be as transient as fleeting clouds.
The kind heart originates in human nature, and virtuous behavior accords with the law of nature.
Perseverance will eventually win the best reward.
The kind heart harbored in the chest has never been in doubt.
Although one has to go through constant hardships, one can still be in frequent touch with truths.
And that's the greatest consolation in life.

This poem promotes kindness and goodness, which are the traits of benevolence as an important moral virtue, in terms of the "heart harbored in the chest". Following Mencius' philosophical tradition, the poet suggests that benevolence is part of human nature, which is originally good and is localized in the heart. Thus, people should "preserve the heart" so as to "cultivate human nature", and "exhaust the heart" in order to "understand human nature" (see Ch. 2). Since benevolence (i.e. being loving and caring and eager to do good) is part of human nature, it is therefore a disposition of the human heart, which is then metonymically referred to as the "container" of benevolence. However, as Mencius argued, the heart of benevolence, as a "valuable object or possession", can get "lost". When the kind or benevolent heart is no longer harbored in our chest, "everyone else is an enemy at hand", and humans would "live for a barbarous existence of animals". In terms of metonymy and metaphor, HEART STANDS FOR HUMAN NATURE and HEART IS A VALUABLE POSSESSION (i.e. an object). Once the heart is lost, human nature is gone, and humans are reduced to lower animals. The metaphor A HUMAN BEING IS AN ANIMAL (fish, mouse) in this poem is part of the Great Chain metaphor (Lakoff and Turner 1989), based on a folk theory of the nature of beings and things, which are placed hierarchically from the top to the bottom of a scale: human, animal, plant, inanimate object. Humans are distinguished from animals by their "higher" faculties, including moral sense and rational capacity, which are traditionally localized in the heart in Chinese culture.

《心锁》

无数心锁，锁住心灵无数秘密。
寻找那把万能钥匙，是人生最重要的事。
人生真真假假，心锁却是实实在在。
没有开锁钥匙，就永远被拒之在外。
虽然居住在家里，但是流浪在心门之外。
看不见的幸福，不是在看得见的家里，
而是在看不见的心里。
打开心锁，里面有人生的真象和真实的人生。
是什么把看不见的心锁住？
又是什么能把心门打开？
一切奥秘的答案，都在时间里。
有的解开的时间短，
有的解开的时间长。

The Heart Locks

Countless heart locks have locked countless secrets in the heart.
The most important thing in human life is to find that omnipotent key.
Human life is a mixture of truth and falsehood, but the heart locks are real and solid.
If you don't have the key to these locks, you will be forever kept outside.
Although you live in your home, you are roaming outside the door of the heart.
Invisible happiness is not in the visible home,
But in the invisible heart.
If you open the heart lock, inside are the truth of human life and the true human life.
What locks the invisible heart?
And what can open the door of the heart?
All the solutions to the mysteries lie in time.
Some take shorter time to solve,
And some take longer.

This poem highlights the metaphorical conceptualization of the heart as the "container" of "countless secrets" that has a "door" that is usually "locked". Inside the heart-container lies what is true and real – "the truth of human life and the true human life". However, it seems that this heart is not always accessible even to the person who owns it because this person does not necessarily have the "omnipotent key" to the "countless heart locks". Without it the person can only be "roaming outside the door of the heart".

The overall image this poem invokes is the "split self": the outer self versus the inner self, the external versus the internal, the physical versus the spiritual, and the false life versus the true life. We are confronted with a dual understanding of the self, but this duality is defined in terms of the exterior versus the interior of the heart as a "container". Central to the poem are the metaphors HEART IS THE CONTAINER OF TRUE SELF and HEART IS THE CONTAINER OF TRUE LIFE. Another important duality is the contrast between "home" and "heart". The "home" is metonymic for the physical and material world, i.e. HOME STANDS FOR THE MATERIAL WORLD, whereas the "heart" represents metonymically one's spiritual and mental world, i.e. HEART STANDS FOR THE SPIRITUAL WORLD. It is emphasized that real happiness, which is "invisible" in nature, lies in the "invisible heart" rather than the "visible home". What is "invisible" may appear mysterious, because it is not easily accessible, but it stands on the side of "time" as being eternal. It can be interpreted that "the solutions to the mysteries" actually come from that "omnipotent key", which is the faith in all the spiritual values, including moral values. That is, FAITH IN SPIRITUAL VALUES IS THE OMNIPOTENT KEY TO COUNTLESS HEART LOCKS. Only when one firmly believes in the spiritual values can one reach into the depth of the heart, or the "invisible heart", where one's true self is located, "the truth of human life and true human life" are stored, and real happiness is felt.

《心泉》

生命是水，心是泉。
本有先天循环，置之不用而枯干。
井无水，为心枯。
清澈见底，为心空。
心枯无用，心空无所不能。
凡心象染缸，把万物染成同一颜色。
圣心象清泉，还原万物本来面目。
心空如手空，只是无事做，不是没有手。

The Heart Wellspring

Life is water and the heart is a wellspring.
Originally it moves in natural cycles, but it may run dry when no longer in use.
When there is no water in the well, the heart is dry.
When the water is so clear that the bottom of the well can be seen, the heart is empty.

Whereas a dry heart is useless, an empty heart is capable of anything and everything.
A worldly heart is like a dye vat that turns ten thousand things into one color.
A holy heart is like a clear wellspring that turns ten thousand things into their original looks.
When the heart is empty, it's similar to the hands that are empty,
Doing nothing because nothing needs doing, not because there are no hands.

This poem again characterizes the heart metaphorically as a "well" or a "wellspring" (HEART IS A WELL), i.e. a water source, and life as water from that source (LIFE IS WATER). In line with the ancient Chinese philosophical tradition, the poet suggests that an "empty heart" is different from a "dry heart". The latter is a "well" running out of water, whereas the former is a "well" with clear and pure water that is both reflective and receptive. The poet makes a further distinction between the "worldly heart" and the "holy heart" by employing two metaphors: WORLDLY HEART IS A DYE VAT (again a "container") and HOLY HEART IS A WELLSPRING (a "container" and a "source"). While the "dye vat" is distorting, imposing, and rejecting, the "wellspring" is clarifying, reflecting, and receiving. These are the metaphorical entailments projected onto the "worldly heart" and the "holy heart" respectively. Ideally, the function of the heart is to understand the world as it truly is. The "worldly heart", however, cannot do it; on the contrary, it only distorts the world with misunderstandings. In contrast, the "holy heart" is capable of "washing" away the "mud" covering the "ten thousand things", and restoring them into their "original looks". This cognitive function of the heart qualifies it to be microcosmic of the universe. With its water source image, this poem brings the heart to the fore as the central faculty of cognition. As a "water well", the heart works at its best in performing its cognitive tasks when it is "empty" and "clear", i.e. when it is "doing nothing", as much as the empty hands.[105] The water image of the heart can be traced back to Zhuangzi and Xunzi over two thousand years ago. The maximal message, one that has been passed down through Chinese philosophical tradition, is: "Use the heart, or it will run dry" (see 2.2.1; 4.6, esp. the discussion on Example 160).

While highlighting the cognitive functions of the heart as knowing and understanding the world, the poem is constructed around a primary metaphor KNOWING IS SEEING (or UNDERSTANDING IS SEEING), which brings

---

105 For a detailed discussion from a cognitive linguistic perspective of Daoist concept of *wuwei* (无为), which literally means "doing nothing", see Slingerland (2003).

into play a cluster of metaphorical entailments (e.g., IMPEDIMENT TO KNOWLEDGE IS BLOCKAGE OF SIGHT, ADDITION TO KNOWLEDGE IS ACCESS TO SIGHT, THOROUGH KNOWLEDGE IS CLEAR SIGHT, SUPERFICIAL KNOWLEDGE IS MURKY SIGHT, DEEP KNOWLEDGE IS INSIGHT). Whether or not one can know or understand the world depends almost entirely on the conditions of the heart, the central faculty of cognition: whether it is a "dry well" or an "empty well", a "dye vat" or a "wellspring". On the one hand, a "dry well" is useless because it is lifeless (LIFE IS WATER), and a "dye vat" is distorting because it imposes one color onto ten thousand things (DISTORTING IS DYEING). On the other hand, an "empty well" is full of clear and pure water that is capable of "reflecting and receiving" the whole universe (KNOWLEDGE IS SIGHT), and a "wellspring" is capable of "washing away and clarifying" which that is covering the truth (TO KNOW OR UNDERSTAND IS TO CLARIFY [IN ORDER TO SEE]).

《心灵》

每个人心中都装着一轮明月，
尽管不是都能照亮自己的眼睛。
既使是萤火之光，也会令人温暖，无法割舍。
心灵是人的圣殿，理应金壁辉煌。
我们把身外的浮云看重，把身内的宝藏看轻。
好象太阳在银河中寻找光明。
地球的昼夜，让光明之源清醒，
原来宇宙在随着自己旋转。
太阳唯一要寻找的光明就是太阳自己，
心灵唯一要寻找的宝藏就是心灵本身。

The Heart (i.e. The Heart-Mind or The Heart-Soul)

In everyone's heart there is a bright full moon,
Even though it cannot illuminate everyone's own eyes.
Even if it's just a glimmering light, it still warms people, who will think it's indispensable.
The heart is the holy palace of the human being, and ought to be resplendent and magnificent.
We take the floating clouds outside our body too heavily, and take the precious treasures inside our body too lightly.
It's like the sun looking for light in the Milky Way.
The day and night of the Earth make the source of light aware
That the universe is revolving around itself.
The only light that the sun should seek is the sun itself;

The only precious treasure that the heart should seek is the heart itself.

This poem evokes several metaphorical images that are connected with one another. Primarily, HEART IS A CONTAINER and HEART IS A SOURCE. As a container, the heart has "a bright full moon" in it that is also a source of light enabling people to "see" things (HEART IS A SOURCE OF LIGHT). As a container, the heart is a "resplendent and magnificent" "holy palace" that ought to be glittering and glistening too. As a container, the heart has "precious treasures" stored or hidden in it (i.e. SPIRITUAL VALUES ARE TREASURES and MENTAL FUNCTIONS ARE TREASURES), and the "precious treasures" are gleaming and glimmering (i.e. "enlightening") as well (cf. 2.2.3). As a source of light, the heart is like the "sun" that shines and radiates, enlightening others around it in the system (cf. 3.2.1). It is the sunlight that makes the earth experience "day and night". The CONTAINER OF TREASURES and SOURCE OF LIGHT metaphors, which have existed for over two thousand years, contribute to the Chinese cultural conceptualization of the heart as the central faculty of cognition. This cultural conceptualization can be summarized by a single ancient saying, which represents a time-honored cultural belief, i.e. "The heart governs the spiritual light" (心主神明), discussed in detail in Chapters 2 and 3. If the human heart is the "sun" (i.e. HEART IS THE SUN), why should it, or the person who possesses it, seek around after "valuable treasures"? According to the poet, material treasures outside the body are simply "floating clouds" whereas spiritual values inside the heart are truly "precious treasures". It is worth noting that the poet, in this poem, talks about the human "heart" in terms of the moon, the sun, the Milky Way, and the universe. This line of thinking reflects the ancient notion of the unity and correspondence between the universe and the human, central to and throughout the history of Chinese thought. In the context of this poem, the connection or correlation between the universe and the human also raises the status of the "heart" to being microcosmic of the universe.

In sum, these poems have a heavy moral component as well as a robust mental component, and they treat the heart as the human agent or human subject, and as the organ of moral judgment. They reflect a cultural conceptualization of the heart housed in the cultural models consisting of numerous propositions, metonymies, and metaphors, which I list below. Note that, the list of metaphors in (8) consists only of those directly involving the "heart", either as the source or the target concept.

(6) Propositions:

a. HEART IS THE CENTRAL FACULTY OF COGNITION
b. HEART IS THE LOCUS OF MORAL SENSES AND VALUES
c. HEART IS THE SEAT OF THE INNER SELF
d. HEART IS THE MICROCOSM OF THE UNIVERSE
e. HEART IS SACRED AND HOLY

(7) Metonymies:

a. HEART STANDS FOR PERSON (PART FOR WHOLE)
b. HEART STANDS FOR MORALITY (CONTAINER FOR CONTAINED)
c. HEART STANDS FOR HUMAN NATURE (CONTAINER FOR CONTAINED)
d. HEART STANDS FOR SPIRITUALITY (CONTAINER FOR CONTAINED, in contrast with HOME STANDS FOR MATERIALITY, or PART FOR WHOLE)

(8) Metaphors:

a. HEART IS A SOURCE (OF WATER, POWER, OR LIGHT)
  HEART IS A WELL
  HEART IS A WELLSPRING
  HEART IS AN ENGINE
  HEART IS THE SUN (AND MOONLIGHT)
b. HEART IS AN OBJECT
  HEART IS AN ORGANISM
    HEART IS A BIRD
  HEART IS A CONTAINER
    HEART IS A BIRD
    HEART IS A HOUSE
    HEART IS A HOLY PALACE
    HEART IS A DYE VAT
c. BEING MORAL IS HAVING A CLEAN HEART
  MORAL IS CLEAN (MORAL IS GOOD + GOOD IS CLEAN)
  HEART FOR MORALITY IS AN OBJECT
d. BEING IMMORAL IS HAVING A DIRTY HEART
  IMMORAL IS DIRTY (IMMORAL IS BAD + BAD IS DIRTY)
  HEART FOR MORALITY IS AN OBJECT

As we can see, this list of propositions, metonymies and metaphors overlaps, significantly, the one formulated for the essay in 5.2. First and foremost, the propositions in (6) are identical with those in (1). Thus, these poems, like the essay, manifest the traditional cultural belief that the heart is the central faculty of cognition (6a). Under this overarching belief, the heart as the seat of thoughts and feelings assumes various mental and emotional functions. Two propositions listed in (6) are HEART IS THE LOCUS OF MORAL SENSES AND VALUES (6b) and HEART IS THE SEAT OF THE INNER

SELF (6c). The proposition (6d) that HEART IS THE MICROCOSM OF THE UNIVERSE finds its strongest expression in the last poem, as discussed above. The proposition HEART IS SACRED AND HOLY is manifested linguistically, for instance, by the expressions "holy heart" and "holy palace". Remember that in ancient Chinese thought the heart was already believed to be the "holy palace" of the "spiritual light" (see Chs. 2–3). The metonymies in (7) are the same as those in (2) except that (7) has one more metonymy, HEART STANDS FOR SPIRITUALITY, which contrasts with HOME STANDS FOR MATERIALITY. The list of metaphors in (8) is longer than that in (3) because it contains more metaphors with concrete source concepts for the "heart". The conceptual network composed of metonymic and metaphoric mappings and entailments involving the "heart" as either the source or the target is illustrated by Figure 9.

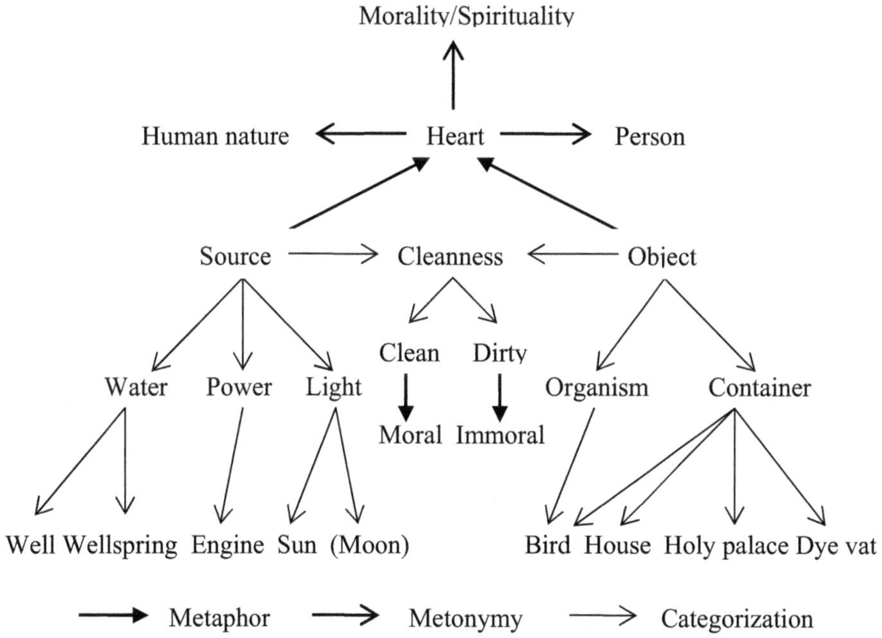

Figure 9. The network of metaphoric and metonymic mappings and entailments in the poems

It is obvious that this figure is more complicated than Figure 8 in 5.2. As indicated in this figure, "heart" still metonymically stands for "Person"

(7a), "Human nature" (7b), and "Morality" (7c), but "Spirituality" (7d), which contrasts with "Materiality" and supersedes "Morality" (i.e. spiritual values include moral values), is added. As in this figure, "heart" itself is conceptualized metaphorically both as a "source", i.e. HEART IS A SOURCE (8a), and as an "object", i.e. HEART IS AN OBJECT (8b). When it is a "source of water", HEART IS A WELL and HEART IS A WELLSPRING. When it is a "source of power", HEART IS AN ENGINE; and when it is a "source of light", HEART IS THE SUN (and in another case it radiates the light of the moon, which it contains). Note that these "source" concepts are related: Both water and light are forms of energy and can be transformed into power. Secondly, when "heart" is an "object", the metaphor has two separate cases: HEART IS AN ORGANISM and HEART IS A CONTAINER. Under the CONTAINER version, HEART IS A HOUSE, A HOLY PALACE, or A DYE VAT. More exactly, HEART IS A DYE VAT should be WORLDLY HEART IS A DYE VAT, which forms a contrastive pair with a SOURCE metaphor, HOLY HEART IS A WELLSPRING. Under the ORGANISM version is the metaphor HEART IS A BIRD, which, together with its related metaphor DESIRES ARE BIRD FOOD and DESIRES ARE FETTERS (see 10 below), activates a series of metaphorical entailments, as listed below in (9):

(9) HEART IS A BIRD
DESIRES ARE BIRD FOOD
DESIRES ARE FETTERS

	SOURCE		TARGET
a.	physical or spatial action	→	mental or intellectual function
b.	bustling on the ground	→	leading a material life
c.	flying in the sky	→	leading a spiritual life
d.	eating more food	→	having more desires
e.	eating less food	→	having fewer desires
f.	getting fat	→	satisfying desires
g.	reducing fat	→	reducing desires
h.	body weight	→	possession
i.	gaining weight	→	gaining possession
j.	losing weight	→	losing possession
k.	a heavier and stouter body	→	more possession
l.	a lighter and slimmer body	→	less possession
m.	ability to fly	→	freedom from possession
n.	inability to fly	→	restriction by possession

It is worth noting that while it is good to have a "big heart", it is not good to have a "fat heart" (see Ch. 4). A "big heart" that is "empty" has much room for the Dao 'Way' whereas this is not true with a "fat heart".

Finally, as shown in the middle of Figure 9, both HEART AS A SOURCE and HEART AS AN OBJECT are characterized by the entailment of "Cleanness", i.e. a "source" or an "object", with its physical existence, can be "clean" or "dirty", and this distinction has to do with morality that originates and exists in the heart. Therefore, (8) contains the following metaphors, which are identical with (3b) and (3c) in the preceding section: BEING MORAL IS HAVING A CLEAN HEART (8c) and BEING IMMORAL IS HAVING A DIRTY HEART (8d). They can of course undergo the same decompositional analysis as in (4) and (5). These metaphors, and those of the heart and emotions and feelings, for instance, result in the following pair of complex metaphors found in one of the poems:

(10) a. A POLLUTED HEART IS THE SOURCE OF PAIN
b. A CLEANED HEART IS THE SOURCE OF HAPPINESS

In this pair, EMOTIONS OR FEELINGS ARE WATER, whereas HEART IS A SOURCE from which emotions or feelings "flow". Whether it is a positive or negative feeling that "flows" out of the heart-source depends on whether this "source of water" is "polluted" by immorality or "cleaned" by morality. In the poem "The Heart Wellspring", the heart is also conceptualized as the source of life, which is understood as water from the heart-wellspring. Thus, a wellspring that has run dry is lifeless and useless.

In addition to the metaphors in (8) that have "heart" as either the source or the target concept, the poems in the series actually involve many more metaphors, as already mentioned in the above discussion. These are given in the list in (11) below:

(11) More Metaphors
a. SPIRITUAL VALUES ARE TREASURES (IN HEART)
b. MENTAL FUNCTIONS ARE TREASURES (IN HEART)
c. MORALITY IS AN ESSENTIAL ELEMENT OR FORCE
MORALITY IS WATER
MORALITY IS BREATH
MORALITY IS EARTH
d. EMOTIONS OR FEELINGS ARE WATER
e. LIFE IS WATER
f. HAVING MORE DESIRES IS HAVING MORE WEIGHT
DESIRES ARE BIRD FOOD
DESIRES ARE FETTERS

g. HUMAN BEING IS A PLANT
   HUMAN BEING IS A TREE
   HUMAN HEART IS THE ROOT
h. HUMAN BEING IS AN ANIMAL
   HUMAN BEING IS A FISH
   HUMAN BEING IS A MOUSE
i. MENTAL FUNCTION IS PHYSICAL ACTION AND SPATIAL MOVEMENT
j. KNOWING OR UNDERSTANDING IS SEEING
   KNOWLEDGE IS SIGHT
   TO KNOW OR UNDERSTAND IS TO CLARIFY IN ORDER TO SEE

These metaphors do not directly involve "heart" as the source or the target concept except HUMAN HEART IS THE ROOT under the metaphor HUMAN BEING IS A PLANT (11g). It needs to be made clear that the list in (11) is not meant to be exhaustive.

5.4. Summary and discussion

As Steen (2002) points out, many cognitive linguists have been concerned with the study of metaphor in language, but not many of them have paid attention to the study of metaphor in discourse and its cognitive processing. In this chapter I have expanded my study into the territory of discourse, as found in an essay and a series of poems. Using the heart as his principal source of metaphors, the essayist Ying-shih Yu (2005) discusses the loss and recovery of traditional moral values in modern and contemporary China. The poet Ming Hushui characterizes the heart as the seat of the inner self, and the organ of moral judgment. They both demonstrate that the heart is indeed conceptualized as the central faculty of cognition that plays various mental and emotional functions. The two different kinds of genres of writing made use of almost the same set of propositions and metonymies. The poems, however, involve many more metaphors (see 8 and 11) than the essay, which is of course not surprising considering the characteristics of the two different genres. Nevertheless, as the two lists (3 and 8) the two figures (8 and 9) show, the essay and the poems share some basic metaphors. Here are some examples of differences and similarities between the two. When the heart is the target concept, it is conceptualized in terms of an object, either an organism or a container, in the essay. In comparison, the heart is understood both as an object – organism or container – and as a source of water, power, or light in the poems.

Other than the aforementioned, there are two important differences between the essay and the poems, as illustrated by (3) on the one hand and (8) and (11) on the other. First, "heart" is the only basic-level concept that serves as a source or target concept in the essay. In contrast, there is a variety of basic-level concepts serving as source concepts for the target concepts in the poems: e.g., tree, fish, and mouse for person; heart, water, breath, and earth for morality; well, wellspring, engine, sun, bird, house, palace, and vat for heart.[106] Basic-level concepts are capable of evoking concrete images characteristic of poetic language. The second important difference, as shown in (3) and (8) and the two figures, is that the entailment of "size" for "object" plays a role in the essay but not in the poems. Thus, the following conceptual metaphors are found in (3) but not in (8):

MORAL IS BIG (MORAL IS GOOD + GOOD IS BIG)
IMMORAL IS SMALL (IMMORAL IS BAD + BAD IS SMALL)
BEING MORAL IS HAVING A BIG HEART (MORAL IS BIG + HEART FOR MORALITY IS AN OBJECT)
BEING IMMORAL IS HAVING A SMALL HEART (IMMORAL IS SMALL + HEART FOR MORALITY IS AN OBJECT)

All four of them are complex metaphors, but the latter two have the first two as their components. In other words, the first two, which are each composed of a proposition and a primary metaphor, are more basic than the latter two, even though they are all considered as complex metaphors. It seems that the first two metaphors still hold in the present-day Chinese language.[107] In contrast, the latter two, while apparently popular in ancient

106 Things are generally categorized into three levels in the hierarchy: the superordinate (e.g. furniture, electronics, automobile), the basic-level (e.g., chair, stool, desk, bed), and the subordinate (e.g. kitchen chair, living room chair, garden chair; or armchair, rocking chair, turning chair). The basic level is where we perceive the most obvious differences among things, and form a single image of the category (e.g. chair vs. stool, desk vs. bed, dog vs. cat, bird vs. fish).

107 For instance, when describing a morally good person I would think of the words 高大 *gao-da* (tall-big) 'lofty; great' or 高尚 *gao-shang* (tall-esteem) 'noble; lofty', and when describing a morally bad person I would think of the words 藐小 *miao-xiao* (petty-small) 'petty; insignificant' or 渺小 *miao-xiao* (tiny-small) 'tiny; insignificant', but not the other way around. In present-day Chinese, the word 小人 *xiao-ren* (small-person) 'a small or petty man' still refers to a morally bad person, inheriting its meaning from ancient times (see

times (see Ch. 2), seem to display very limited linguistic manifestation in contemporary Chinese. The essayist makes use of them when he tries to "restore" what he thinks is a "lost" tradition in ancient Chinese thought.

I have to note that in the limited space of this chapter, I have merely done a textual analysis of a tiny drop of samples out of the seas and oceans of contemporary discourse in Chinese. As I mentioned earlier, these texts were chosen because I found them centered on the concept of "heart" so that I could look closely into a relatively small section of discourse and find out how the authors of the texts, both prosaic and poetic, actually perceive and conceive the notion of "heart" within their separate "conceptual universes" (Freeman 2000, 2002, 2006). Therefore, the findings of my analysis in this chapter are significant only relative to my limited samples, which are representative only to the extent they actually are. That being said, I have found that the cultural conceptualization of the *xin* 'heart' outlined in the previous chapters is reinforced, in one way or another, by the results of my analysis presented in this chapter. These results are summarized by the lists of propositions, metonymies, and metaphors in (1–3) and (6–8, 11), and by Figures 8 and 9, respectively for two different genres. It is not surprising to see a scholar of Chinese philosophy and history, who argues for the restoration of what he thinks are the "lost" values of traditional Chinese thought, to use more or less the same or similar terms in his essay as those well-known ancient philosophers did. His intent and effort are, after all, to promote the traditional conceptualization in Chinese culture. What is interesting to observe is the fact that the "nameless" online poet, who composed a series of poems in description of the "heart", has also, by and large, fallen into the general thinking template of traditional Chinese thought in his poetic creativity. As I already pointed out, there are two major differences between the essay and the series of poems. First, the poet resorts to much more concrete imagery than the essayist, which of course is expected as a genre difference between argumentative or persuasive discourse, on the one hand, and poetic discourse, on the other. Second, the poems do not manifest the pair of complex metaphors BEING MORAL IS HAVING A BIG HEART and BEING IMMORAL IS HAVING A SMALL HEART present in the essay, which, according to my observation, may coincide with a change in the

---

2.3.3). It is worth mentioning that, other than the two pairs of MORAL metaphors discussed in this chapter, i.e. MORAL IS CLEAN and IMMORAL IS DIRTY, and MORAL IS BIG and IMMORAL IS SMALL, there should exist another pair, i.e. MORAL IS HIGH/UP and IMMORAL IS LOW/DOWN, which conceptualizes subjective judgments and abstract values in spatial terms.

cultural conceptualization that has been reflected in the language as well (see Chs. 2 and 4). Despite the differences, we can say that both the essay and the poems are situated within the Chinese cultural models for the concept of "heart", which I attempted to outline in Chapters 2–4. The implication for the study of literary discourse is that, as Cognitive Stylistics or Cognitive Poetics has argued (Semino and Culpeper 2002a; esp. Freeman 2002; Shen 2002; Tsur 2002; see also Yu 2003b), writers, poets included, are cognitively constrained in terms of what they can do originally and creatively. Although they may try to push their originality and creativity beyond conventionality for aesthetic and artistic purposes, they are still restrained by a number of factors: the boundaries of their minds that are fundamentally embodied, the shapes of the cultural models that are historically constructed and modified, as well as the communicative goals that they intent to attain.

Finally, the discussion of the findings of this chapter brings us back to the question: To what extent are the sample texts under study in this chapter representative of present-day Chinese discourse that reflects the underlying conceptualization of the "heart" in Chinese culture, both historically and contemporarily? This is an empirical question that cannot be answered without many more studies being done. I certainly hope that more studies will pursue a more satisfactory answer to this question. All I have achieved in this chapter is to have added another dimension or perspective to the studies that I presented in Chapters 2–4. Next, in Chapter 6, I will attempt to add still another dimension or perspective to my research, that is, a cross-linguistic and cross-cultural dimension and perspective.

Chapter 6
The HEART in cross-cultural comparison

6.1. Introduction: An external viewpoint

In the previous chapters, I investigated the Chinese concept of "heart", encoded in the word *xin* 'heart', from different angles. In the diachronic dimension, I studied the conceptions of the heart in ancient Chinese philosophy (Ch. 2) and traditional Chinese medicine (Ch. 3). I found that the heart was treated as the central faculty of cognition and the central organ of the person in ancient Chinese thought. In this respect, traditional Chinese medicine, which is vitally and profoundly influenced by ancient Chinese philosophy, is not very different at all. As noticed, even today the cognitive functions of the brain are still not fully acknowledged by Chinese medicine, and are understood within, and incorporated into, the physiological system of a heart-centered body. In the synchronic dimension, I studied conventionalized expressions involving *xin* 'heart' in the present-day Chinese language (Ch. 4) and analyzed sample prosaic and poetic texts from contemporary Chinese discourse (Ch. 5). I found that the cultural conceptualization of the heart, as outlined by a systematic analysis of linguistic evidence, is largely rooted in the cultural soil conserved, cultivated, and enriched throughout the history of China, despite the fact that it has lost some of its old twigs and branches, and gotten new ones instead, due to the impact of climatic changes.

In this chapter, the question that I want to ask is: How does the Chinese conceptualization of the heart, as delineated in the previous chapters, stand in comparison with the Western conceptions formulated and developed in the history of Western civilization? However, a systematic comparison between the two cultural traditions is really beyond what I can achieve in this chapter. My limited goal here, a more realistic one, is therefore to set up an external viewpoint so that the discussions of the Chinese concept of "heart" in the previous chapters can be viewed in a new light, within a larger reference frame and a comparative context. In the following sections, I first survey the conceptions of "heart", and "brain", as they are constructed and reconstructed through the cultural history of the Western world (section 6.2). This is an attempt to gain some insights from a review of history. I then take a comparative look at the concepts of "heart" and "brain" in English and Chinese, with reference to their definitions in some English and Chinese dictionaries (section 6.3). As brief and concise as they are, dictionary definitions can shed some contrasting highlights on the objects under comparison. Finally, I take a historical approach and compare the cultural contexts of English and Chinese with a focus on the four-humor theory in the West and the five-element or five-phase theory in China (section 6.4). In both of these cultural systems the heart occupies an important position in relation to other parts of the body and in connection between body and nature.

6.2. Conceptions of the heart and brain in the West

In this section I provide a brief survey of the conceptions of the heart, in relation to the brain, in the West from classical antiquity to the early modern period. My historical review here is by no means meant as symmetrical to the studies of the Chinese conceptions of the heart presented in Chapters 2 and 3. Instead, it merely provides a Western "point" of reference from which the discussions of the Chinese conceptions of the heart can be viewed from a comparative perspective. For detailed diachronic studies of Western conceptions of the heart, readers are referred to the following references on which this survey is based: Clarke and O'Malley (1968), Crivellato and Ribatti (2007), Doueihi (1997), Erickson (1997), Foolen (2008), Godwin (2001), Hillman (1992), Høystad (2007), Jager (2001), Le Goff (1989), Marti (1991), Sharifian et al. (2008a), Stevens (1997), Wetherbee (1990), and others. It appears from these studies that throughout Western history from antiquity to the modern period the heart and the brain in the head have been the two contenders vying for the dominant position "ruling" the rest of the body. According to Høystad (2007), as early as in the fifth century BC, the heart (and the liver) already began to be challenged for pride of place by the brain, as a result of the first scientific dissections carried out by ancient Greek physician Alkmaeon of Croton (c. 5th century BC), who claimed that both the senses and reason reside in the brain (see also Crivellato and Ribatti 2007: 329–330). As Clarke and O'Malley (1968: 1) put it, "Throughout antiquity, and to some extent up to the end of the eighteenth century, there was controversy on the question of which organ was the seat of the soul, the intellect, the passions, and the guiding force in the control of the motor and sensory phenomena of the body". In his article titled "Sacred Heart and Secular Brain", however, Stevens (1997: 265) points out that it is easy to fall into a false dichotomy when discussing the respective roles of brain and heart, "but such a split would grossly oversimplify the complex and heterodox systems of meaning ascribed to each organ over the centuries".

In the West, the heart, as well as the brain, has taken a prominent position in the understanding of the person and the self. Centrally located in the body, the heart has been regarded as the "seat of soul and intellect" (Crivellato and Ribatti 2007: 331), the "vital center of being", the "microcosm of the self" (Jager 2001: xv), the "secret chamber" or the "most intimate part" of a person (Hillman 1992: 26). As Jager (2001: xiv) points out, different moral, religious, or philosophical conceptions of the human being, entailed by cultural changes, have associated the self with three parts of the person, namely "the ancient (Neoplatonic) 'soul', the medieval (Christian) 'heart', and the modern (secular) 'brain'". Of these three, the soul, though understood in contrast with the body, is believed to reside in the body, and particularly in the heart, the brain, and the liver, which were said to be the "three principal members" of the body (Stevens 1997: 266).[108] However, the liver seems never to have been a real contender as "the source of the self", and the question then is which one should be in command of the others, the heart or the head (p. 267).

In Western history, it is said (cf. Jager 2001), two traditions were founded during the time of ancient Greek philosophy and medicine, distinguished by a psychology and anthropology centered on the heart or the head. These two traditions can be labeled as "cardiocentrism" versus "cerebrocentrism" (or "cephalocentrism", "encephalocentrism") (see Clarke and O'Malley 1968; Crivellato and Ribatti 2007; Foolen 2008; Sharifian et al. 2008b; section 1.1). Both heart and brain were listed as critical organs of the body in the ancient Greek theory of the four humors. Although earlier civilizations such as those of the ancient Egyptians and Hebrews had selected the heart as the central organ, the Greeks were divided on this matter, between those who selected the brain and those who preferred the heart (Clarke and O'Malley 1968; Crivellato and Ribatti 2007).[109] The question

---

108 See Bremmer (1983) for a study of the early Greek concept of "soul", and Wierzbicka (1989, 1992) for semantic analyses of "soul" in the Anglo-Saxon context. See also section 1.1.

109 According to Høystad (2007), for instance, the heart played an important religious function for the Egyptians, who made every effort to find a technique that could preserve the physical heart and prevent it from rotting within the mummy. After they embalmed the body, the heart was the only inner organ to be replaced in it while the rest were placed in jars and laid next to the mummy

Greek philosophers asked is: Where is the body's ruling principle (*archē*), its controller (*hegemonikon*)? "Plato and Diogenes championed the supremacy of the brain, while others like Aristotle pushed the heart's hegemony" (Kuriyama 2002: 160; see also Crivellato and Ribatti 2007). This controversy can be found in the writings of the Hippocratic physicians (see Clarke and O'Malley 1968: 4; Foolen 2008). For instance, the brain was considered as the most powerful organ of the body in one writing, *The sacred disease* (Clarke and O'Malley 1968: 4–5; Crivellato and Ribatti 2007: 330), but the same power was ascribed to the heart as the center of intellectual activity in another, *De corde* (Erickson 1997: 199; see also Jager 2001). For this reason, Hippocrates is labeled contradictorily as representing both the cerebrocentric (e.g., Clarke and O'Malley 1968; Crivellato and Ribatti 2007; Robinson 1998) and the cardiocentric tradition (e.g., Erickson 1997; Jager 2001).[110]

Erickson (1997: 20) summarizes the interaction of these two traditions from the classical antique to the early modern period in terms of "thinking brain" and "thinking heart", as follows:

> Counterpoised against the Platonic-Galenic tradition of the thinking brain in Greek physiology is the tradition, beginning perhaps with the "Hippocratic" *De corde*, of the heart as the center of intellectual activity, and extending to Aristotle's view of the heart as the source of sensation, memory, and imagination. The trope of the "thinking heart" was an important alternate paradigm to that of the thinking brain from the ancient world through the early modern period.

One of the earliest ancient Greeks interested in the nervous system was Alcmaeon (c. 5th century BC), whose most striking contribution was the recognition of the brain as "the central organ of sensation and thought" (Clarke and O'Malley 1968: 3; see also Crivellato and Ribatti 2007: 330). His ideas are known to have influenced later Greek writers such as Hippocrates and Plato. Plato (c. 427–347 BC) believed that the brain was the most important organ of the body, and for him the soul was made up of three

---

in the grave. "The brain was seen as unimportant and was thrown away" (p. 25).

110 Jager (2001: 151–152) refers to the former as "the Platonic-Galenic tradition", which "located the rational soul in the head", and the latter as "the Aristotelian-Hippocratic one", which "favored the heart" as the central organ with the same function.

parts, and the most important part, the rational, was assigned to the head or the brain in the head. In his words, the head is "the divinest part of us and lord over all the rest" (Clarke and O'Malley 1968: 6), and the brain may be "the originating power of the perceptions of hearing and sight and smell" (p. 7). He placed "the immortal soul" and reason in the head and encased "the mortal soul" and passion in the breast; for him the heart is just "the knot of the veins and the fountain of the blood" set as a guard to channel the whole power of feeling in the body (Erickson 1997: 1). Stevens (1997), however, believed that almost no part of the Platonic model is based on biological observation.

The cerebrocentric view that the brain was the body's primary organ was only "the minority opinion" of the time whereas the opposing cardiocentric view was supported by, among others, its most distinguished advocate, the great Greek philosopher and biologist Aristotle (Clarke and O'Malley 1968: 7). Championing the heart's pride of place in his natural philosophy and anatomy, Aristotle (384–322 BC) regarded the heart as "the origin of the other organs in the development of the body" (Høystad 2007: 52). Since the heart is the basis for the production of blood, all organs filled with blood grew out of it. He argued that the heart was "the chief organ of the body and the center for thought and the appreciation of sensation", whereas the brain "was secondary to it and functioned only as a means of cooling the heart's heat" (Clarke and O'Malley 1968: 8; see also Crivellato and Ribatti 2007: 330–331). He laid stress on the heart as "the location of the soul", which as "the vital force and source of human agency" is "found throughout the whole body" but "emanates from the heart" (Stevens 1997: 265–266). For Aristotle, the *psyche* or soul controls the body from the heart; soul and heart are thus intimately interconnected. The reason why the heart can be the center of life is because the soul is located there. The upgrading of the heart by Aristotle was an important reason why it retained the central position almost into the modern age (Høystad 2007).[111]

From the very beginning of Greek medicine, the heart was thought to be the source of heat in the body while heat was the source of life and nutrition (Erickson 1997). Little wonder, this organ would come to be understood, in both physiological and poetical terms, as the "sun of our body"

[111] According to Erickson (1997: 4), however, "Aristotle placed sensory knowledge, memory, and imagination (but not intelligence) in the heart. For Aristotle, intelligence or *nous* was not located in any physical organ, but this distinction became blurred in early modern discussions of the Aristotelian heart".

and the "fountain of life" (Jager 2001: 151).[112] The Hippocratic physicians, whose writings are often attributed to Hippocrates (c. 460–377 BC), based their interpretations of the human body in health and in disease on the theory of the four elements (water, earth, fire, air) and of the four humors (phlegm, black bile, yellow bile, blood). As already mentioned, their writings do not seem to be consistent as to whether the heart or the brain was the body's dominant organ. According to Erickson (1997: 199), the Hippocratic heart was "a strong muscle with a large hot chamber housing the intelligent ruling principle of the soul". That is, as "the chief" of the body, the heart, rather than the brain, was "the place of mental functioning" (p. 3).

As Clarke and O'Malley (1968: 4–5) note, however, in *The sacred disease*, the brain is interpreted as the organ responsible for human emotions, perceptions, moral judgments, and intelligence in terms of the four-humor theory (see also Robinson 1998: 145). For instance, in the following passage, the brain is related to the element of air for its intellectual functions (Clarke and O'Malley 1968: 5):

> I consider the brain to be the most powerful organ of man's body, for when it is healthy it is our interpreter of the impressions produced by the air; now, the air gives it intelligence. The eyes, the ears, the tongue, the hands, the feet, act according to the brain's understanding; in fact, the whole body participates in the intelligence in proportion to its participation in the air; now, the brain is the messenger for the intelligence. When man draws breath into himself, this breath first arrives at the brain, and it is in this way that the air disperses itself through the rest of the body, leaving in the brain its most active part, the part that has intelligence and understanding.

---

112 Høystad (2007: 170) points out that the "connection between the sun and the heart recurs in a number of cultures". While the heart is "the life-center" of the microcosm that animates the entire body in the same way as the sun gives life to the earth and the macrocosm, the other human organs correspond to the planets round the sun, which is "the heart of the world" (p. 171). See also Crivellato and Ribatti (2007), Doueihi (1997), and Godwin (2001) for the conceptions of the heart as the "sun of human life", the "body's sun" or the "inner sun" in various ancient cultures, where "the heart-sun-enlightenment connection is paramount in value, though the means of expressing that value evolves from visceral to chemical to symbolic" (Godwin 2001: 16). Erickson (1997: 15) suggests that "the heart's expulsive power was repeatedly compared to a fountain, maintaining the vital economy of the body. In fact, the comparison of the heart to a fountain is perhaps the primary image of the heart in ancient and early modern discourse".

Galen (129–199), who greatly expanded the Greek notions of four humors and their effect on the human body, was the "most vocal opponent" of Aristotle, who was "the foremost proponent of the cardiocentric theory" (Clarke and O'Malley 1968: 15). By placing the governing part in the brain, not the heart, he "established perception and cognition as functions of the brain" while leaving the emotions localized in the heart (Jager 2001: xv). For him, "the brain is the *hegemonikon*, the ruling principle and the regent part of the body" (Crivellato and Ribatti 2007: 334). Making use of experiment, reasoning, and analogy, he marshaled an imposing array of arguments to demolish the ancient belief and to establish his own that "the seat of intelligence, motion, and sensation is the brain, not the heart" (Clarke and O'Malley 1968: 15). He refuted those who upheld the cardiocentric view that the source of nourishment of human beings is in the heart and therefore the power of reason and intelligence is located in it. The heart was still the central organ of life for Galen, but he reinvigorated the Platonic doctrine of three souls simultaneously governing and serving the body. These are the rational soul presiding over the rational thought and causing sensation and motion, the vital soul governing the emotions and providing the life force, and the natural soul controlling nutrition, which are respectively seated in the brain, the heart, and the liver (Erickson 1997). He asserted that the brain alone was responsible for sensation and voluntary motion, which are the two main attributes of the rational soul. "He based his view on the claim that the brain and the spinal cord were the only sources of the nerves, an assertion strongly contrasted by cardiocentrists, who maintained that the heart was the origin of all body nerves" (Crivellato and Ribatti 2007: 334). The Galenic model, in which three principal members controlled three separate but necessarily interconnected systems within the body, "put the brain on a higher level than Aristotelian physiology had" (Stevens 1997: 266). In his anatomy, Galen "postulated a three-part division of power, as he traced the nerves to the brain, the arteries to the heart, the veins to the liver; but the problem of ultimate rule remained central to his thinking. The three sources were by no means equal: as the seat of reason, the brain reigned supreme" (Kuriyama 2002: 161). To Galen, in short, the brain is "the great king" of the body whereas all the senses that the head encloses are "the servitors and satellites" (Clarke and O'Malley 1968: 17).

In Roman thought, however, the conception of the heart as "the body's main source and center of physical and spiritual energy" gained much acceptance (Marti 1991: 145). It was conceived of as "a rich locus of thought, feeling, and memory" in Latin literature (Jager 2001: 8). Furthermore, "classical Latin commonly used the heart (*cor*) as a synonym for thought, memory, mind, soul, and spirit, as well as for the seat of intelligence, volition, character, and the emotions" (p. xv). The biblical allusions to the heart show how all the organs of the body from top to bottom, from outside to inside – the eye, the ear, the bowels, the kidneys, the genitals – connect significantly with the heart as "the vital center of bodily life and thought" (Erickson 1997: 50). The Bible also suggests a vital relation between language and the heart, by which the heart is "both the source and the instrument of language" (p. 50).

In the Middle Ages, "the heart regained its nominal primacy over the other principal members" (Stevens 1997: 266). As one of the most outstanding Moslems who were active in preserving and, in some instances, extending the Greek medical learning, Avicenna (980–1037) attempted to reconcile Aristotelianism and Galenic medicine, but on the whole sided with Aristotle (Clarke and O'Malley 1968; Stevens 1997). The following passage is cited from his work (Clarke and O'Malley 1968: 21):

> Many philosophers, and all physicians who follow Galen, consider that each faculty has its own principal member, which forms its storehouse, and from which its functions emerge. On this view the rational faculty resides in the brain, and its functions proceed from the brain. … Now the great philosopher Aristotle believes that the heart is the source of all these functions, though they are manifested in the several principal organs.

Repeating Aristotle, Avicenna thought that "the first organ to develop in the embryo was the heart and that it influenced the growth of other organs, including the brain" (p. 21). Avicenna's work was the primary source for most medieval scholars of the body (Stevens 1997).

Discussing the heart versus brain controversy during the Middle Ages, Clarke and O'Malley (1968: 25) note that the controversy over the relative merits of the heart or the brain as the central organ of the body continued throughout the medieval period; many individuals felt that there was sufficient evidence to support the argument in favor of the cardiocentric theory. During this period, the Bible was a preeminent authority representing a heart-centered Christianity. In the Bible, according to Erickson (1997: 26), the term "heart", the most significant word pertaining to the relationship between deity and humankind, "connotes the inner resources of the whole person, especially the mind and will, with somewhat less emphasis on the emotions", bringing together "mind and emotion, body and soul, human and divine".

In biblical physiology the heart is "the center of understanding and feeling" (Erickson 1997: 20) and "an emblem of the totality of the human personality" (Marti 1991: 140). Scripture "equated the heart with the innermost self, including conscience, memory, and volition" (Jager 2001: xv). From scriptural sources "the heart emerges as both the center and synecdoche of the body", becoming "the most important medieval symbol of corporeal and spiritual interiority" (Marti 1991: 145). In language, for instance, the wordplay on the terms *cor* and *corpus* and the sentential expression *He is all heart* are archetypical examples of synecdochic figuration stressing the heart's microcosmic implication (Jager 2001: 88; Marti 1991: 140). While the human body is the microcosm of the entire world, the human heart functions "as a microcosm within a microcosm", and it is thus said that the heart is sometimes figured as "a miniature human body" and "a microcosm of the microcosmic body of man" (Erickson 1997: 14–15; see also Barkan 1975; O'Neill 1985).

The most important figures in the development of Western Christianity all held to a heart-centered psychology. Saint Paul embraced the Hebraic notion of man as a fleshly being whose heart denotes "the center of the person as a rational, emotional and volitional being" – the "hidden core of the self" (Jager 2001: 12–13). For Saint Augustine, the inner person and interior life were centered in the heart, understood in its biblical sense as "the moral and spiritual core of the human being", or as "the center of moral and intellectual life, including conscience, understanding, the affections, volition, and memory"; as he put it, "My heart is where I am whatever I am". In his best-known work, the *Confessions,* "heart" (*cor*) is the most common term for "the innermost self and the scene of interior life". The heart also remained "the center of language" as he foregrounded the heart's role in the activities of reading and writing and "the heart's configuration as a 'text' of memory, understanding, and affective response" (Jager 2001: 28–29; see also Hillman 1992: 26–37).

A commonplace in the history of man's self-perception, as Marti (1991: 132) points out, is "the observation that man's center has migrated, since the Renaissance, from the heart to the head". This migration, attributed to "Western man's growing trust in reason" (p. 2), is of course a long process and can be traced back to long before the Renaissance. A forerunner in this migration is Bernardus Silvestris (c. 1085–1178), a medieval Platonist philosopher. In his *Cosmographia*, he placed the human intellect and wisdom in the head and expounded human cognition as below (Wetherbee 1990: 123):

> Belief holds that wisdom chose the head as its seat, and divided it into three chambers. In these three is placed the threefold power of the soul; each part fulfills its function in an unalterable sequence. The recollective faculty is placed at the rear, the speculative power is foremost, and reason exercises its power at the center. All share in the work when the five attendant senses inform them of the external events which they perceive. A messenger of sense enters and arouses the tranquil mind to confirm the matter by sure judgment.

As we can see, the "soul" is still tripartite, but its three parts exist in the "three chambers" within the head rather than the "three principal parts" of the body, the brain, the heart, and the liver. Although the brain is placed above the heart in Silvestris' hierarchical conception of the body, the heart is still conceptualized metaphorically as the "king" of the body, among other things, as the following quote clearly illustrates (p. 125):

> The heart is second in dignity to the brain, though it imparts to the brain the source of its vitality. It is the animating spark of the body, nurse of its life, the creative principle and harmonizing bond of the senses; the central link in the human structure, the terminus of the veins, root of the nerves, and controller of the arteries, mainstay of our nature, king, governor, creator. It is a noble lord journeying abroad through all the state of the body, to the limbs and the ministering senses, each of whom it maintains in the function assigned to it. Its sacred shrine is within the breast, its royal palace and imperial throne; its form is such as its brother element, fire, provides, whose crown tapers upward to a point.

Here, even though the brain is above the heart "in dignity", the heart as the "source of vitality" for the brain and the whole body is still the "king" of the body, with its "sacred shrine" within the chest.

In fact, the heart-king metaphor was a common one of the time owing to the heart's attributed physical and psychological functions as the "vital center of the being". Conversely, however, "the heart's physical centrality also lent itself to political metaphor in the Middle Ages: as the heart was the 'king' of the body, so the king was the 'heart' of the body politic" (Jager 2001: xv).[113] This phenomenon is characterized by a pair of concep-

---

113 While the KING AS HEART metaphor was the dominant one of the body politic of the time, it was not the only one. For instance, in his book of political science and philosophy produced in the early Middle Ages (1159), John of Salisbury, English author, diplomat and bishop, asserted that the state is a body within which the prince occupies the place of the head, which is "governed by

tual metaphors: BODIES ARE SOCIETIES and SOCIETIES ARE BODIES.[114] Therefore, there are bodily metaphors for the political use, as well as political metaphors for the bodily use. Le Goff (1989: 14), studying medieval Christianity's application of bodily metaphors to politics inherited from Greco-Roman antiquity, believes that the "Christian system of bodily metaphors is based chiefly upon the pair *head/heart*".[115] Thus, the Church, as a community of the faithful, is a *body* of which Christ is the Head and believers are multiple limbs connected through Christ to the unity of a single body. That is, the Church is commonly known as "the mystic body of Christ", whose head, according to Saint Paul, is God (see note 6, Le Goff 1989: 24).

According to the New Testament, the heart is not only the "seat of vital forces" but also the "source of intellectual thoughts, of faith, of comprehension" and the "center of decisive things, of the moral conscience, of unwritten law, of encounters with God" (Dufour 1975: 171; quoted in Le Goff 1989: 16). A good example of the king-heart metaphor is found in an anonymous treatise, *Rex pacificus*, written in 1302 in the context of the polemic between King of France, Philip the Fair, and Pope Boniface VIII. The treatise, written by one of the king's supporters, speaks of man, "the microcosm of society", as having two principal organs: the head and the heart. Whereas the pope is the head, from which emanate the nerves that bind the limbs to one another and to their head, the prince is the heart, from

---

the soul", whereas the senate occupies the place of the heart, "which gives good and bad deeds their impulses" (Le Goff 1989: 17). In addition, his STATE AS BODY metaphor also maps the sense organs such as the eyes, the ears, and the tongue onto the judges and the provincial governors, the hands onto the officers and soldiers, the flanks onto the regular assistants, the belly and the intestines onto the quaestors and the registrars, and the feet onto the peasants.

114 The reciprocal metaphorical mappings between BODY and SOCIETY should be attributed to the fact that these two concepts are viewed as microcosm and macrocosm of each other. See Chapter 2 and Yu (2007a).

115 According to Le Goff (1989: 16), the liver is a "loser" in the metaphorical configuration of medieval Christianity, whose "rejection of all forms of pagan divination had completely effaced the prestige given the liver in augury, which was already an archaic practice and which the Romans had always considered 'foreign'". Besides, the liver had "acquired a markedly pejorative physiologico-symbolic status" as the "seat of voluptuousness and concupiscence". "The liver/belly, or intestines, had been cast *down*, below the belt, to the region occupied by the shameful parts of the body, where it became the seat of lewdness, of the concupiscence that Christianity had been persecuting and repressing ever since Paul and Augustine".

which emanate the veins that distribute the blood to all parts of the body. That is, in the macrocosm, from the king emanate ordinances, laws and customs that have the force to carry the nourishing substance, i.e. justice, into every part of the social organism. "Since blood is the vital element par excellence, indeed the most important element of the whole human body, it follows that the veins are more precious than the nerves, and that the heart wins out over the head"; the king is, therefore, superior to the pope (Le Goff 1989: 21). However, the author of the treatise concludes that the king and the pope should autonomously cohabit, fulfilling their own separate functions, so that the one does not encroach upon the duties of the other. As Le Goff (1989: 22) interprets it, the structure and the functioning of the social body are conceptualized and explained in terms of "a double circuit" within the human body: the circuit of nerves emanating from the head and the circuit of veins and arteries branching out from the heart. This conception corresponds closely to the medieval physiological knowledge strengthened by the symbolic and metaphorical promotion of the heart during the Middle Ages. It is interesting to note that Philip the Fair's surgeon, Henry of Mondeville, wrote the following in a treatise on surgery: "The heart is the principal organ par excellence...which gives vital blood, heat and spirit to all other members of the entire body. It is located in the very middle of the chest, as befits its role *as the king in the midst of his kingdom*" (from Le Goff 1989: 23; italics in the original). When asked who the Sovereign of the body is, he replied unequivocally: the heart, that is, the king.

As Le Goff (1989: 23) points out, however, the head would remain or once again become "chief of the body politic". Thus, a theorist on the monarchy wrote in the fifteenth century that the "mystical or political body of the kingdom" must obey the head, which represents the essential unifying principle and assures order within society and the state. It is "the principal member" that the other members must obey, and since a two-headed society would be monstrous and anarchic, the pope is merely "a secondary head". That is, with "the migration of the body's perceived center from the heart up to the head" (Marti 1991: 2), the head at the top of a vertical hierarchy was to replace the heart in the middle of a centrality schema, taking up the dominant position in the political and physiological characterizations in the early modern period.

With the fast development of anatomy and physiology in the sixteenth century, medical science was coming to recognize the brain as the center of the human self as it underwent "the movement toward a psychophysical parallelism that would come to locate all mental activity – intellect and affect alike – in the brain" (Stevens 1997: 264). On the other hand, the church continued to prefer the heart over the brain as the locus of self, elevating the heart as a metaphor for person, in the face of growing physiological evidence to the contrary. A survey of the development of the conceptions concerning brain and heart function would attest to “the heterodox tradition that existed as the Renaissance approached” (p. 267). As Stevens puts it, “there was a myriad of published opinions on the human mind and body circulating in the seventeenth century. Any attempt to reduce these theories to an either-or situation would be facile” (p. 270).

The author of *Anatomy of Melancholy*, Robert Burton (1577–1640), drew on traditional metaphors of the body politic to explain the organization of the “principal members” of the body. He called the brain in the upper regions of the body a “Privy Counselor” to the heart as the “King”, who keeps his “Court” in the chest and communicates life to the whole body by his arteries (Stevens 1997: 269–270). In the middle region of the body, he said, “the principal part is the heart, which is the seat and fountain of life, of heat, of spirits, of pulse and respiration, the sun of our body, the king and sole commander of it, the seat and organ of all passions and affections”. It “lives first and dies last in all creatures” (from Erickson 1997: 75). However, according to Burton, the brain “is the most noble organ under heaven, the dwelling-house and seat of the soul, the habitation of wisdom, memory, and in which man is most like unto God” (Stevens 1997: 270).

The year 1628 saw the publication of William Harvey’s best-known work *The Motion of the Heart* (*De motu cordis*), which is one of the greatest and most famous contributions to physiology in the century. A royalist, Harvey (1578–1657) wrote a dedication (“To the most Illustrious and Invincible Monarch”) to King Charles I, who was the “heart” of his commonwealth for Harvey and Burton and their generation of the 1620s. He chose the king as the royal champion of his new doctrine of the heart and blood, and wrote this dedication in part to show the king that “the workings of the heart are a model for the proper relationship of king and commonwealth” (Erickson 1997: 65; see also Godwin 2001: 112–115; Hillman 1992: 18–25). He began the dedication as below, quoted from Erickson with minor modifications (2001: 65):

> Most Gracious King, The Heart of creatures is the foundation of life, the Prince of all, the Sun of their Microcosm, on which all vegetation does depend, from whence all vigor and strength does flow. Likewise the King is the foundation of his Kingdoms, and the Sun of his Microcosm, the Heart of his Commonwealth, form whence all power and mercy proceeds.

It is interesting to note that Harvey allowed his original dedication to King Charles to stand unchanged at the beginning of the English version of his *The Motion of the Heart*. The reciprocal mappings reflect the conceptual equation between the king and the heart. Going with the shift from the organicist model toward a mechanistic understanding of the universe and the human body in early modern science and philosophy, Harvey would then see the heart as "a muscle best understood as a pump" (Stevens 1997: 273) – "a place of motion, not emotion" (Jager 2001: 151). As Eisenstein (1979) suggests, the new technology of the age may have encouraged a parallel mechanization of the human body and the use of the same visual devices to delineate machine parts and human organs may have encouraged new analogies between pump and heart or between mechanical piping and plumbing and human venous or arterial systems (quoted in Jager 2001: 154). Emphasizing the importance of the heart "as the first organ in the body to live and the last to die", John Norris resorted to a different mechanical image and compared the heart to "a main component of the 'Humane Machine'" in *The Theory and Regulation of Love* (1688). As he said, "the Heart is the great Wheel of the Humane Machine, the Spring of all Animal and vital Motion, and the Head-fountain of Life ... and that its Motion is the First and Leading Motion of all, that it begins as soon as the Flame of Life is Kindled" (quoted in Erickson 1997: 186). That is, the heart is compared metaphorically to the "great Wheel of the Humane Machine", and the mechanical "Spring" of vital motion, in addition to its more traditional images of the "Head-fountain of Life" and the "Flame of Life".

If Harvey helped to vindicate the Galenic physiology by redefining the heart as a pump, René Descartes (1596–1650) extended Platonic anthropology by locating the soul not just in the brain but specifically in the pineal gland, which is in the middle of the brain (Jager 2001). However, as Stevens (1997: 269) points out, Descartes did not necessarily locate the soul or mind ("soul" and "mind" he used interchangeably) in the pineal gland to the exclusion of the rest of the body. Instead, he merely considered the brain and, specifically, the pineal gland as the physiological sites of interaction between mind and body, and viewed the soul or mind as existing throughout the human frame. In fact, he was profoundly reluctant to equate the self with the bodily "machine", i.e. the brain, as he said, "One thing is certain: I know myself as a thought and I positively do not know myself as a brain" (p. 277). The much discussed Cartesian dualism, characterized by a "disembodied rational mind", should be a "mind-brain split" as well as the "mind-body split" (pp. 268–269). In Descartes' dualistic philosophy, the body, from which the mind was separated, was "constructed like a machine" and the functioning of the nerves was explained "based upon mechanical phenomena" (Clarke and O'Malley 1968: 156). This aspect of his work was characteristic of one trend in the seventeenth century "to explain biological phenomena on the basis of physical laws" (p. 156). For him, as much as for Harvey, "the heart is simply a motor, a mechanical pump that controls the circulation of the blood and manages its distribution in the human body" (Doueihi 1997: 134). In the same trend, the English philosopher Thomas Hobbes (1588–1679) says: "What is the heart, but a spring; and the nerves but so many strings; and the joints but so many wheels, giving motion to the whole body" (quoted in Synnott 1993: 22–23). "It is ironic that Hobbes, and others, used the inorganic metaphor of machines to explain the body, and the organic metaphor of the body to explain politics" (p. 23).

In the context of cultural change, and especially with "a split between medical and theological faculties", the heart would be discussed as "a muscle in material terms and the seat of the soul in what would be seen increasingly as metaphoric terms" (Stevens 1997: 273). "As scientists and philosophers transferred more and more of the human subject from the metaphysical to the material side of the ledger, the brain became a logical last resort of the self, soul, or essential 'person'" (Jager 2001: 152). Although it was generally considered as the center of the self at this time, the brain was never represented as a metaphor of the self. That is perhaps why these two rival "principal parts" of the body are respectively referred to as "Sacred Heart" and "Secular Brain" (Stevens 1997). Most Westerners today still live their lives under the influence of the "great rift between heart and head", which fractured seventeenth-century thought, utterly changed the landscape of human relations, and split people into "divided kingdoms of intellect versus feeling" and a host of other "either/or" dualities (Godwin 2001: 112).

In short, in the West, it seems that the heart has been the metaphorical center of the self whereas the brain's signification as the center of the self remains in the physical realm. Stevens (1997: 276–277) has suggested the reason why this is the case. Now that we know that "a heart can be transplanted from one body to another, it makes the uniqueness of one's heart metaphorical rather than physical"; on the other hand, the uniqueness of the brain "as the site of our consciousness (and thus our selves) is inescapably physical". The brain is always "the sign of its own materiality". The heart, in contrast, "seems often on the verge of losing its materiality in discourse". As a physical object and metaphor, it signifies on many levels despite "medical science's conviction that it is a muscle, a pump". Once known that it is not the locus of mental activity, the heart is "paradoxically freed from a 'scientific' discourse of the self" and "no longer available for a purely physiological explanation of consciousness (as is the brain)". Instead, it is "allowed to reoccupy a metaphoric space in which it operates as a symbol of the conjunction of body and soul". Besides, the heart remains "an enduring link between past and present" with its "enduring centrality in the discourse of affect".

By way of conclusion, Stevens (1997: 278) further argues that "Reading the symbolism of the body, in parts or whole, allows us to acknowledge that materialist and metaphorical discourses occupy not parallel but exclusive realms". The body is often their most immediate site of interaction. The heart has proven an enduring symbol of both the spiritual and physical worlds, allowing us to exist in both worlds at once. The brain, on the other hand, seems tied to its own physicality and materiality, oddly separate from the term "mind". Perhaps the brain remains taboo due to the fear that understanding the brain would be equal to possessing power over the mind. "In this age of organ transplants and synthetic parts, the brain may seem to be our last irreplaceable organ – a part uniquely 'us'". We want to protect the singularity of an individual brain because we fear that a deeper understanding of its functions will reduce mental life to "a biological phenomenon" and not to "a spiritual mystery".

In summary, it seems that in the West there have been two perceived centers of the self, the heart and the head or brain, ever since the time of Greek antiquity. The two perceived centers are represented as cardiocentrism versus cerebrocentrism. Their interaction through Western cultural history displayed an early upper-handedness of cardiocentrism, which was to become the dominant theory during the Middle Ages, before cerebrocentrism had taken over by the early modern period.

In the West, as has already been shown to a certain degree, the heart has been conceptualized in various metaphorical terms. The source-domain concepts include, for instance, the predominant image schema of container. Thus the heart-container, with "chambers" or "rooms" inside, is a "two-story house" or "apartments", the "dwelling place of Christ" or the soul, the "home" of blood, and the "storehouse of secrets, memories, or lived experience" (see, e.g., Erickson 1997: 15–16, 81). The heart is also "a microcosmic building within the temple of the body" and "God's Spirit" can enter a person's body "through the 'door of the heart', transforming the structure of his belief from the inside" (Marti 1991: 176). In terms of the figure-ground relation, the heart is "the center of the self", "the moral and spiritual core" (Jager 2001: 28–29), and "the vital center of bodily life and thought"

(Erickson 1997: 50). With "chambers" and "strings" inside it, the heart is "musical instruments" which need "putting in tune" and whose "beating" produces "melody" in them; it is "a multiplex, resonating receptacle for all kinds of impressions from the outside world and from inside the body" (p. 16). As "the source of vitality", the heart, with its "expulsive power", is "a fountain, maintaining the vital economy of the body" (p. 15); it is also the "sun of our body", the "source of 'treasure'" of blood and heat as nutrients of the body (pp. 75–76). The heart being the "fountain" and the "sun" is also interpretable as the source of knowledge and wisdom, from which ideas spring and intelligence emanates (see, e.g., Erickson 1997: 24, 49). It is because the heart is believed to have mental functions and to be capable of being reflective and contemplative that it is metaphorically compared to a "mirror" (p. 66). In agrarian terms, the heart is "the ground, earth, or soil", which is receptive to the "seeds" of words and thoughts. Little wonder it is said that the "heart of a Christian is Christ's garden" (p. 17). Shifted into mechanical terms, the heart has been understood as a "pump" transporting vitality to all parts of the body through veins and arteries as its piping and plumbing system (Jager 2001: 154; see also Doueihi 1997; Stevens 1997). Furthermore, it has been conceived of as "a strong engine or a mechanical spring" (Erickson 1997: 200), and a great wheel of human machine and a spring of vital motion (p. 186), with the human body operating like "a clockwork automation" (p. 20). In intellectual terms, when the inner person or self is understood as a kind of "text", the heart has been respectively conceptualized as the ancient "scroll", "writing tablet" or "tabula rasa", the medieval "manuscript codex", and the modern "printed book" (Jager 2001; see also Erickson 1997; Marti 1991). However, as Jager (2001: 157–159) points out, "the book of the heart was gradually displaced by the book of the mind or brain" in keeping with a modern brain-centered psychology. As he further points out, "A conceptual revolution in the cognitive sciences has enshrined the computer as the dominant metaphor for the human psyche, completing the break with a long tradition of textual metaphor that stretches back to antiquity" (Jager 2001: 157; see also Sternberg 1990: Ch. 6). Finally, the heart was also believed to exercise "rulership" (Marti 1991: 138) over the body's other members as the king, the prince, the lord, the chief, the commander, and so forth (e.g., Clarke and O'Malley 1968; Crivellato and Ribatti 2007; Erickson 1997; Jager 2001; Le Goff 1989; Stevens 1997).

6.3. A comparative perspective from English

Having surveyed the literature on the historical development of and interaction between the concepts of "heart" and "brain" in the West, I now take a comparative look at the English and Chinese conceptualizations focusing on their definitions in some English and Chinese dictionaries. Dictionary definitions, brief and concise as they are, are expected to throw some highlights on the objects under comparison, and provide some useful clues to the English and Chinese conceptualizations of the heart and brain and to the overarching cultural models that organize them. It is hoped that a comparative perspective from English will add a new dimension to my study in Chinese.

In his book titled *The Language of the Heart, 1600–1750*, Erickson gives a brief yet comprehensive summary on the multi-faceted nature of *heart* as a polysemous word in English. He says the following, where the emphatic italics are in the original (Erickson 1997: 11):

> By the early modern period, the word "heart" had come to mean a variety of things: the center of all vital functions, the source of one's inmost thoughts and secrete feelings or one's inmost being, the seat of courage and the emotions generally, the essential, innermost, or central part of anything, the source of desire, volition, truth, understanding, intellect, ethics, spirit. *It was the single most important word referring both to the body and to the mind.* No other word performed what "heart" did, and no other word today quite replaces it.

That is, historically, the English *heart* has been assigned comprehensive affective and cognitive functions, in a way quite similar to the Chinese *xin* 'heart', in spite of the fact that the brain or head was already the other serious contender for the "rulership" of the body early on. In what follows, we look at this issue more closely.

I start with the definitions of *heart* provided in the *Longman Dictionary of Contemporary English* (LDCE 1978). Here are the first two meanings listed under the word *heart*:

1. the organ inside the chest which controls the flow of blood by pushing it through the blood vessels;
2. the same organ when thought of as the center of the feelings, esp. of kind feelings (as the brain is the center of thought).

As can be seen in sense 2, there is a perceived division of labor in contemporary English for the heart and the brain.[116] The former is "the center of the feelings, especially of kind feelings" whereas the latter is "the center of thought". This division of labor is, however, still a cultural conceptualization, which is not necessarily consistent with the scientific definition, as becomes obvious in light of the first meaning listed under the entry *brain*: "*med* the organ of the body in the upper part of the head, which controls thought and feeling".[117] It is obvious that the medical definition of *brain* contradicts sense 2 of *heart* in that the brain is supposed to control both thought and feeling, i.e., the division of labor suggested by sense 2 of *heart* does not exist in scientific terms. In sense 2, *brain* is defined as the "mind". The brain and the mind are the "two sides of one coin", functioning respectively as "hardware" and "software" of a computer.[118] In sum, the inconsistency of the definition of the heart as the center of feelings and that of the brain as the center of both feelings and thoughts, in a single English dictionary, demonstrates the difference between cultural understanding and scientific understanding, which are coexistent in the minds of English speaking people. The difference between cultural definition and scientific (medical) definition parallels the difference between metaphoricality and physicality or materiality in the understanding of the heart and the brain, reviewed in the previous section.

Now let us turn to Chinese temporarily. The following are the first two senses listed under *xin* 'heart' in *Xiandai Hanyu Cidian* (Modern Chinese Dictionary, XDHYCD, 1996; my translation here and hereafter), which is one of the most popular dictionaries in China:

---

116 The LDCE (2003) has made some noticeable changes in wording or definition. The second sense of *heart* now refers to "EMOTIONS/LOVE" with the definition "the part of you that feels strong emotions and feelings". That is, the heart is where emotions and feelings are actually felt.

117 The LDCE (2003) defines *brain* as "the organ inside your head that controls how you think, feel, and move". That is, the function of controlling movement is added to the brain. With regard to its difference from the heart, the brain controls feelings whereas the heart feels them. Defined as an "ORGAN", the brain is the central faculty of cognition in general; defined as "INTELLIGENCE", it represents "the ability to think clearly and learn quickly", i.e., it specializes in thinking and learning as the seat of intellect.

118 See also Dirven (2002), Lakoff (1999), Lakoff and Johnson (1999). Readers are referred to Dirven (2002) for a discussion of the relationship between *head, brain,* and *mind*, and the metonymic chain *head* → *brain* → *thinking* → *mind* → *thoughts* → *intelligence.*

1. the organ inside the body of human beings and other higher animals that gives impetus to the circulation of blood. The heart of a human being is in the center, a little to the left side, of the thoracic cavity, with the shape of a circular cone and the size of one's own fist. Inside the heart there are four cavities, of which the upper two are called atriums and the lower two called ventricles. The diastoles and systoles of the atriums and ventricles circulate blood to all parts of the body. The heart is also called "the heart organ";
2. usually also refers to the organ for thinking, and to thoughts, feelings, etc.

Obviously, sense 1 is more of a scientific definition of the "physical heart" when it defines the heart as a bodily organ in terms of its physiological function and structure. Sense 2, on the other hand, represents more of a cultural conception of the "mental heart". Significantly, the heart is conceptualized in sense 2 as "the organ for thinking". Remember that Mencius said, about 2,300 years ago, that "the organ of heart is for thinking" (心之官则思) (see 2.2.1). This heritage of cultural conceptualization has been passed down to the present day. In sense 2, *xin* 'heart' can also refer to both "thoughts" and "feelings" by the conceptual metonymy CONTAINER FOR CONTAINED. According to a popular Chinese-English dictionary (H-YCD 1995), the word *xin* is given these two English senses supposed to be equivalent to senses 1 and 2 in XDHYCD (1996): (a) "the heart"; and (b) "heart; mind". That is, the Chinese word *xin* 'heart' comprises what are known as "heart" and "mind" in English, even today, whereas the English word *heart* does not have that meaning any more (see also Godwin 2001: 61–68).

That sense 2 of *xin* 'heart' in XDHYCD (1996) reflects the Chinese cultural model for the concept of "heart", which is not consistent with scientific knowledge, as becomes obvious in light of the definitions for *nao* 'brain' in the same dictionary. The two meanings given below are relevant to what is under discussion:

1. the organ in the human body that is in charge of consciousness and movement of the whole body, and of such mental activities as thought and memory; the main part of the nerve system, composed of forebrain, midbrain, and hindbrain;
2. the capability of thinking, memorizing, etc.

Apparently, the brain is seen in Chinese as the organ of thinking, and the seat of intellect, in scientific terms.[119] In *Hanyu Da Cidian* (HYDCD 2000), notably, it is pointed out that, because the ancients took the heart as the thinking organ, the term *xin* 'heart' has been traditionally used to refer to the thinking function even though modern science ascribes this function to the brain.

In comparison between English and Chinese in terms of meanings assigned to the body-part terms for the heart in the contemporary stage, I outline the following similarities and differences in summary. First, the Chinese conception of the heart, as reflected in sense 2 of XDHYCD, is culturally constructed, as much as the English one reflected in sense 2 of LDCE. Both are inconsistent with modern scientific knowledge, as reflected respectively in sense 1 of *nao* 'brain' in XDHYCD, and of *brain* in LDCE. Secondly, and very significantly, the Chinese heart is conceptualized as the organ of thinking, but the same thinking function has been attributed to the mind, associated with the brain, in English. The dichotomies between body and mind, heart and head, in English do not exist in traditional Chinese thought. Traditionally, the "part" that enables a person to think and know, namely the "mind" as known in English, is located in the "heart" in Chinese, as analyzed in the previous chapters. Thirdly, and very interestingly, the heart in present-day Chinese is conceptualized as the organ of all feelings as well as thoughts, whereas the heart in present-day English is conceptualized as the organ of feelings only. Scientifically, however, we now know that both thoughts and feelings originate from the brain rather than the heart.

As Wierzbicka (1992: 47–48) points out, the "heart" is seen in English as "the organ of emotions" or "the emotional heart", it is "perceived as more closely related to the body than either *soul* or *mind*". However, it is not viewed as a seat of all emotions, but only of emotions that are seen as either "good" or "bad". Thus, one can say "His heart was full of joy, bitterness, or sadness" but hardly "His heart was full of surprise, amazement, or interest". Also, although a "heart" can feel both "good" and "bad" things such as joy and sorrow, it can contain only "good things" such as admiration or gratitude but not "bad things" such as hatred, jealousy or contempt. A person can be "kind-hearted" or "warm-hearted", but not evil-hearted" or "vicious-hearted". This suggests that a heart is seen as not only an organ of feelings, good or bad, but also an organ of empathy and benevolence, i.e.

---

[119] Interestingly, emotions or feelings are not mentioned here in relation to the functions of the brain in either sense 1 or sense 2 of the word *nao* 'brain'.

good feelings for others. Thus, Wierzbicka formulated the following explication of "heart" in terms of Natural Semantic Metalanguage (NSM):

heart
a part of a person
one cannot see it
one can imagine that it is a part of a person's body
  (in the middle of the upper half of the body
  one can hear its movements)
because of this part, a person can feel good things and bad things
because of this part, a person can feel good things toward other people

In short, it seems that English has undergone the change leading to the separation of "thinking" from "feeling", represented by the dichotomies between head and heart, or more generally between mind and body.[120] Let us trace the change back in history and get some diachronic glimpses at the conceptualization of the English heart by referring to *Shorter Oxford English Dictionary on Historical Principles* (SOED, 5th ed., 2002) and *Oxford English Dictionary* (OED, 2nd ed., 1989). There, it appears that the English heart used to be conceptualized as a comprehensive structure in which all human faculties are unified and integrated some time in history. In Old and Middle English, the heart, other than being the bodily organ regarded as the center of vital bodily functions or seat of life, is also the "seat of feeling and thought" (SOED) or the "seat of feeling, understanding, and thought" (OED). More specifically, in the older strata of English, the word *heart* is defined as having, among others, the following meanings adapted from OED:

1. = MIND, in the widest sense, including the functions of feeling, volition, and intellect
2. the seat of one's inmost thoughts and secret feelings; one's inmost being; the depths of the soul; the soul, the spirit
3. intent, will, purpose, inclination, desire
4. disposition, temperament, character

---

120 Western dualism represented by Descartes believes that the mind is "disembodied" whereas the brain, or the pineal gland inside the brain, merely serves as the physiological site of interaction between mind and body (Stevens 1997). In this sense the Cartesian mind is not only "disembodied", but also "disembrained".

5. the seat of the emotions generally; the emotional nature, as distinguished from the intellectual nature placed in the *head* (in earlier use often referring to the physical organ; in later mostly figurative)
6. more particularly, the seat of love or affection; kindly feeling; cordiality, heartiness; susceptibility to the higher emotions; sensibility or tenderness for others; feeling
7. the seat of courage; hence, courage, spirit; the source of ardor, enthusiasm, or energy
8. the seat of the mental or intellectual faculties; often = understanding, intellect, mind, and (less commonly) memory
9. the moral sense, conscience

Of course, most of these senses are regarded as archaic or obsolete today. In present-day English, they either do not exist at all, or exist to a very limited extent. For instance, *heart* can mean "intent", "will", etc., only in *after one's own heart*, and "memory" only in *learn by heart.*

Table 5. Differences between English and Chinese in the cognitive functions ascribed to the heart and the brain

Cognitive functions	Old/Middle English	Ancient Chinese	Modern English	Modern Chinese
thinking	heart (brain)	heart	brain	heart (brain)
feeling	heart	heart	heart (brain)	heart

The above comparison between Chinese and English has led to the finding that the Chinese conceptualization of the heart as the seat of feelings and thought appears to be quite similar to that found in the Old and Middle English periods, when the English *heart* was also conceptualized as the center of thought, as well as feelings. That is, the separation of the mind from the heart, or of thinking from feeling, is a later development in English.[121] In contrast, it seems, the conceptualization of the heart as the seat of both feelings and thought has been more persistent in Chinese. The histori-

121 In English, as Dirven (personal communication) points out, this view of the heart as center of higher faculties may have co-existed to some extent with an equally important folk view of the head as being in command of everything else. This point is fully consistent with the review of the conceptions of the heart and the head/brain in the West presented in the previous section. See also Niemeier (2008), Foolen (2008).

cal differences between the two cultures and languages in the cognitive functions ascribed to the heart and the brain may be presented in Table 5, where the parentheses indicate that the organ inside is assigned a relatively small part in the cultural conceptualization of the cognitive function, but this part has been growing owing to the increasing influence of scientific knowledge. This table, I have to stress, is very simplistic in nature, merely sketching out a possible trajectory of historical development. In effect, as the survey in the previous section suggests, the cognitive functions of the brain was already recognized in the West as early as in Greek antiquity, at least by some philosophers and physicians, such as Plato and Galen, even though the cerebrocentric view was "the minority opinion" back then (Clarke and O'Malley 1968: 7). As Stevens (1997: 278) points out, unlike the heart, which has been "an enduring symbol of both the spiritual and physical worlds", the brain seems to have been "tied to its physicality" in medicine in particular and in science in general. This difference is certainly reflected in the language as a window of cultural conceptualizations.

Now, the question to ask is: If there really is a difference between Chinese and English conceptualizations of the heart, what caused this difference? The answer lies, it seems, in the general trends of philosophical thought. In English, the divorce between the mind and the heart in cultural conceptualization took place in response to the rise of the mind-body dualism in Western thought, as promoted and championed by Descartes (see, e.g., Damasio 1994; Lakoff and Johnson 1999). Dualism, for instance between soul and body, mind and matter, had been a long tradition in Western thought before it gained its special prominence with Descartes and the spread of rationalist philosophy in the eighteenth century (Sharifian et al. 2008b).[122] As a result, the mind came to be seen as "disembodied". In contrast, Chinese thought, dominated by Confucianism and Daoism throughout history (and Buddhism does not seem to be much different from them in this respect), has always held the belief that the "heart governs the spiritual light". That is, the "mind", as known in English, has always been "embodied" in the heart in Chinese thought and cultural conceptualization. In other words, the change in the philosophical trend in the Western world has caused the change in the concept of "heart" in English, as reflected in the change in meaning of the word *heart*. On the other hand, the notion of the heart as the center for all emotional and intellectual activities, and as the

---

122 According to Høystad (2007), dualism between body and soul first emerges in the work of the Greek philosopher Democritus (c. 460–370 BC), and is therefore older than Plato.

central faculty of human cognition, has been held relatively stable in Chinese thought and cultural conceptualization. This relative stable conception of the heart is also reflected in the Chinese language accordingly.

Language change reflects the development of cultural history. Niemeier (2000, 2008) has studied the metonymic and metaphorical expressions involving *heart* in present-day English from a cognitive linguistic point of view. In her (2000) study, she focuses on the cultural model of the heart as the site of emotions as it exists in the English language. She notes that "English is particularly rich in both metonymic and metaphorical expressions making use of the concept *heart* to speak of emotional issues" (Niemeier 2000: 195–196). This is, she points out, grounded in the most basic bodily experiences:

> people have a heart and they can feel it acting differently according to the emotions they experience: the heartbeat quickens, slows down, stops altogether, etc. Already in ancient times emotions were assumed to reside in the most conspicuous body organ … and the heart was taken as a metonymy for the whole body and thus it stands for the whole person experiencing a specific emotion. It is on the basis of this archetypal metonymy that the other understandings could arise and flourish. (Niemeier 2000: 209–210)

Niemeier (2008) then moves on to study the head-heart dichotomy in present-day English, which reflects, metonymically and metaphorically, the existing cultural models of the heart as the locus of emotions and feelings (e.g. *warm-heartedness, a heart overflowing with gratitude, the heart filled with joy*) and the head as the locus of intellect and rational thought (e.g. *to keep a cool head, to have no head for figures, to lose one's head*). She argues that this dichotomy in English relates to a specific period in language and thought development, starting from the seventeenth century, when Descartes and his successors propagated the latent dualism between emotions and reason. Niemeier's study shows that the conceptualizations of *head* and *heart*, as related to their underlying cultural models, are far from being arbitrary, but reflect the concepts that are or were at a certain historical stage present in English culture. "Even if today's advanced medical knowledge does not agree anymore with these traditional concepts, linguistic expressions that are so deeply entrenched that they have come to belong to unconscious knowledge far outlive such a change in conscious knowledge and still function as a basic demarcation line in allocating the locus of both faculties" (Niemeier 2008).

Discussed here as manifested in English and Chinese, the two cultural conceptualizations of the two critical organs of a person – the heart and the brain inside the head – in terms of the locus of the cognitive functions of thinking and feeling are indeed constructed through their respective cultural histories and embedded within their respective cultural contexts. In the next section, we will look at two cultural systems consisting of complicated networks of biological and cosmological relations that connect the body and the universe as microcosm and macrocosm of each other.

6.4. Four humors and five elements

In this section, I take a comparative look at two folk theories: the theory of the four humors in Western culture and the theory of the five elements (or five phases) in Chinese culture. The four-humor theory stemmed from ancient Greek medicine and philosophy and dominated Western thought until the seventeenth century. The five-element theory figured prominently in ancient Chinese philosophy, and it has been a guiding doctrine in traditional Chinese medicine. The heart takes an important position in both cultural systems because it is perceived in them as the radiating and converging center of the biological and cosmological relationships between microcosm and macrocosm, human and nature, and body and universe. While the human body is the microcosm of its natural environment and the whole universe, the human heart, as understood by ancient Greeks and Chinese, is not only the engine of that physiological body, but also the locus of cognitive agency, the "great fulcrum of the cosmos" (from Godwin 2001: 44), which makes the whole micro-macrocosm relationship meaningful.

It is suggested that Hippocrates (c. 460–377 BC) laid the foundations of the humoral doctrine but Galen (129–199 AD) gave it its classical form that dominated the Middle Ages (Geeraerts and Grondelaers 1995: 156–157). The five-element theory should have existed before Confucius (c. 551–479 BC), who referred to it in his works.[123] What I present below as a comparison between them is just an initial look and is doomed to be fairly general, merely pointing out some differences and similarities on the surface between these two cultural systems. As mentioned above, the heart organ has an important place in both systems. Looking at the systems provides us

123 Yin and yang and the five elements are recurring themes in the *Yi Jing* (or *I Ching*) 'Book of Changes', the oldest of Chinese classical texts, dating back to the Western Zhou dynasty (c. 1100–771 BC), which describes an ancient system of cosmology and philosophy at the heart of Chinese cultural beliefs (Zhang 1993).

with a better understanding of the cultural models of the conceptualizations of the heart under discussion.

Both the four-humor and the five-element theories are analogical in nature. They are cultural systems of categorization, establishing interrelationships with perceived correspondences within and between the human body and nature. What is of special interest is that as cultural systems they have historically exerted their influence on the English and Chinese languages respectively (see, e.g., Geeraerts and Grondelaers 1995; Fernando 1996; Yu 1995, 1998). The two systems are shown respectively in Table 6 (from Geeraerts and Grondelaers 1995: 158) and Table 7 (adapted from Wang et al. 1987: 14; repeated from Ch. 3 for convenience).

Table 6. A system of humoral correspondences

	Phlegm	Black bile	Yellow bile	Blood
Characteristic	cold and moist	cold and dry	warm and dry	Warm and moist
Element	water	earth	fire	air
Temperament	phlegmatic	melancholic	choleric	sanguine
Organ	brain/bladder	spleen	liver/stomach	heart
Color	white	black	yellow	red
Taste	salty	sour	bitter	sweet
Season	winter	autumn	summer	spring
Wind	North	West	South	East
Planet	moon	Saturn	Mars	Jupiter
Animal	turtle	sparrow	lion	goat

A fundamental difference between these two systems is that the four-humor theory is primarily a medical theory, based however on a philosophical theory of the four basic elements (Høystad 2007), whereas the five-element theory is embedded within a broader philosophical theory. Thus, in the former, the four "head" categories, under which other categories of correspondences are organized, are the four humors – phlegm, black bile, yellow bile, and blood – in the body. According to the humoral doctrine, physiologically, the four humoral fluids "regulate the vital processes within the human body"; psychologically, they "define four prototypical temperaments, i.e., a person's character is thought to be determined by the preponderance of one of the four vital fluids in his body" (Geeraerts and Grondelaers 1995: 156).

Table 7. A system of five-element categorization

Elements	Wood	Fire	Earth	Metal	Water
Nature					
Location	east	south	center	west	north
Season	spring	summer	long summer	autumn	winter
Climate	windy	hot	humid	dry	cold
Planet	Wood Pl. (Jupiter)	Fire Pl. (Mars)	Earth Pl. (Saturn)	Metal Pl. (Venus)	Water Pl. (Mercury)
Animal	chicken	sheep	ox	horse	pig
Crop	wheat	millet	foxtail millet	rice	bean
Life Cycle	birth	growth	ripeness	harvest	storage
Odor	rancid	scorched	fragrant	fishy	putrid
Flavor	sour	bitter	sweet	spicy	salty
Color	blue/green	red	yellow	white	black
Human					
Zang Org.	liver	heart	spleen	lung	kidney
Fu Org.	gallbladder	small intestine	stomach	large intestine	bladder
Sense Org.	eyes	tongue	mouth	nose	ears
Tissue	tendons	vessels	flesh	skin/body hair	bones
Emotion	anger	joy	overthinking	grief	fright
Indicator	nails	complex-ion	lips	body hair	hair
Expression	shouting	laughing	singing	wailing	moaning
Spirit	ethereal soul	spirit	purpose	corporeal soul	will

For the humoral theory, "the basic therapeutic rule" is "to restore the balance of the humors, given that a disturbance of their well-balanced proportion is the basic cause of the pathological situation" (p. 156). According to Høystad (2007: 53), Hippocrates developed his four-humor theory analogous to the four elements (water, earth, fire, air) of Empedocles the Elder (c. 483–423 BC), who claimed that "man could sense and perceive the world because he himself was made up of the same four basic elements as the rest of the universe".

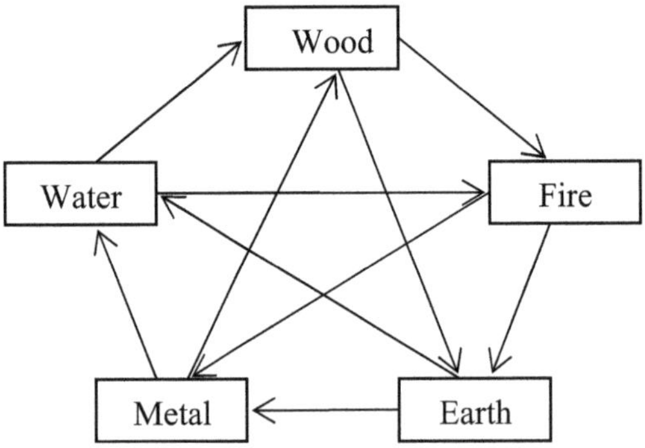

Figure 10. Relation of mutual promotion and restraint between the five elements

The five-element theory, together with the yin-yang theory, is a cosmological doctrine meant to account for the formation and operation of the universe in ancient Chinese philosophy. For that reason, its "head" categories, wood, fire, earth, metal, and water, are thought to be the five basic elements that compose the universe. These five elements are in a relation of mutual promotion and restraint, as shown in Figure 10 (adapted from Chen 1989b: 1000; repeated from Ch. 3 for convenience). In this figure, the lines forming the outer pentagon indicate the relation of promotion, and the lines forming the inner five-pointed star indicate the relation of restraint, with arrowheads indicating directions of promotion or restraint (see also Yu 1995, 1998). It is with this relation of mutual promotion and restraint among the five elements that the balance of the universe is achieved. The balance of the universe is destroyed when the balanced proportion of the five elements is lost, and that results in ecological problems or natural disasters such as floods and droughts. The theory of the five elements has its own conceptual schematization in categorization. For instance, "wood" is associated with "spring", the beginning season of the year when it is "windy", and with the "east", the location from which the sun greets the beginning of a new day. It is associated with the "green" color of new leaves and the "sour" taste of unripe fruit (see Wiseman and Feng 1998: 205–207 for a more detailed discussion of the correspondences in the five-element categorization).

It is interesting to note that both theories under discussion are medical and cosmological at the same time, seeking systematic correlations between the microcosm of the body and the macrocosm of the universe, although they go in opposite directions, as specified above. In the case of the five-element theory, Chinese medicine has borrowed it from Chinese philosophy, as a reasoning tool of analogy, to study the human body and its relationship with its natural environment. It starts with the five basic elements of the universe, and all categories of things under them fall into the pattern of five. For instance, instead of four seasons in a year, there are five, including a "long summer", in this system. Also, the six fu organs are reduced by one, the triple heater, to fit into this five-element schema. In contrast, the humoral theory starts with the four basic fluids in the body, and the things that come under them all fall into the pattern of four. For instance, its basic elements of the universe are water, earth, fire, and air, in contrast with the Chinese five-element categorization, i.e. wood, fire, earth, metal, and water.[124] As can be seen, both systems include adjectival modifiers such as "cold", "hot", and "dry". However, because of the difference in the starting point, the humoral theory uses them to characterize the humoral fluids whereas the five-element theory uses them to characterize the climatic patterns.

It needs to be mentioned that not all categories of correspondences in each theory are included in the two tables given above. For instance, a different table in Fernando (1996: 123) lists two categories, "physiognomy" and "attributes", which are absent from Table 6. Table 7 has left out a few

[124] It is worth mentioning that the element of air, called "qi" in Chinese, is not completely out of the picture of cosmology of ancient China. On the contrary, it was regarded as a more fundamental substance than the five elements: "since ancient times the Chinese have conceived of *qi* as something indispensable to all existence, the fundamental substance from which all things rise and upon which everything depends for survival" (Zhang and Rose 2001: 26). In fact, the universe started with the undifferentiated substance of *yuan qi* 'original qi', which then divided into two opposite forces of yang and yin, separately forming Heaven and Earth. The eternal interplay between yin and yang gave rise to qi 'air', and gave life to ten thousand things. This is what the founder of Daoism Laozi (c. 571–480 BC) meant in his *Daode Jing* when he said: "Dao gives birth to One. One gives birth to Two. Two gives birth to Three. Three gives birth to Ten Thousand Things" (see Zhang and Rose 2001: 25–27). It is also said that in Chinese philosophy the universe consists of Heaven and Earth, Heaven being made of *qi* and Earth being made of the five elements.

categories from the original one in Wang et al. (1997: 14): "sound", "number", "symptomatic location", and "stress response".

In addition to those differences noted above, there are still the following differences between the two systems:

1. There are some categories that are in the one system but not in the other. Notably, the humoral theory emphasizes the correspondences between the "temperaments" and the humors. The five-element theory, however, establishes the correspondences between the internal and external organs, and between these organs and the "emotions" and "spirits". This theory also places more emphasis on agriculture, including the categories of "crop" and "life cycle" modeled on farming seasons.
2. Although the two systems share some categories, they may have different items in those categories. Interestingly, for the category of animal, the humoral theory has all the wild animals whereas those corresponding to the five elements are home-raised animals, typically seen in the agricultural setting in China. For the planets, only the medically-based humoral theory includes the moon, which influences the tides of the sea in nature and the menstruations in women's bodies, whereas the theory of the five elements includes five major planets, named in modern Chinese after the five elements. For the internal organs, saliently, the humoral theory already includes the brain whereas the five-element theory does not. This difference represents the contrast between the traditional heart-dominating Chinese body and the Western body that has alternated between two centers in the heart and in the head. As noted in section 6.2, ancient Greeks started to recognize the mental functions of the brain about 2,500 years ago, although the cerebrocentric view did not get the upper hand until the early modern period in its interaction with cardiocentrism. In contrast, the mental functions of the brain are either not acknowledged at all or taken as part of the heart-centered physiological and mental system of the person even in Chinese medicine today. Also, the four-humor theory pairs the brain and bladder, and the liver and stomach, placing them in the same cell, but the theory of the five elements pairs the zang with the fu organs, emphasizing their close functional relationship as pairs.
3. There are major crossings or crossovers in correspondences between these two systems. For instance, in the humoral theory, the heart is associated with air, sweetness, spring, east, and Jupiter. In the five-element theory, however, the heart is associated with fire, bitterness, summer, south, and Mars, known as the Fire Planet in Chinese. Interestingly, the liver in the humoral doctrine corresponds to fire, bitterness, summer, south, and Mars, which are all aligned with the heart in the theory of the five elements.

There are other similarities and differences between the two systems that cannot be discussed one by one here. The question of interest to ask is: Were these two systems in any way related or connected to each other back in history? In other words, did the one in any way influence the other, or did they influence each other at certain points in history? These are questions that call for further research.[125] No matter whether or not they have crossed paths back in history, these two systems of categorization for medical and cosmological purposes exhibit remarkable similarities despite their differences. They may represent the common heritages of human cognition in different developmental stages of different civilizations in the world. The highlights of these two systems, which are of special and central interest for my study, are the bodily organs that are perceived as the central faculties of human cognition. The indisputable center in the heart of one system and the heart-brain coexistence as two potential centers of the other symbolize, as I see it, an important difference between two major civilizations of the world that has lasted through history and lingered until the present day: the heart-centering holism and the heart-head dualism. This is, of course, a difference in cultural conceptualization rather than scientific knowledge.

6.5. Summary and discussion

The survey provided in 6.2 traces the diachronic contour of the conceptions of the heart and the brain developed in the West. As Clarke and O'Malley (1968) point out, although earlier Western civilizations had chosen the heart as the central organ, the ancient Greeks were divided between the cardiocentric and cerebrocentric view, with the latter being the minority opinion. It might as well be the case that the cerebrocentric view, being a new theory of the human body, the self, and the cognitive agent, was still limited to some philosophers and physicians like Plato and Galen, and yet

---

125 As noted, the four-humor theory is based on the theory of the four elements in ancient Greece. According to Wikipedia, the Greek theory of the four elements may have been modeled on Buddhist theory of classical elements in India. It is said that the Buddha's teaching of the four elements predates Greek teaching of the same four elements and that Buddha sent 60 disciples to the known world to spread his teaching. The Chinese theory of the five elements originated in Daoism and can be traced back to early religious thought in the Yin (c. 1400–1100 BC) and Western Zhou (c. 1100–771 BC) dynasties (see Zhang 1993: 8–11).

to enter the minds of the general public. It is not so hard to imagine why cardiocentrism preoccupied cultural conceptualizations early on and got the upper hand in its wrestling with cerebrocentrism in Greek antiquity when the choice was made between a "loud" heart and a "quiet" brain. The "sacred" heart, rather than the "secular" brain, then would continue to be dominant during the medieval period when the Catholic Church revived the religious symbolism of this "divinest" organ of the body in the spiritual world. After the Middle Ages, the perceived center of the human being migrated up from the heart, the figure of a centrality configuration, to the head, the top of a hierarchical structure, as medical science was gaining more and more "insights" into the human body in early modern times. The rise of rationalism led to or, rather, further separated the dichotomy between the head or brain on the one hand as the center of reason, intellect and thought, and the heart on the other as the seat of feelings, passions and emotions. The Cartesian dualism, characterized by "a disembodied rational mind", which merely interacts with the body in the brain, even attempted a mind-brain split as well as the mind-body split. That is, this rational mind is not only disembodied, but "disembrained" as well. This general intellectual climate represented by dualism has persisted in the cultural models and scientific theories in the Western world up to the present day (Sharifian et al. 2008b).

As the survey in 6.2 shows, the heart in the West has been conceptualized in various metaphorical terms throughout the history from the classical antiquity to the early modern period. The metaphorical images include that of a "container" such as a "dwelling or storage place" for mental and emotional entities, processes, and activities. As a "source" of both physical and mental vitality, the heart is a "musical instrument" producing the melodic sound of the soul, a "fountain" or "spring" supplying the flow of vital life forces to the whole body, or the "sun" emitting the heat and light that the rest of the body needs for its energy or guidance. As an "object" with a reflexive function, the heart is a "mirror" capable of reflecting the external world. In agrarian terms, the heart is the "ground", "earth", or "soil" out of which the "seeds" sowed will grow into "plants" that will bear "grains" or "fruits" in due time. In mechanical terms, the heart is a "pump", an "engine", a "motor", a "spring", or a "wheel" that is part of a larger mechanical structure. As natural products of an age of industrialization propelled by the rapid development of science and technology in the West, such mechanics metaphors gave rise to the understanding of the heart as the "source of energetic forces" that are more "mechanical" than mental. In intellectual terms, the heart is understood through metaphors related to the "text" ranging from the ancient "scroll" or "codex" to the modern "printed book". In terms of a "ruler" over the rest of the body, the heart is the "king", "prince", "lord", or "commander" that has power over the other parts. The metaphorical source-domain concepts are very suggestive and informative of the ways in which the heart has been conceptualized, and the cultural models for the concept of "heart", over the history in the West.

In Old and Middle English, the heart appeared to be the center of both feelings and thought. Present-day English, however, regards the heart as the center of feelings and the brain as the center of thought, whereas in scientific terms the brain controls both thought and feelings, as well as movement. That is, the current English conceptualization of the heart as the center of feelings is still cultural, not scientific, according to the definition of Western medicine. In contrast, Chinese medicine today still considers the heart as commanding the rest of the body, including the brain, even though it has gained a better understanding of the cognitive functions of the brain.

The study finally compares two folk theories in Western and Chinese cultures, namely the theories of the four humors and the five elements. It is shown that they are both cultural systems of schematization and categorization, establishing correspondences within and between body and nature. There are important differences between them, however. Most importantly, the four-humor theory started as a medical doctrine, but no longer holds its ground in Western medicine; the five-element theory started as a philosophical doctrine, and still serves as a guiding and reasoning theory in Chinese medicine, although its limitations are noted (Wiseman and Ellis 1996: 13–14; see also the relevant discussion in Ch. 3). If the change of philosophical trend in Western thought has caused the separation of the mind from the heart in the English-speaking culture, the lack of such change in Chinese thought probably accounts for the relatively stable conceptualization of the heart as the central faculty of cognition in Chinese culture. Science will certainly cause conceptual change, but this kind of change takes place in a very slow and long process and scientific advancement is only one of the interactive factors in the process, others including philosophy, religion, arts, literature, and language.

Another important difference between the four-humor and five-element doctrines is the presence and absence of the brain. The absence of the brain from the five-element categorization and schematization reflects a heart-centered, heart-dominated cultural tradition that has been relatively stable and persistent through Chinese history. The presence of the brain, along with the heart, in the humoral doctrine epitomizes the interaction between the cardiocentric and cerebrocentric views that started back in Greek antiquity.

Chapter 7
Conclusion

7.1. Looking back in perspective: Some highlights

Ruiz de Mendoza Ibáñez and Peña Cerval (2005b: 4) suggest that there are two general topics that will have wide-ranging implications for the future of research in Cognitive Linguistics: (i) the relationship between the embodied nature of language, cultural models, and social interaction; and (ii) the role of metaphor and metonymy in inferential activity and as generators of discourse links. My studies presented in the preceding chapters stand within the boundaries of both topics. Having presented the topics in separate chapters, I now want to take a step back and cast a perspective look at them as a whole.

The focus of this book is on a single concept, that of "heart". The heart is central to our life because it is simultaneously "the organ and symbol of the most basic and yet crucial manifestations of life" (Doueihi 1997: 17). In his recent book, *The Meaning of the Body: Aesthetics of Human Understanding* (2007), Johnson argues that the body's "visceral connections to life", including all bodily processes, perceptions and movements, are the deepest and most profound sources and roots of human meaning, understanding, and reasoning. The human heart, without a doubt, stands at the very *heart* of all the visceral depths and origins of meaning. Little wonder its conceptualizations are the main subject of a number of books published in the past two decades (e.g., Doueihi 1997; Erickson 1997; Godwin 2001; Hillman 1992; Jager 2001; Høystad 2007; Marti 1991; see also Sharifian et al. 2008a). The conception of the human heart is an important and essential part of the conception of the human body. Our body, although such a fundamental and intimate thing to us, does not give rise to a uniform understanding. On the contrary, it invokes markedly different conceptions across cultures.[126] As Synnott (1993: 262) concludes, "every culture constructs its own body differently". Cultures construct their bodies differently because, largely, they conceptualize how the "mind" (i.e. the cognitive functions of

[126] There are different conceptions of the body, especially of its internal organs, even within cultures, for instance, over different periods of history (see, e.g., Sharifian et al. 2008a; section 6.2).

thinking and feeling, etc.) is related to, or located in, the body differently. Thus, there exist different perceived centers of the human body in different cultures. The Western body, for instance, has split centers in the head (or the brain inside the head) and the heart, the former being the center of thought and the latter the center of feelings. The Chinese body, in contrast, is centralized around and dominated by the heart, which is the perceived central faculty of cognition.[127] The conceptualization of the heart, therefore, plays a prominent role in the understanding of mind, self, and person.

In this book, I have studied the cultural conceptualization of the heart in Chinese, which has hitherto received relatively little scholarly attention. I have systematically explored the heart as a part of the body regarding what it can potentially mean and why and how it means what it means in the Chinese language and culture. While my focus is on the Chinese concept of "heart", my exploration extends along both diachronic and synchronic dimensions, which are respectively the vertical and horizontal axes of a coordinate crossing each other at the focal point. An adequate analysis of the motivation behind cultural conceptualizations and linguistic expressions that manifest them has to take into account the diachronic dimension since cultural models, in which cognition and language are rooted, are constructed in and renovated through history (see Geeraerts and Grondelaers 1995).

Along the diachronic axis, I have explored both ancient Chinese philosophy and traditional Chinese medicine because the concept of "heart" lies at the core of both of these important domains in Chinese culture. In ancient Chinese philosophy, i.e. both Daoism and Confucianism, the heart is believed to be the central faculty of cognition hosting all cognitive activities, mental, intellectual, emotional, and moral. Thus, the heart feels, thinks, contemplates, examines, infers, understands, knows, reasons, and judges. Because the heart is culturally believed to be the locus of the "mind" (i.e. THE HEART IS THE LOCUS OF THE MIND), it is metaphorically characterized as the "ruler" commanding the rest of the body (i.e. THE HEART IS THE RULER OF THE BODY). This metaphor is not isolated, but part of a larger metaphor system in ancient Chinese thought that perceives parallel relationships between the microcosm and the macrocosm:

---

[127] There are also cultures that maintain an abdomen-centered or, more specifically, liver-centered body (see, e.g., Sharifian et al. 2008a).

Microcosm		Macrocosm
Body/Person	↔	Country/Society
Heart	↔	Ruler
Mental Power	↔	Political Power
Other Organs	↔	Officials

These parallel relationships are expressed by the following metaphors with reciprocal mappings: A BODY/PERSON IS A SOCIETY/COUNTRY and A SOCIETY/COUNTRY IS A BODY/PERSON; THE HEART IS THE RULER OF THE BODY and THE RULER IS THE HEART OF THE COUNTRY; MENTAL POWER IS POLITICAL POWER and POLITICAL POWER IS MENTAL POWER. That is to say, a human body is seen as analogous to a country with its social structure, and the person's mind or mental power, localized in and attributed to the heart, is compared to the supreme political power of the ruler of the nation, and vice versa. These bi-directional metaphors reflect the fundamental belief in the unity and correspondence between the universe and the human as expression of humanism in ancient Chinese philosophy. Under this cosmological view of Chinese thought, the heart is the "center" of the body whereas the human is the "heart" of the universe. Therefore, the heart is the focal point of the whole universe.

Traditional Chinese medicine extensively incorporates the cosmological theories of yin-yang, the five elements, and the qi in ancient Chinese philosophy to account for physiological functions and pathological changes of the human body. According to this medicine, the heart is regarded as the center of the body's operating system, which consists of five functional subsystems represented by the five zang organs. As the psychological as well as physiological center of the body, the heart governs the "spiritual light" or mental power. Traditional Chinese medicine inherits the central metaphor in Chinese thought that understands the heart as the "ruler" (monarch, emperor, master, etc.) of the body and applies it as part of a GOVERNMENT metaphor system. This metaphor system characterizes the body as an operating system in which the functions of the internal organs are conceived of as the roles played by governmental officials under the ruling of the heart-emperor (see 3.2). It is interesting to note that the brain, called the "marrow sea", is designated as one of the "extraordinary fu organs" (brain, marrow, bones, vessels, gallbladder, and uterus), which are taken as less important than either zang or fu organs. The two main functions of the brain, according to Chinese medicine, are (i) to store the marrow, and (ii) to control the movement of the four limbs. Although its cognitive functions are recognized, the brain can at best be incorporated into an operating system dominated by the heart (see 3.4). The interesting phenomenon in China today is that, while Chinese medicine has been very much marginalized in its medical system, which is dominated by Western medicine, it still receives popular support, more so as a cultural heritage, I think, than as a medical science (see the relevant discussion in 3.5).

The study of two important aspects of Chinese culture along the diachronic dimension sets up the stage for a thorough synchronic study of the Chinese *xin* 'heart' as a key word of Chinese culture. Along the synchronic axis, I have made a systematic analysis of conventionalized expressions that reflect the underlying cultural models and conceptualizations and that manifest the underlying conceptual metaphors and metonymies. Furthermore, I have also attempted to reveal the present realities of these underlying cognitive structures by means of analyzing prosaic and poetic texts from present-day Chinese discourse. The analysis of a large number of conventionalized expressions, including compound words, idiomatic phrases, and proverbial sayings, shows that the present-day Chinese language, which has undergone enormous change since ancient times, still echoes the conceptions of the heart in ancient Chinese philosophy and traditional Chinese medicine of two millenniums ago. The linguistic evidence shows that the Chinese heart is culturally conceptualized as the central faculty of cognition, as the seat of both mental and emotional lives, and as the locus of human nature and true self. It is simultaneously mental, spiritual, moral, intellectual, rational, volitional, temperamental, as well as emotional. It is noted that all the images evoked by the conventionalized expressions stem from a traditional cultural belief, i.e. THE HEART IS THE CENTRAL FACULTY OF COGNITION, which can be traced back to ancient Chinese thought. According to this belief, the heart is the home of the inner self, the residence of personal disposition, the abode of moral character, the center of thought, the seat of emotions, and so forth.

It has been noted in section 4.6 that the present-day Chinese terms *tounao* 'head-brain' and *nao* 'brain' are also conceptualized as the seat of the intellect and the locus of the "mind". This brings about an apparent clash between the brain and the heart as the locus of the "mind" in Chinese. Nonetheless, it is also noted that the brain as the locus of the "mind" is manifested only in a very small number of compound words in contrast with the vast quantity of conventionalized expressions involving *xin* 'heart' discussed in Chapter 4. The word *xin* 'heart' plays a far more prominent and important role in Chinese phraseology than the word *nao* 'brain'. The tremendous difference between them in quantity distinguishes *xin* 'heart' as a key word of Chinese culture, separating it from *nao* 'brain'. Also, the use of *nao* 'brain' in the sense of being the locus of the "mind" is limited, as far as my studies show, to modern Chinese, reflecting the influence of modern science. I would attribute the relatively strong presence of the heart and weak presence of the brain in the conceptualizations of cognitive functions, both mental and emotional, to the shaping and molding force of the cultural models based on ancient Chinese thought and traditional Chinese medicine, which are the most influential and important components of traditional Chinese culture. Ancient Chinese philosophy largely ignored the brain, at least as far as I can see it (Ch. 2). Traditional Chinese medicine, which was as philosophical as it was medical, also relegated the brain to the peripheral (Ch. 3). Even in Chinese medicine today, the questions of what cognitive functions the brain performs and how it relates to the heart in performing those functions are still topics under discussion (see Wang et al. 1997; section 3.4).

In general, one's cultural conceptualization may very well clash with one's scientific knowledge, but the two of them may co-exist, I argue, in two separate "minds" of a person, i.e. the largely unconscious "cultural mind" and the more conscious "scientific mind", which occupy different domains in one's conceptual system and make sense in different contexts (see 4.6). While the conscious "scientific mind" grows through one's education and intellectual activities, the largely unconscious "cultural mind" is molded within one's culture, which includes such aspects as philosophy, religion, music, arts, literature, as well as language. When people are brought up in the midst of conventionalized expressions that suggest that the heart "thinks" and "feels", they would to some extent take it as a cultural belief or assumption. The overwhelming number of such expressions as shown in Chapter 4 (and in Appendix 1) is likely to have a shaping and molding impact on the formation of the cultural conceptualization of the heart in Chinese. Both cultural conceptualizations and scientific knowledge can partially construct and shape a set of multiple, and sometimes contradictory, cultural models which members of a cultural group hold onto (Pritzker 2007). What I am dealing with in this book is the Chinese cultural conceptualization of the heart. In such a conceptualization, the brain could still be incorporated into a heart-centered operating system, if a COMPUTER metaphor is applied, as the "processor" that "fetches" instructions on what to perform, "decodes" and "executes" them, and then "writes back" the results for storage. The heart, however, is the "hard disk drive" where the software programs are preinstalled and the data are permanently saved.[128]

My synchronic investigation is not limited to the study of conventionalized expressions in the Chinese language. It expands into the territory of textual analysis of present-day Chinese discourse, critically scrutinizing an essay and a series of poems. The essayist discusses the loss and recovery of traditional moral values in modern and contemporary China in terms of the heart, which, perceived as the locus of moral character, serves as the principal source of metaphors. The poet characterizes the heart as the seat of the inner self and the organ of moral judgment, employing some basic metaphors that are to some extent similar to those utilized in the essay. The detailed analysis of the texts of different genres shows that the heart is indeed conceptualized as the central faculty of cognition performing various mental and emotional functions, thus further confirming the cultural conceptualization of the Chinese heart already established. What is of special interest is the fact that even poetic originality falls into the general thinking template of traditional Chinese thought.

Finally, I have stepped beyond Chinese and looked at the Western cultural history, focusing on the development of its conceptions of the heart and the brain from the ancient Greek to the early modern period. While earlier Western civilizations had regarded the heart as the central organ of the body, or as the center of both thought and feelings, the ancient Greeks started to develop two conflicting views regarding whether the heart or the brain is the cognitive center of a person, i.e., cardiocentrism and cerebrocentrism. The cardiocentric view dominated the classical and the medieval

---

[128] While using a COMPUTER metaphor to account for the functions of the brain in relation to the heart, I am aware that the COMPUTER metaphor originally emerged from earlier cognitive science where it is used to characterize or describe the human brain, i.e. THE BRAIN IS A COMPUTER. However, as Damasio (1994) points out, this metaphor implies Cartesian dualism positing a disembodied mind. That is, mind and brain are related only in the sense that the mind is the software program run in a piece of computer hardware called brain, and brain and body are related only in the sense that the former cannot survive without the life support of the latter. It is also worth mentioning in passing that the reversed metaphor THE COMPUTER IS A BRAIN also exists. For instance, the Chinese word for "computer" is literally "electrical or electronic brain" (电脑 *diannao*). Its "twin" (if not "elder sister") name is literally "computing machine" (计算机 *jisuanji*), which, apparently a direct translation from "computer", has largely dropped out of popular use and is limited to more technical context.

period until the early modern period when the growing trust in reason and the rise of rationalistic thinking led to a double dualistic understanding of the human being: that of the mind versus the body, and that of the brain versus the heart. These dualities have lasted into the present-day Western world. While the brain came to be seen as the center of thought and the seat of the intellect, the heart remained the center of feelings and the seat of emotions.

My studies presented in the previous chapters show that the heart is conceptualized metaphorically in both Chinese and Western cultures. A glance at the source-domain concepts for "heart" touched upon in this book reveals some interesting similarities and differences. These source concepts form clusters falling into a number of conceptual domains. Both Chinese and Western cultures resort to the RULER metaphor, emphasizing the heart as the central or dominant organ of the body, although the "ruler" could mean different things with different implications in different political systems and in different cultural contexts. For instance, a Chinese "emperor" and a Western "king" trigger off very different images with different sets of political and cultural meanings. Also, as already noted, both cultural worlds conceptualize the heart as a CONTAINER, especially as a dwelling place for the soul, spirit, emotion, thought, etc. (e.g. palace, residence, house, room, chamber, storehouse, nest), and as a SOURCE for heat, light, water, sound, and so on (e.g. sun, lamp, fire, spark, mirror, well, wellspring, water spring, fountain, fountainhead, instrument). These metaphors apparently have a very general bodily basis resulting from the anatomical structures and physiological functions of the heart, as a "hollow" organ that "pumps" the blood to all parts of the body. They also have to do with the heart being conceptualized as the central faculty of cognition, which "governs" and "commands" the rest of the body, and as the central organ of the life force, serving as the body's ultimate "source" of heat and nutrient. Another domain that gives rise to source concepts for "heart" in both cultural worlds is AGRICULTURE. Thus, we find some concepts (e.g. soil, field, land, earth, ground, plant, water) in this domain used in one or the other or in both cultural contexts. For instance, "soil", is the one utilized in both cultures for "heart", in which thoughts and feelings can grow, like "seeds", into "plants" and bear "fruits". It seems, however, that the AGRICULTURE metaphor is more elaborate in Chinese culture than in Western cultures.

Of course, both Chinese and Western cultures also exhibit differences with respect to source concepts for the metaphors of the heart. Some of these differences are especially significant as "stamps" or "imprints" of specific periods in the social history of the culture concerned. For instance, as Jager (2001: xv) notes concerning Western conceptualizations, the "book of the heart is a quintessentially medieval trope in that it combines the central symbol of medieval textual culture, the manuscript codex, with a psychology and anthropology that were centered on the heart rather than the head". The source concepts for the metaphors of the heart include "text", "scroll", "writing tablet", "tabula rasa", "manuscript codex", as well as "printed book". Another interesting difference between Chinese and Western cultural conceptualizations lies in the utilization of the MECHANICS metaphors. With the advancement of scientific knowledge in the early modern period in the West, a "mechanistic turn" took place in the understanding of the universe and the human body. Thus, the heart is understood as various machine parts and components, such as a "pump" (and venous or arterial systems as mechanical piping and plumbing), an "engine", a "mechanical spring", a "wheel", or as "clockwork". On the other hand, Chinese seems to lack this kind of MECHANICS metaphors for the heart. This difference in the use of metaphors, as pointed out above, really reflects different social and historical backgrounds in the West and in China. In China, a traditionally agrarian country, industrialization is very much delayed; it did not really take place until the twentieth century. In my study of the Chinese heart, I came across only one instance of the MECHANICS metaphor, i.e. THE HEART IS AN ENGINE, which occurs in one of the poems analyzed in Chapter 5. It is worth repeating that those are contemporary poems first posted online only a few years ago.[129]

Having surveyed the conceptions of heart and brain in the West, I also turned to a comparison of the definitions of the words for "heart" and "brain" in English and Chinese dictionaries. I take such dictionary definitions as "highlights" of the objects under scrutiny that can give us certain insights, especially if they provide a historical perspective. This comparison shows that both dualism in Western cultures and the heart-centering tradition in Chinese culture have found their own expressions in the respective languages. Looking at the two ancient cultural systems – the four-humor theory in the West and the five-element theory in China – we see the evidence of different understandings of the bodily organs and loci of human agency and cognition that characterize different civilizations in the world. Over two thousand years ago, the ancient Greeks already acknowledged the brain as a critical organ of the body on a par with the heart, thus

[129] It is of course likely that there exist other instances of the MECHANICS metaphor of the heart that I have missed in my study. In this case, any future study taking a corpus linguistic approach may be useful.

initiating the interaction between cardiocentrism and cerebrocentrism and laying the foundation for dualism in modern Western cultural history. The ancient Chinese, on the other hand, largely left the brain out of the picture while focusing on the heart as the "grand master" of the five zang and six fu organs. The indisputable dominance of the heart as the sole center of the Chinese system and the heart-brain coexistence as two potential centers of the Western system symbolize an important difference between two major civilizations of the world caught in our label as heart-centering holism versus heart-head dualism.

7.2. Bringing into focus: Holism and dualism, heart and head

As Kuriyama (2002: 180) points out, Western commentaries on Chinese medicine and philosophy frequently stress the holistic unity of the Chinese body and self, which is often viewed against Western dualisms, e.g., "the radical oppositions of divine spirit and corrupt flesh, of immaterial mind and material body". Not finding these dichotomies in Chinese thought, however, has often resulted in a failure to recognize the distinctions that the Chinese did make. For example, one such distinction, and a critical and fundamental one, is that between 形 *xing* 'form' and 神 *shen* 'spirit', which bears a certain degree of resemblance to the Western dichotomies between body and soul in antiquity, and body and mind in modern times. What really distinguishes Chinese medicine and philosophy is, however, their "holistic view of *xing* and *shen* as being mutually dependent" (形神相倚的整体观 Wang et al. 1997: 57). Thus, *xing* 'form' and *shen* 'spirit' are "a holistic construct of life activity, dependent upon, and inseparable from, each other" (p. 56). According to this view, there does not exist a "formal body" (形体 *xingti*) without "spiritual activity" (精神活动 *jingshen huodong*) operating in it or "spiritual activity" without a "formal body" to reside in. It is the qi, however, that plays a mediating and unifying role between form and spirit. As an ancient medical text, *Generalized Essentials on Various Diseases*, says:

> 人禀天地阴阳之气而生，借血肉以成其形，一气周流于其中以成其神，神形兼备，乃谓全体。《杂病广要》(Wang et al. 1997: 57)
> Man is born from the qi of yin and yang between Heaven and Earth, and is composed of blood and flesh that form his body. The qi circulates inside his

> body to transform into his spirit. Only when man possesses both spirit and form can he have a whole body.[130]

That is, the qi is the key to the interaction and unity between form and spirit. It is the life force for the congenital transformation and the postnatal generation of the essential qi. As the *Elementary Questions* states, "the form is substantiated by the qi, and when the qi is exhausted, the form will fall ill; the spirit stands leaning on the qi, and when the qi gathers, the spirit will exist" (形以气充，气耗形病；神依气立，气合神存 Wang et al. 1997: 57). Another medical source says that "when the qi is waning, the spirit will disperse; when the spirit is dispersing, the form will deteriorate" (气衰则神散，神散则形坏 p. 57).

Primitive as it is, as we can see, this "holistic view" of *xing* 'form' and *shen* 'spirit' as being dependent on each other, in ancient Chinese thought and medicine, is in sharp conflict with what Damasio (1994: 247–252) refers to as "Descartes' error", i.e., "the abyssal separation between body and mind". An "emblem for a collection of ideas on body, brain, and mind that in one way or another remain influential in Western sciences and humanities", Descartes asserted a dualist notion with which he "split the mind from brain and body" (p. 247). The Cartesian idea of a disembodied mind is well represented by a famous statement of his: "I think, therefore I am". It treats thinking as an activity quite separate from the body, and celebrates the separation of mind, the "thinking thing", from the "nonthinking body" (p. 248). Yet, as Damasio (1994: 248) argues, humanity must have evolved from a simple being to a being with an elementary consciousness, and from a simple mind with an elementary consciousness to a more complex mind with the possibility of thinking and, even later, of using language to communicate and organize thinking better:

> For us then, in the beginning it was being, and only later was it thinking. And for us now, as we come into the world and develop, we still begin with being, and only later do we think. We are, and then we think, and we think only inasmuch as we are, since thinking is indeed caused by the structures and operations of being.

---

130 Note that in Chinese thought yin and yang form a primary pair of binary distinction at the cosmological level, but the two of them also form a "unity of opposites" that not only oppose each other, but also depend on each other and even transform into each other under certain circumstances.

In brief, the human brain is body-minded. While "the mind itself depends on brain-body interactions" (p. 225), "the body provides a ground reference for the mind" (p. 223), contributing "a *content* that is part and parcel of the workings of the normal mind" (p. 226). This is what a more recent trend in cognitive science calls the thesis of "the embodied mind", based on its scientific findings on the mind as arising from the relation and interaction between brain and body, and between organism and environment (e.g., Damasio 1994; Gibbs 2006; Johnson 1987, 2007; Lakoff and Johnson 1999). Our minds, which are capable of abstract reasoning, are nonetheless "shaped critically by the peculiarities of our human bodies, by the remarkable details of the neural structure of our brains, and by the specifics of our everyday functioning in the world" (Lakoff and Johnson 1999: 4). According to this view, the human "mind" and "body" are but two aspects of "one organic process", and all our meaning, thought, and language emerge from the "aesthetic dimensions of this embodied activity", which include "qualities, images, patterns of sensorimotor processes, and emotions" (Johnson 2007: 1). In sum, the ancient Chinese "holistic view", as part of the dialectical thinking tradition characteristic of Chinese thought and philosophy, stresses the mutual dependence of *xing* 'form' and *shen* 'spirit' as a pair of binary opposites unified by the qi. In contrast, modern cognitive science takes on an evolutionary view of "embodied cognition" that emphasizes the dependence of mind on body based on modern scientific discoveries of the functions and structures of the human brain and its neural and physiological connection and interaction with the rest of the human body. Both theories, however, take into account the impact of specific environments on human cognition as "embodied" in the physical world, which is inevitably a social and cultural world as well (see, e.g., Frank et al. 2008; Gibbs 2006; Ziemke, Zlatev, and Frank 2007).

It is worth mentioning that the Chinese "view of the body-mind unity" (and in Chinese it would literally be the "view of the body-heart unity" 身心统一观 *shenxin tongyi guan*) also takes a unified look at humans' mental and emotional life, which form another binary distinction. Thus, one's mental life and emotional life are intimately related: The former causes the latter and the latter manifests the former (see Wang et al. 1997: 56–57). That is, on the Chinese view, one thinks and therefore one will feel emotions; one feels emotions because one thinks. Therefore, on this view, thinking and feeling, or thought and emotion, are two sides of one coin that cannot be completely separated from each other. Therefore, the dualism between heart and head, which is a popular cultural belief in the West, does not exist in Chinese, where "heart" and "mind" are believed to be a holistic one that is the combination of "form" and "spirit". The so-called "mind" as known in English is localized or "embodied", so to speak, in the heart in Chinese. The heart as the "ruler" of the body is that part of the body that governs the "spiritual light", or the mental power that controls one's thought, feeling, and action, although "spirits" (神 *shen*) and "emotions" (情 *qing* or 志 *zhi*) are separately related to and stored in all five zang organs, namely the liver, heart, spleen, lungs, and kidneys. This conceptualization has a certain degree of similarity, in spirit, with Aristotle's cardiocentric view that the heart is the source of the soul, which however is manifested separately in the principal organs of the body (see section 6.2). Since the soul controls the body from the heart, the heart and the soul are thus intimately interconnected.

As discussed in section 6.2, the notion of "principal organs" of the body in the West refers to the heart, brain and liver, and this reference can be traced back to the classical Greek period. However, the liver was never a serious contender for pride of place, and therefore the two competing theories were cardiocentrism and cerebrocentrism. Since the early modern period, the so-called Cartesian dualism, which splits body and mind, has been dominant in the West, resulting in the popular cultural belief in the dichotomy between heart and head. The heart is the center of feelings whereas the head, which contains the brain, is the center of thought. In an age and culture that revere rational thinking, free from emotions, the head is naturally promoted whereas the heart is necessarily demoted. As Gail Godwin, an American novelist and short story writer, points out in her nonfictional book titled *Heart* (Godwin 2001: 16):

> It has been said by many thoughtful people that our era, or the era we are just completing, has represented the nadir of the heart. Since the onset of the Industrial Revolution, we have lived in a culture that increasingly worships decisions of the head alone.

Today in the West, despite all the advancement in cognitive science, and especially in neuroscience, which has enormously increased the knowledge about the brain, people like Godwin still believe, out of a cultural rather than scientific conviction, that it is necessary to have "a *uniting of head and heart*" (p. 45). "It is vital to keep one's head, of course; but it is wrong to be so cold-blooded as to prevent the whole person, with heart and head together, from coming into action and being profoundly moved" (see Godwin 2001: 45). As Godwin sees it, it is always "beneficial in heartening the human in us and humanizing the heart in us" (p. 26). That is why the heart is both the organ and the symbol of what it means to be human and humane.

Of course, "a uniting of head and heart" is simply a convenient way of speaking, symbolically or metaphorically, of a cultural conceptualization or conviction that represents the latest "turn" away from the Cartesian disembodiment dominant in the past few centuries in the West. Scientifically, however, it takes a lot more to prove "Descartes' error". As Damasio (1994) shows, cognitive science has revealed that the feelings of human emotions stem from the interaction between brain and body, and from the activation of "neural signals" and "chemical signals" that travel back and forth via "neural circuits" and via the "bloodstream" between the brain and the rest of the body. Furthermore, and more importantly, emotions and thought are intimately correlated since the essence of emotions is "the combined perception of certain body states with whatever thoughts they are juxtaposed to" (p. 146). It is therefore not sensible to leave emotions and feelings out of any overall concept of mind, and the view that emotions and feelings are elusive entities unfit to share the stage with the tangible contents of thoughts is indeed too narrow-minded. Thus, according to Damasio (1994: 245), "feelings are a powerful influence on reason", and "the brain systems required by the former are enmeshed in those needed by the latter". That is to say, feelings are very relevant in the process of reasoning. While reasoning depends on specific brain systems, some of these systems happen to process feelings also. In other words, one cannot but have "a passion for reasoning". This means that the Western dualist view that emotions and reason do not mix does not hold true, nor does the corresponding dichotomy between heart and head.

It is worth noting that the cultural belief in the dichotomy between heart and head has different variants of interpretation in the West. In the above, we focused on a popular one that the heart is the center of feelings whereas the head is the center of thought. This is, however, not the sole interpretation. Here is another one that reflects the existence of multiple and contradictory cultural models for the understanding of the person and the self in the West. Hill (in press) studies the everyday language of White racism in the United States. She notes a "folk psychology" of "head" and "heart" that emerges in three propositions:

1. the meanings of a person's words are determined by intentions that reside in a stable core of belief and thought, the heart;
2. the meanings of a person's words are inherent in the words themselves and speakers can be assumed to choose words that reflect their beliefs;

3. certain circumstances interrupt this connection between belief and meaning and can produce talk that reflects only an unstable and error-prone animating psychological locus, the head. These include careless inattention to speech, but also "light talk" and joking.

As we can see, the dichotomy here is between "a stable core of belief and thought, the heart" and "an unstable and error-prone animating psychological locus, the head". Thus, after the Republican Senator Trent Lott was severely criticized for making some remarks with racist implications in 2002, he made an apology by saying that he had made "a mistake of the head, not of the heart", and then elaborated it saying, "I take full responsibility for my remarks. I can't say it was prepared remarks. As a matter of fact, I was winging it" (see Hill, in press). *Winging it* means "speaking without careful preparation", and that is the "mistake of the head, not of the heart". Despite his apology, repeated again and again by the media, Trent Lott was forced to resign as the Majority Leader of the U.S. Senate. Hill (in press) interprets the logic of the dichotomy implied in his apology as follows:

> Alongside the "heart", where "heartfelt" beliefs reside, folk psychology also provides a second intentional locus, the "head". The head is a site of superficial views, associated with the moment-to-moment conduct of communication instead of deep and lasting beliefs. The "head" is invoked in proposals that the meaning of words has been disengaged from deep and consistent belief. ... In summary, the folk psychology ... holds that language that comes from the "heart" is the authentic voice of a person's intentional core, but when we hear the "head" we hear only superficial and fleeting expressions that can include "mis-speaking", "blundering", "mistakes", and "poorly chosen words".

As can be seen, the dichotomy here is actually reminiscent of the older cardiocentric view in the West that the heart is the real source of the soul, which is however manifested through the principal organs including the brain. In short, the heart so viewed is the "hard core" of the self, or the locus of one's true self. The mistake made by the head is just a "malfunction" of the brain as the mere "processor". To a certain degree, this conception resembles the cultural conceptualization of the heart in Chinese where the heart is the central organ whereas the brain is more of an auxiliary one.

Today, indeed, the Chinese share all the scientific knowledge about the brain, but this scientific knowledge about the brain has not nudged aside their cultural conceptualization of the heart, which is the subject of my book. As I suggested earlier, scientific knowledge of the brain and cultural conceptualization of the heart are both part of the Chinese cultural models of the self and cognitive agency. They can coexist in Chinese people's conceptual systems, probably in different domains, and they may be separately retrieved to make different senses for different purposes in different contexts. Undoubtedly, scientific knowledge will affect cultural conceptualization, but this can be a very long process. Considering the fact that the Chinese conceptualization of the heart has not changed much during the last two thousand and five hundred years, we can predict that it will probably not change much for many years to come, in spite of the fact that China now is undergoing rapid and fundamental changes of modernization, economically, scientifically, politically, and necessarily conceptually.[131]

Finally, let me summarize the main difference between Western and Chinese cultures concerning the present status of the "heart" or "heart" metaphor. I would say that in the West the heart has largely become a cultural symbol or a mere metaphor, pointing to a long history of significance now left behind, whereas in Chinese the view of the heart is still, to a large extent, a cultural belief, carrying along and continuing a long history of significance. I would also say that, in spite of this difference, there is room for a common view of the brain: The West and China share the scientific knowledge that it is the brain that controls the human body and the whole person. Although scientific knowledge serves as part of cultural models, it does not do so overnight: the West has already incorporated the new status of the brain in its cultural conceptualization, whereas Chinese has not and still fully associates mental and intellectual life with the heart.

---

131 It is perhaps relevant to mention that, historically, feudalism lasted through many dynasties over two thousand years in China. Many blame Confucianism for China's long-lasting feudal system because it promoted a stable social structure and ethical codes favored by the ruling class. The Republican Revolution that overthrew the last feudal dynasty broke out nearly a century ago, but real modernization has been under way for about two decades only. It would be interesting to see how rapid modernization will bring about conceptual changes in China. As I discussed in section 3.5, the proposal to eliminate Chinese medicine from China's public health system for being "a folk theory and practice without real scientific grounding", and the national debate triggered by it regarding not only the future of Chinese medicine but also the attitude toward the heritages of traditional Chinese culture at large, are just examples of such changes and the tension that they may cause.

7.3. Looking beyond: Methodological issues

As for the research method used in this book, I have mainly leaned on a qualitative approach. That is, I have explored the field along three dimensions: a diachronic one, a synchronic one, and a cross-culturally comparative one. My research has, of course, the kinds of limitations that qualitative studies have in that they cannot produce the kinds of verifiable findings that quantitative studies do produce. Discussing the methodological issues in Cognitive Linguistics, Geeraerts (2006d: 44–46) argues that linguistics in general and Cognitive Linguistics in particular need to make a radical methodological turn, moving more toward various forms of quantitative and empirical research such as experimental, corpus-based, and statistical approaches. But he also points out that empirical research does not mean restricting the investigation to one kind of method or technique. Rather, it means using the quantitative methods in combination with qualitative methods such as analytical and interpretative approaches in the empirical cycle of successful research. Qualitative and quantitative methods in linguistics or, more generally, in the social sciences and the humanities, are complementary to each other. They are each good at addressing certain issues, solving certain problems, and obtaining certain findings. They each, however, are also limited in addressing some other issues, resolving some other problems, or getting some other findings. Therefore, as I see it, both qualitative and quantitative approaches can be very informative to each other and provide each other with insights lacked by the other. Fully aware of the limitations of my studies presented in this book, I hope that the scope of my studies will be both expanded and deepened by studies that are methodologically complementary to mine. Pritzker's (2007) recent article titled "Thinking hearts, feeling brains: Metaphor, culture, and the self in Chinese narratives of depression" presents a study that is in one way complementary to mine, especially with its quantitative findings.[132]

In this article, Pritzker (2007: 251) explores "the heart and brain metaphors used in the meaning-making efforts of Chinese individuals diagnosed with depression". To do this she looks at "spontaneously generated speech" recorded while interviewing 49 Chinese depression patients in various

[132] Pritzker (2007) uses my paper "The Chinese heart as the central faculty of cognition" (Yu 2008c) as one of her main references. My paper was first presented at the 9th International Cognitive Linguistics Conference held at Yonsei University, Seoul, Korea in 2005. Therefore, it is listed as Yu (2005) in her paper.

medical contexts in Beijing, although in this particular article she looks closely into three patients' narratives solicited by the interviewer. Her finding is that, of the 49 participants in the study, 45 (92%) used "metaphors of the heart" to express both thinking and feeling, and 18 of the 45 (37%) also used "brain metaphors" to express both thinking and feeling; no informants solely referred to their brains in their narratives (p. 257). Based on this finding, Pritzker argues that cultural understandings of the self can be multiple. "The use of a combination of heart and brain metaphors to describe experience by 37% of the participants in the study" suggests that "Chinese individuals can and do simultaneously hold various models from which they can draw upon in understanding and expressing their experience" (p. 252).

I truly appreciate Pritzker's empirical study that found out the percentages of the 49 depression patients that referred to the heart or brain in talking about thinking and feeling, although I do not necessarily agree with her use of such terms as "heart and brain metaphors" and "metaphorical models of the self" in the situation described. I will explain why and how below. As I see it, the fact that 92% of the patients referred to the heart when expressing thinking and feeling really reinforces, from a different viewpoint and a different approach, my central claim in this book for the cultural conceptualization of the Chinese heart as the central faculty of cognition. But what about 37% of the patients also referring to the brain when talking about thinking and feeling? This does not really surprise me, especially because Pritzker's study was conducted in a medical context, and I completely agree with her argument that the Chinese hold multiple cultural models of the self. As a matter of fact, it would have surprised me if the percentages had been reversed, i.e., if 92% had referred to the brain, whereas only 37% of them would have referred to the heart, under the same circumstances. It would be interesting to find out what corresponding percentages there would be in the same situation in a Western context, but my speculation is that we are likely to see such a reversal. When I argued that the heart is conceptualized as the central faculty of cognition in Chinese culture, I meant that it is perceived by the Chinese as the main, but not the sole, faculty of cognition. In section 4.6, as well as in Yu (2008c), I noted that the brain is also manifested in Chinese as the seat of thought, memory, and intellect, and hence as the locus of the "mind", too. I also cited two examples, from Feng (2003) and Gu (2005), which appear to present contradictory views regarding whether the brain or heart is regarded as the cognitive agent, or the locus of "mind", of a person. My argument is that the Chinese actually believe both, holding them simultaneously and separately in what I referred to as "scientific mind" and "cultural mind". Schemas of scientific knowledge and cultural knowledge exist in different domains of individuals' conceptual systems, playing different roles in different contexts at both local and more global levels. In other words, people may hold different, and sometimes contradictory, cultural models, as Pritzker (2007) argues.

In studying idiomatic expressions involving *xin* 'heart' and *nao* 'brain' in Chinese phraseology, using commonly-used dictionaries as a sort of data corpus and examples collected from actual discourse, I found that those involving the latter are incomparably fewer in number than those involving the former (see Ch. 4 and Appendix 1). My argument is that *xin* 'heart' is a key word (in the sense of Wierzbicka 1997a) of Chinese culture but *nao* 'brain' is not. This argument is not based on a linguistic study of idiomatic expressions alone. Instead, my synchronic study (Ch. 4) is built on and extended from my diachronic studies of both ancient Chinese philosophy (Ch. 2) and traditional Chinese medicine (Ch. 3), and is complemented by textual analyses of contemporary Chinese discourse (Ch. 5). The findings of all these studies, from different viewpoints, support the same argument that the Chinese conceptualize the heart as the central, though not the sole, faculty of cognition. While language reflects its cultural context, it also exerts an influence on its users' cognition. Scientific knowledge will, beyond doubt, influence and change human cognition, but this may be a long process affected by many other factors such as philosophy, religion, arts, literature, and language. All of these factors, interacting with one another, determine the landscape of cultural conceptualizations in particular and of cultural models in general. Only when one factor has become so big and strong as to be able to change other factors will it bring about a significant change to the landscape of individual conceptual systems and collective cultural models of a group.

Now, I turn and look at Pritzker's Chinese data, provided below as examples (from Pritzker 2007: 257–258). I would call into question her claim that the Chinese patients were using "heart and brain metaphors" to express thinking and feeling or to refer to their mental experience:

我心里就这么想

Wo	***xinli***	*jiu*	*zheme*	***xiang***
I	heart-inside	then	like-this	think

'In my heart I think like this'

我心想，我是妈妈
Wo ***xin*** ***xiang,*** *wo shi mama*
I heart thinks I am mother
'My heart thinks, "I am a mother"'

这脑子里老想这个
Zhe ***naozi*** ***li*** *lao* ***xiang*** *zhege*
this brain inside always think this
'In my brain I always think of this'

脑子想的事太多了
Naozi ***xiang*** *de shi tai duo le*
brain thinks MOD troubles too much PRT
'My brain thinks too much of my troubles'

I agree that in these cases the heart or brain is understood metaphorically as a container, but I would be hesitant to call them "heart and brain metaphors" for the thinking and feeling self. Look at the following propositions:

1. THE HEART IS THE RULER OF THE BODY
2. THE HEART IS THE LOCUS OF THE MIND
3. THE HEART IS THE LOCUS OF THE SELF

I would treat the above three propositions differently. I would call the first one a metaphorical proposition, or a conceptual metaphor, as is generally known in Cognitive Linguistics. I would, however, prefer to regard the second and third as nonmetaphorical propositions, or cultural beliefs and assumptions that are not meant as metaphorical by people who believe or assume them, especially in the Chinese cultural context.[133] All three of them, nonetheless, serve as parts of the Chinese cultural models for the concepts of "heart" and "self". I want to clarify my position here because, according to Pritzker (2007: 256), she was following me (Yu 2008c) in classifying "heart and brain metaphors" into "three major categories".

As I said earlier, the heart has long become "a cultural symbol" or "a cultural metaphor" in the West, but it is still "a cultural belief" in Chinese. As for the reference to the brain in these instances, it reflects modern scientific knowledge about the brain. Of course, scientific knowledge can be part

133 Readers are referred to Dirven (2002) for a subtle division and classification of the points along a conceptual continuum at various levels, such as literal and nonliteral; nonfigurative and figurative; literal, metonymic (consisting of different types of metonymy), and metaphorical.

of the cultural models. Those examples involving *nao* 'brain', as well as *xin* 'heart', do reflect the Chinese cultural models of the self, but these are not "metaphorical models of the self" (Pritzker 2007: 252). Cultural models can be and often are composed of nonmetaphorical or literal propositions.

Having said the above, I really believe that Pritzker (2007) has made an important contribution to the Chinese conceptualization of the self and person with her valuable findings, despite the fact that her paper also contains some deficiencies.[134] She quantified her data collected from depression patients' spontaneously generated speech. That is a perspective that I do not have in the studies presented in this book. In Chapter 5, I analyzed some sample texts from contemporary Chinese discourse, but those are the texts carefully generated by an essayist and a poet. It is because of her different approach from mine that Pritzker (2007) was able to arrive at some findings and conclusions that are complementary to mine. Based on her quantified findings, her point that people may draw from multiple, sometimes

---

[134] There is one more thing that I want to point out here. That is, Pritzker (2007: 258) says in her article, "Yu's (2005) suggestion that the use of brain metaphors to describe thinking relate to Western philosophical framework prompted me to examine how and if the use of brain metaphors reflected a more 'Westernized' orientation in terms of age, sex, urban versus rural residence, education, or employment". That is a mis-citation of my paper. In fact, what I claimed in that paper is the opposite. First of all, I would not characterize those instances as "brain metaphors". Furthermore, I argued that, while the rise of Cartesian dualism in the early modern period had an impact on the dichotomy between heart and head in the West, the lack of such a philosophical change in Chinese thought (Daoism, Confucianism, etc) makes the cultural conceptualization of the heart as the central faculty of cognition more stable and persistent. My point is that the brain plays a relatively small part in the Chinese cultural conceptualization of cognitive functions of thinking and feeling, "but this part has been growing owing to the increasing influence of scientific knowledge". I attributed the increasing role of the brain in Chinese to modern science, rather than to the influence of Western philosophy. If the cultural conceptualization of the heart as the central faculty of cognition in Chinese has not changed much during the past two thousand and five hundred years, how can one find significant differences in this regard between, say, the older and younger of the present time? I assume, however, that in the future the brain's role will continue to increase, though slowly, in the Chinese cultural conceptualization of the self, due to increasing scientific influence.

contradictory, cultural models is especially well taken.[135] As she notes, while others "focus on broad culturally salient trends", her own approach "advocates supplementing such analyses with a focus on the specific ways in which cultural trends are and are not enacted in the daily lives of individuals", and the two perspectives or approaches are "fully complementary" (p. 269).

In general, it is important to realize and acknowledge the complementary nature of various research methodologies since each of them, applying a PAINTING metaphor, can see merely one aspect of the object under scrutiny from a particular angle with a specific viewpoint in space. Only when the object is examined from all angles can its real shape and structure be revealed and understood. Usually, researchers are only trained to approach the object from one angle, or they are perhaps only interested in looking at it from one viewpoint. This is fine, but they need to be aware that they are viewing only one aspect of the object instead of the whole thing. Hopefully, others will take different approaches to looking at the same object so that all its aspects will be viewed in full.

7.4. Emerging from it: Afterword

In this book, I have at least attempted to look at more than one aspect of the object of my study – the Chinese *xin* 'heart' – from more than one angle. It was not until I had fully embarked on and delved into this book project that I began to realize that a comprehensive study of this single Chinese concept of *xin* 'heart' was perhaps too ambitious a goal for me to achieve; and that it could as well be something beyond my grasp. I have been more than gratified, as well as humbled, by my experience during the last few years working on it or wrestling with it, in bright or dim light, and sometimes in total darkness, before finally emerging from it now. I have to leave it at that, at least for the time being, and now prefer to see it as a preliminary rather than comprehensive study, and hope to conduct or see further empirical studies that complement it in one way or another.

---

[135] The example of Trent Lott (Hill, forthcoming) cited in section 7.2 is another good example illustrating that there exist multiple and contradictory cultural models for conceptualizing heart and head in a Western context.

Appendix 1
Additional idiomatic expressions involving *xin* 'heart'

I. Compound words

心盛 *xin-sheng* (heart-vigorous/energetic) 'in high spirit; enthusiastic'
心传 *xin-chuan* (heart-pass) '(Buddhism) mind-to-mind instruction from master to disciple (without the aid of scriptures); a doctrine or theory passed on from generation to generation'
心死 *xin-si* (heart-die) 'one's will dies within one – see the futility of one's attempt'
心胆 *xin-dan* (heart-gallbladder) 'will and courage'
心腹 *xin-fu* (heart-belly) 'trusted subordinate; reliable agent; henchman; bosom friend; confidential'
心身 *xin-shen* (heart-body) 'mind and body'
心力 *xin-li* (heart-strength) 'mental and physical efforts'
心脏 *xin-zang* (heart-organ) 'the heart; the central or most vital part of anything'
心战 *xin-zhan* (heart-war) 'psychological warfare'
甘心 *gan-xin* (sweet/willing-heart) 'do sth. willingly; be ready and willing; be reconciled to; resign oneself to; be content with'
钻心 *zuan-xin* (drill-heart) '(of pain, itching, etc.) unbearable'
芳心 *fang-xin* (fragrant-heart) 'the heart of a young woman'
春心 *chun-xin* (spring-heart) 'thoughts of love; stirrings of love; budding love; desire for love; longing for love'
安心 *an-xin* (set at ease/calm-heart) 'feel at ease; be relieved; set one's mind at rest; keep one's mind on sth.'
塌心 *ta-xin* (fall down-heart) '*dial.* settle down to sth; set one's mind at ease'
闲心 *xian-xin* (idle-heart) 'leisurely mood'
唯心 *wei-xin* (only-heart) 'idealistic'
戒心 *jie-xin* (guard against-heart) 'vigilance; wariness'
疑心 *yi-xin* (suspicious-heart) 'suspicion; suspect'
吃心 *chi-xin* (eat-heart) '*dial.* be oversensitive; be suspicious; be absorbed in sth.'
多心 *duo-xin* (more [than enough]-heart) 'oversensitive; paranoid'

过心 *guo-xin* (exceed-heart) '(*dial.*) oversensitive; paranoid'
祸心 *huo-xin* (disaster-heart) 'evil intent; evil intention; malice'
信心 *xin-xin* (confident-heart) 'confidence; faith'
空心 *kong-xin* (empty-heart) 'hollow inside'
满心 *man-xin* (full-heart) 'have one's heart filled with'
中心 *zhong-xin* (middle/central-heart) 'center; heart; core; hub'
重心 *zhong-xin* (heavy-heart) 'center of gravity; heart; core; focus'
核心 *he-xin* (core-heart) 'nucleus; core; kernel'
轴心 *zhou-xin* (axle-heart) 'axle center; axis'
圆心 *yuan-xin* (circle-heart) 'the center of a circle'
天心 *tian-xin* (heaven-heart) 'God's will; the will of Heaven'
攻心 *gong-xin* (attack-heart) 'attack the mind; make a psychological attack'
归心 *gui-xin* (return-heart) 'thoughts of returning home; homesickness'
收心 *shou-xin* (get back-heart) 'get into the frame of mind for work or study; concentrate on more serious things; have a change of heart'
问心 *wen-xin* (ask-heart) 'examine oneself; examine one's conscience'
扪心 *men-xin* (touch-heart) 'touch or feel one's heart by hand; examine one's conscience'
偏心 *pian-xin* (inclined to one side-heart) 'partiality; bias'
平心 *ping-xin* (flat/level-heart) 'in all fairness; being fair, impartial'

心上人 *xin-shang ren* (heart-on person) 'person of one's heart; one's beloved'
寻开心 *xun kai-xin* (seek open-heart) '*dial.* make fun of; poke fun at; joke'
责任心 *zeren-xin* (responsibility-heart) 'sense of responsibility'
有心人 *you-xin ren* (have-heart person) 'a person who sets his mind on doing sth. useful; a person with high aspirations and determination; an observant and conscientious person'
心头肉 *xin-tou rou* (heart-head flesh) 'a dearly loved person or a treasured possession'
主心骨 *zhu-xin gu* (manage-heart bone) 'backbone; mainstay; pillar; a definite view; one's own judgment'
心腹事 *xin-fu shi* (heart-belly matter) 'a secret in the depth of one's heart'
心腹话 *xin-fu hua* (heart-belly words) '(tell sb.) sth. in strict confidence'
心气高 *xin-qi gao* (heart-qi high) 'have high aspirations'
心气窄 *xin-qi zhai* (heart-qi narrow) 'narrow-minded'

II. Idiomatic phrases

心地善良	*xin-di shan-liang* (heart-land kind-good) 'good-natured; kind-hearted'
心地单纯	*xin-di dan-chun* (heart-land simple-pure) 'simpleminded'
心地坦白	*xin-di tan-bai* (heart-land flat-white) 'candid; open'
心地光明	*xin-di guang-ming* (heart-land light-bright) 'upright and pure in mind; always open and aboveboard'
心地狭窄	*xin-di xia-zhai* (heart-land narrow-narrow) 'be narrow-minded; have a mean heart'
心神不宁	*xin-shen bu-ning* (heart-spirit not-peaceful) 'be anxious and pre-occupied; agitated; be on tenterhooks; be distracted; feel ill at east; feel restless; fidgety; have no peace of mind; in a state of discomposure; wandering in thought'
心神不安	*xin-shen bu-an* (heart-spirit not-peaceful) 'not to feel easy in one's mind; be disconcerted; be confused and worried'
心神不定	*xin-shen bu-ding* (heart-spirit not-settled) 'be anxious and preoccupied; be agitated; feel restless'
心神不羁	*xin-shen bu-ji* (heart-spirit not-restrained/controlled) 'difficult to concentrate one's mind on sth.; with one's mind running wild'
心神颠倒	*xin-shen dian-dao* (heart-spirit upside-down) 'be utterly confused; go off into raptures or ecstasies'
心神恍惚	*xin-shen huanghu* (heart-spirit in-a-trance) 'be ill at ease and full of dread; perturbed in mind; spellbound'
心荡神驰	*xin-dang shen-chi* (heart-wave spirit-gallop) 'feel excited; go into ecstasies over sth.; go into raptures over sth.; distracted'
心荡神迷	*xin-dang shen-mi* (heart-wave spirit-enchanted) 'be in ecstasies; go into ecstasies'
心荡神摇	*xin-dang shen-yao* (heart-wave spirit-rock) 'feel very excited; go into ecstasies'
心照神交	*xin-zhao shen-jiao* (heart-illuminate spirit-cross) 'have a tacit mutual understanding'
心驰神往	*xin-chi shen-wang* (heart-gallop spirit-go) 'one's thoughts fly to (a place or person); have a deep longing for'
心旷神怡	*xin-kuang shen-yi* (heart-vast/spacious spirit-joyful/cheerful) 'relaxed and joyful; carefree and happy'
心领神会	*xin-ling shen-hui* (heart-get/understand spirit-meet) 'understand tacitly; readily take a hint'
心潮起伏	*xin-chao qi-fu* (heart-tide rising-falling) 'one's heart seems to rise and fall like the waves; the tide in one's heart rises and falls'

心潮澎湃 *xin-chao pengbai* (heart-tide surging) 'feel an upsurge of emotion; one's thoughts surge like the tide; one's mind is flooded with memories; one's mind is in a turmoil'

心绪万千 *xin-xu wan-qian* (heart-thread ends; ten thousand-thousand) 'in an emotional turmoil'

心手相应 *xin-shou xiang-ying* (heart-hand mutually-respond) 'the hand responding perfectly to the mind – amazingly skilful; mind and hand in accord; what the mind wishes the hands are able to do'

心慕手追 *xin-mu shou-zhui* (heart-admire hand-chase) 'admire greatly and do one's utmost to imitate the skill; what one's heart admires the hands follow'

心胆俱裂 *xin-dan ju-lie* (heart-gallbladder both-split) 'be so frightened that one's heart and gall burst; be frightened out of one's wits; be terror-stricken'

心殒胆落 *xin-yun dan-luo* (heart-die gallbladder-fall) 'be scared to death'

心血来潮 *xin-xue lai-chao* (heart-blood come-tide) 'be prompted by a sudden impulse; be seized by a whim; have a sudden inspiration'

心宽体泰 *xin-kuan ti-tai* (heart-broad body-safe) 'carefree and healthy'

心气不顺 xin-qi bu-shun (heart-qi not-smooth [in circulation]) 'in a bad mood'

心平气和 *xin-ping qi-he* (heart-flat/even qi-mild) 'even-tempered and good-humored; calm; be in a calm mood; calm of spirit and even of temper'

心余力绌 *xin-yu li-chu* (heart-surplus strength-inadequate) 'one's ability falls short of one's wishes; the spirit is willing, but the flesh is weak'

心余力拙 *xin-yu li-zhuo* (heart-surplus strength-awkward) 'though one still cherishes high aspiration, one's strength falls short of his wishes; more than willing but lacking the power to; bite off more than one can chew'

心投意合 *xin-tou yi-he* (heart-agree thought-get along) 'of the same opinion; hit it off perfectly'

心满意足 *xin-man yi-zu* (heart-full desire-sufficient) 'be perfectly content or satisfied; to one's heart content; be fully satisfied and content'

心明眼亮 *xin-ming yan-liang* (heart-bright eye-shiny) 'see and think clearly; be sharp-eyed and clear-hearted'

心灵手巧 *xin-ling shou-qiao* (heart-quick hand-skillful) 'clever and deft; quick-witted and nimble-fingered; clever in mind and skillful in hand'

心回意转 *xin-hui yi-zhuan* (heart-return thought-turn back) 'change or alter one's mind; change one's views; a change of heart; come around; repent'

心猿意马	*xin-yuan yi-ma* (heart-ape thought-horse) 'a heart like a capering monkey and a mind like a galloping horse – restless; perturbed'
心虔意诚	*xin-qian yi-cheng* (heart-pious wish-sincere) 'with pious wishes'
心口如一	*xin-kou ru-yi* (heart-mouth like-one) 'say what one thinks; speak from the heart; be frank and forthright'
心拙口笨	*xin-zhuo kou-ben* (heart-awkward mouth-dull) 'dull-witted and slow-tongued'
心毒口辣	*xin-du kou-la* (heart-poisonous mouth-peppery/vicious) 'be vicious with a sharp, quick tongue'
心丧气沮	*xin-sang qi-ju* (heart-lost qi-depressed) 'the heart mourns and spirit spoils'
心如滚潮	*xin-ru-gun-chao* (heart-like-rolling-tide) 'like tossing waves in one's heart; one's mind is in a tumult'
心如古井	*xin-ru-gu-jing* (heart-like-ancient-well) 'one's heart is as tranquil as an old well; call forth no response in sb.'s breast'
心如枯井	*xin-ru-ku-jing* (heart-like-dry-well) 'one's heart is as tranquil as an old well; call forth no response in sb.'s breast'
心如止水	*xin-ru-zhi-shui* (heart-like-still-water) 'one's mind settled as still water'
心如冰炭	*xin-ru-bing-tan* (heart-like-ice-coal) 'be heartless and cold as ice'
心如刀刺	*xin-ru-dao-ci* (heart-like-knife-pierce) 'feel as if a knife were piercing one's heart; feel as if one's heart were pierced by daggers; feel as though a knife were sticking into one's heart'
心如刀扎	*xin-ru-dao-zha* (heart-like-knife-stab) 'one's heart seems pierced with a knife'
心如刀割	*xin-ru-dao-ge* (heart-like-knife-cut) 'like a dagger had cut deep into one's heart; one feels as though one's heart were cut in many pieces.
心如刀绞	*xin-ru-dao-jiao* (heart-like-knife-twist) 'feel as if a knife were being twisted in one's heart'
心如针扎	*xin-ru-zhen-zha* (heart-like-needle-prick) 'feel as if needles were pricking one's heart; feel greatly distressed as though one's heart pricks'
心如火焚	*xin-ru-huo-fen* (heart-like-fire-burn) 'one's heart is afire; burning with impatience; the heart burns like fire; torn by anxiety for'
心如火烧	*xin-ru-huo-shao* (heart-like-fire-burn) 'one's heart is afire; burning with impatience; the heart burns like fire; torn by anxiety for'
心如铁石	*xin-ru-tie-shi* (heart-like-iron-stone) 'have a heart of iron; be stony-hearted; be hard-hearted'
心如蛇蝎	*xin-ru-she-jie* (heart-like-snake-scorpion) 'one's heart is as poisonous as any viper or scorpion; have the heart of a devil'

心如石沉 *xin-ru-shi-chen* (heart-like-stone-sink) 'one's heart sank like a stone'

心如死灰 *xin-ru-si-hui* (heart-like-dead-ash) 'one's heart is like dead ashes – hopelessly apathetic; utterly dissipated'

心怀鬼胎 *xin-huai gui-tai* (heart-conceive ghost-fetus) 'have evil intentions; have sinister motives; conceive mischief; entertain dark schemes'

心怀不善 *xin-huai bu-shan* (heart-conceive not-kind) 'cherish evil thoughts'

心怀不轨 *xin-huai bu-gui* (heart-conceive not-on [right] track) 'harbor evil designs'

心怀不满 *xin-huai bu-man* (heart-conceive not-satisfied) 'nurse a grievance; be filled with resentment; have a grievance against; harbor feelings of dissatisfaction'

心怀不平 *xin-huai bu-ping* (heart-conceive not-level) 'have a grievance against; feel aggrieved'

心怀二意 *xin-huai er-yi* (heart-conceive two-thoughts/intentions) 'harbor disloyal sentiments; have two faces'

心怀叵测 *xin-huai po-ce* (heart-conceive impossible-measure) 'harbor unfathomable evil designs; have sinister intentions'

心悦诚服 *xin-yue cheng-fu* (heart-happy sincerely-convinced) 'be completely convinced; feel a heartfelt admiration'

心劳计绌 *xin-lao ji-chu* (heart-labor scheme-inadequate) 'rack one's brains in vain; be at one's wit's end'

心劳日拙 *xin-lao ri-zhuo* (heart-labor day-by-day-dull) 'fare worse and worse for all one's scheming'

心劳力拙 *xin-lao li-zhuo* (heart-labor strength-dull) 'feel tired in mind and exhausted in strength'

心乱如麻 *xin-luan ru-ma* (heart-messy like-hemp) 'one's mind confused like entangled hemp; have one's mind all in a tangle; be utterly confused and disconcerted; be terribly upset'

心头火起 xin-tou huo-qi (heart-head fire-rise) 'burn with anger'

心急如火 xin-ji ru-huo (heart-impatient like-fire) 'be afire with impatience; burn with impatience; his heart burns with anxiety; be very impatient as if being set on fire'

心照不宣 *xin-zhao bu-xuan* (heart-illuminate not-declare) 'have tacit understanding'

心向往之 *xin xiangwang zhi* (heart oriented to it) 'yearning for sb. or sth.'

心无二用 *xin-wu-er-yong* (heart-no-two-uses) 'one cannot keep one's mind on two things at the same time; one should concentrate on one thing at a time'

心眼活泛 *xin-yan huofan* (heart-eye flexible) 'have a supple mind; be quick-witted'
心中无数 *xin-zhong wu-shu* (heart-middle not-have-numbers) 'have no idea of how things stand; not know for certain'
心中有数 *xin-zhong you-shu* (heart-middle have-numbers) 'know the score; have a pretty good idea of how things stand; know fairly well'
心路不正 *xin-lu bu-zheng* (heart-road not-straight) 'harbor bad intentions'
心有余悸 *xin-you yu-ji* (heart-has lingering-fear) 'one's heart still fluttering with fear; have a lingering fear'
心胸豁达 *xin-xiong huo-da* (heart-chest open-understanding) 'with a great heart; broadminded'
心腹之患 *xin-fu zhi-huan* (heart-belly MOD-disease) 'disease in one's vital organs – danger from within; serious hidden trouble or danger'
心腹之交 *xin-fu zhi jiao* (heart-belly MOD friend) 'a very intimate friend; a bosom friend'
心里打鼓 *xin-li da-gu* (heart-inside beat-drum) 'have butterflies in the stomach; feel diffident'
心心念念 *xin-xin nian-nian* (heart-heart think/thought-think/thought) 'longingly; yearningly; keep thinking about; constantly think of; anxiously longing for'
心心相印 *xin-xin xiang-yin* (heart-heart mutually-print) 'have mutual affinity; be closely attached to each other'
心心相连 *xin-xin xiang-lian* (heart-heart mutually-connected) 'hearts are linked together'
归心似箭 *gui-xin si-jian* (return-heart like-arrow) 'with one's heart set on speeding home; impatient to get back; anxious to return'
收心归正 *shou-xin gui-zheng* (get back-heart return to-right) 'give up evil ways and return to the right path; get into the right frame of mind'
平心静气 *ping-xin jing-qi* (level-heart quiet-qi) 'calmly; dispassionately'
问心无愧 *wen-xin wu-kui* (ask-heart no-shame) 'feel on qualms upon self-examination; have a clear conscience'
问心有愧 *wen-xin you-kui* (ask-heart have-shame) 'feel a twinge of conscience; have a guilty conscience'
扪心自问 *men-xin zi-wen* (touch-heart self-ask) 'examine or search one's conscience'
扪心无愧 *men-xin wu-kui* (touch-heart no-shame) 'feel that one has not done anything wrong; feel no qualms upon self-examination; have a good or clear conscience'
直心眼儿 *zhi xin-yan-er* (straight heart-eye-SUB) 'open; frank; straightforward'

实心眼儿 *shi xin-yan-er* (solid heart-eye-SUB) 'honest and serious-minded; having a one-track mind; an honest and serious-minded person'
死心眼儿 *si xin-yan-er* (dead heart-eye-SUF) 'be bent on one purpose; be too pig-headed; stubborn; obstinate and simple-minded; person with a one-track mind'
耍心眼儿 *shua xin-yan-er* (play with heart-eye-SUB) 'exercise one's wits for personal gain; be calculating; pull a smart trick'
斗心眼儿 *dou xin-yan-er* (fight heart-eye-SUB) 'fight a battle of wits; rival in trickery'
诚心诚意 *cheng-xin cheng-yi* (sincere-heart sincere-intention) 'earnestly and sincerely'
真心实意 *zhen-xin shi-yi* (true-heart actual-intention) 'genuinely and sincerely; truly and wholeheartedly'
实心实意 *shi-xin shi-yi* (actual-heart actual-intention) 'honest and sincere'
真心诚意 *zhen-xin zheng-yi* (true-heart sincere-intention) 'wholeheartedly; wholeheartedness; in good faith; with all one's heart'
真心好意 *zhen-xin hao-yi* (true-heart good-intention) 'good intentions'
真心善意 *zhen-xin shan-yi* (true-heart kind-intention) 'sincerely and with good intentions; open and truehearted; with sincerity and good intentions'
全心全意 *quan-xin quan-yi* (whole-heart whole-intention) 'put one's heart and soul into sth.; heart and soul; put one's whole heart into sth.; wholeheartedly; with all one's heart'
同心同意 *tong-xin tong-yi* (same-heart same-thought) 'be hand and glove; be heart and hand; be of the same mind; be of one mind; with one heart and mind'
三心二意 *san-xin er-yi* (three-hearts two-thoughts) 'be of two minds; shilly-shally; be half-hearted; double-minded; change one's mind constantly'
遂心如意 *sui-xin ru-yi* (satisfy-heart accord with-wish) 'be perfectly satisfied'
回心转意 *hui-xin zhuan-yi* (return-heart turn around-thought) 'change one's mind; have a change of heart; turn back one's heart and change one's mind'
锦心绣口 *jin-xin xiu-kou* (splendid-heart beautiful-mouth) 'elegant thought; flowery speech – a fine literary style; elegant and refined; beautiful writing'
随心所欲 *sui-xin suo-yu* (follow-heart be resigned to-desire) 'follow one's inclinations; have one's way; do as one pleases'
从心所欲 *cong-xin suo-yu* (follow-heart be resigned to-desire) 'have whatever one's heart desires; do as one pleases; free-wheeling'

遂心所欲	*sui-xin suo-yu* (satisfy-heart be resigned to-desire) 'to one's liking; follow what the heart desires; have one's will; satisfy one's desire'
苦心孤诣	*ku-xin gu-yi* (bitter-heart solitary-attainment) 'try hard to (do); make a notable achievement after extraordinarily persistent and painstaking efforts; toil single-heartedly; work with a bitter heart and make progress single-handed'
苦心钻研	*ku-xin zuanyan* (bitter-heart research) 'do painstaking research; serious study and investigation'
苦心经营	*ku-xin jingying* (bitter-heart manage) 'mastermind with painstaking effort; manage painstakingly; painstakingly build up (an enterprise, etc.); rack one's brains for ways and means to try making the enterprise a success'
苦心致志	*ku-xin zhi-zhi* (bitter-heart devoted-will) 'by faithful devotion and constancy of purpose'
一心为公	*yi-xin wei-gong* (one-heart for-public) 'devote oneself to the public interests; be heart and soul devoted to public interests'
一心向往	*yi-xin xiang-wang* (one-heart look-to) 'give one's heart completely to'
同心协力	*tong-xin xie-li* (same-heart joint strength) 'work in full cooperation and with unity of purpose; work together with one heart; make concerted efforts'
同心并力	*tong-xin he-li* (same-heart combined-strength) 'unite all efforts for common purpose'
尽心尽力	*jin-xin jin-li* (exhaust-heart exhaust-strength) 'strain every nerve; do one's utmost; exert one's heart and strength to the utmost'
费心劳力	*fei-xin lao-li* (cost-heart take-strength) 'take a lot of trouble'
忠心耿耿	*zhong-xin genggeng* (loyal-heart devoted) 'loyal and devoted; most faithful and true'
野心不死	*ye-xin bu-si* (wild-heart not-die) 'cling to one's ambitious designs'
贼心不死	*zei-xin bu-si* (thief-heart not-die) 'refuse to give up one's evil designs'
安心不善	*an-xin bu-shan* (install-heart not-kind) 'harbor/have evil intentions'
安心不良	*an-xin bu-liang* (install-heart not-good) 'harbor ill intentions/thoughts; harbor thought of injuring others'
居心不良	*ju-xin bu-liang* (store up-heart not-good) 'harbor ill intentions'
居心叵测	*ju-xin po-ce* (store up-heart impossible-measure) 'with hidden intent; with ulterior motives'

用心良苦 *yong-xin liang-ku* (use-heart very-bitter) 'have really given much thought to the matter; have expended much care and thought on sth.'

用心险恶 *yong-xin xian-e* (use-heart dangerous-evil) 'have vicious intentions; harbor sinister motives'

用心竭力 *yong-xin jie-li* (use-heart exhaust-strength) 'attentively and diligently; exhaust one's brain and energy'

处心积虑 *chu-xin ji-lü* (store-heart accumulate-thought) 'deliberately plan (to achieve evil ends); incessantly scheme; brood over a matter for a long time'

钩心斗角 *gou-xin dou-jiao* (hook-heart fight-horn) 'intrigue against each other; jockey for position; engage in petty intrigue and try to get the better of each other; maneuver for positions against rivals; scheme and plot against one another'

狼心狗肺 *lang-xin gou-fei* (wolf-heart dog-lung) 'rapacious as wolf and savage as a cur; cruel and unscrupulous; brutal and cold-blooded; heartless and ungrateful; wicked-hearted'

缺心少肺 *que-xin shao-fei* (miss-heart lack-lung) 'heartless; conscienceless; mean; wicked'

没心没肺 *mei-xin mei-fei* (have no-heart have no-lung) 'heartless; conscienceless; wicked'

痛心入骨 *tong-xin ru-gu* (pain-heart into-bone) 'feel deeply grieved; with deep hatred and resentment'

铭心镂骨 *ming-xin lou-gu* (engrave-heart carve-bone) 'imprint on the heart and engrave on the bones – remember forever with gratitude; be wholeheartedly grateful to sb.'

镂心刻骨 *lou-xin ke-gu* (carve-heart engrave-bone) 'inscribe a debt of gratitude on one's mind or in one's heart'

赏心悦目 *shang-xin yue-mu* (delight-heart please-eye) 'find the scenery pleasing both to the eye and the mind; gladden the heart and please the eye'

得心应手 *de-xin ying-shou* (get-heart respond-hand) 'what the heart wishes one's hands accomplish; with facility; with high proficiency; serviceable; handy'

推心置腹 *tui-xin zhi-fu* (push-heart place-belly) 'repose full confidence in sb.; confide in sb.'

师心自用 *shi-xin zi-yong* (master-heart self-use) 'be opinionated; not willing to listen to advice; act and show overconfidence in oneself; act with self-assurance'

丧心病狂 *sang-xin bing-kuang* (lose-heart illness-wild) 'frenzied; frantic; perverse'

瞒心昧己	*man-xin mei-ji* (hide from-heart conceal from-self) 'deceive oneself; blot out one's conscience; deceive and muddle oneself'
匠心独运	*jiang-xin du-yun* (craftsman-heart uniquely-exercise) 'consummate craftsmanship; exercise one's inventive mind; show one's own ingenuity'
匠心独具	*jiang-xin du-ju* (craftsman-heart uniquely-possess) 'have great originality'
别出心裁	*bie-chu xin-cai* (distinctly-show heart-planning) 'create new styles or fashions; adopt an original approach; try to be different; depart from established practice'
独出心裁	*du-chu xin-cai* (uniquely-show heart-planning) 'create new styles or fashions; be original; show originality'
一个心眼	*yi-ge xin-yan* (one-CL heart-eye) 'have one's heart set on sth.; devotedly; stubbornly; be of one mind'
一门心思	*yi-men xin-si* (one-CL heart-thought/thinking) 'concentrate one's mind on'
挖空心思	*wa-kong xin-si* (dig-empty heart-thought/idea) '*derog.* rack one's brains'
脸软心慈	*lian-ruan xin-ci* (face-soft heart-kind) 'be shy and kind; kind-hearted'
眼明心亮	*yan-ming xin-liang* (eye-light heart-bright) 'see and think clearly; be sharp-eyed and clear-headed'
煞费心计	*sha-fei xin-ji* (very much-spend heart-scheme) 'cudgel one's brains; rack one's brains'
眼花心乱	*yan-hua xin-luan* (eye-blurred heart-messy) 'one's eyes not clear and one's heart confused'
胆颤心惊	*dan-chan xin-jing* (gallbladder-quiver heart-startle) 'strike terror into the heart of; tremble with fright'
胆战心惊	*dan-zhan xin-jing* (gallbladder-tremble heart-startle) 'tremble with fear; be terror-stricken'
胆破心惊	*dan-po xin-jing* (gallbladder-break heart-startle) 'be scared to death'
沁人心脾	*qin-ren xin-pi* (seep into-people's heart-spleen) 'gladdening the heart and refreshing the mind; mentally refreshing; refreshing'
费尽心力	*fei-jin xin-li* (cost-all heart-strength) 'make much ado about'
枉费心力	*wang-fei xin-li* (in vain-cost heart-strength) 'hatch plots in vain; scheme to no avail; rack one's brains in vain'
人面兽心	*ren-mian shou-xin* (human-face beast-heart) 'the face of a man but the heart of a beast – a beast in human form'

佛口蛇心 *fo-kou she-xin* (Buddha-mouth snake-heart) 'a Buddha's words and a serpent's heart – malicious; a villainous hypocrite; a Buddha's mouth but a viper's heart – honeyed words but evil intent'

苦口婆心 *ku-kou po-xin* (bitter-mouth old lady-heart) '(admonish) earnestly and maternally; do one's best to convince sb.; admonishing words and kind feelings; advise in earnest words and with good intentions'

低首下心 *di-shou xia-xin* (bow-head lower-heart) 'bow and scrape; be obsequiously submissive'

诸事顺心 *zhu-shi shun-xin* (all-things go in the same direction-heart) 'all is well (lit. all the things are going with, not against, the heart)'

狼子野心 *lang-zi ye-xin* (wolf-cub wild-heart) 'a wolf cub with a savage heart – have a wolfish nature; be full of wild ambitions'

满怀信心 *man-huai xin-xin* (full-bosom confident-heart) 'be fully confident; have full confidence in; with full confidence'

刻骨铭心 *ke-gu ming-xin* (carve-bone engrave-heart) 'be engraved on one's bones and heart – be remembered with deep gratitude'

怵目惊心 *chu-mu jing-xin* (frighten-eye startle-heart) 'strike the eye and rouse the mind; be shocked at the sight of; be shocked to witness'

利欲熏心 *li-yu xun-xin* (profit-desire smoke-heart) 'be obsessed with the desire for gain; be overcome by covetousness; be blinded by greed'

漠不关心 *mo bu-guan-xin* (indifferent not-involve-heart) 'indifferent; unconcerned; indifferent and apathetic'

别有用心 *bie-you yong-xin* (other-have use-heart) 'have ulterior motives; have an axe to grind'

无所用心 *wu-suo yong-xin* (without-PRT use-heart) 'not give serious thought to anything; be indifferent to anything; have an empty head; without using the brain'

昧己瞒心 *mei-ji man-xin* (conceal from-self hide from-heart) 'do evil against one's conscience; play treacherous tricks against one's conscience'

别具匠心 *bie-ju jiang-xin* (distinctly-possess craftsman-heart) 'show ingenuity; have originality'

独具匠心 *du-ju jiang-xin* (uniquely-possess craftsman-heart) 'have great originality; have an inventive mind; show unique ingenuity'

独具慧心 *du-ju hui-xin* (uniquely-possess intelligent-heart) 'have a special understanding'

木人石心 *mu-ren shi-xin* (wood-person stone-heart) 'a body of wood and a heart of stone – insusceptible; unfeeling; insensitive'

十指连心 *shi-zhi-lian-xin* (ten-fingers-link-heart) 'the fingers are linked to the heart – what happens to children is of vital interest to parents; be like a man's ten fingers, so closely linked to one's heart'

高下在心 *gao-xia zai-xin* (high-low at-heart) 'do as one pleases; do whatever one wants; go or get one's own way; follow one's bent; follow one's own inclinations; at one's own sweet will'

万箭穿心 *wan-jian chuan-xin* (ten thousand-arrows pierce-heart) '(as if) ten thousand arrows have pierced the heart – in extreme grief'

动魄惊心 *dong-po jing-xin* (move-soul startle-heart) 'struck with fear; heart-shaking; shocking; soul-stirring; profoundly affecting'

提溜着心 *diliu-zhe xin* (carry-DUR heart) 'have one's heart in one's mouth'

敢布腹心 *gan-bu fu-xin* (dare-voice belly-heart) 'venture to air some of my views'

触目惊心 *chu-mu jing-xin* (strike-eye startle-heart) 'startling; shocking; horrifying; strike the eye and rouse the mind'

镂骨铭心 *lou-gu ming-xin* (carve-bone engrave-heart) 'engrave on the bones and imprint on the heart – remember forever with gratitude; be wholeheartedly grateful to sb.'

力不从心 *li-bu-cong-xin* (strength-not-follow-heart) 'ability falling short of one's wishes; unable to do as much as one would like to; strength not equal to will'

戮力同心 *lu-li tong-xin* (united-strength same-heart) 'unite in a concerted effort; make concerted efforts'

利禄熏心 *li-lu xun-xin* (profit-emolument smoke-heart) 'be enthusiastic about wealth and emolument'

III. Proverbial and other idiomatic sayings

世路窄狭，人心叵测。
Shi-lu zhaixia, ren-xin po-ce.
life-road narrow, people-heart impossible-measure
'Life's road is narrow and people's hearts are hard to fathom.'

眼睛是心灵的窗户。
Yanjing shi xin-ling de chuanghu.
eyes are heart-soul MOD windows.
'The eyes are windows into the mind.'

心窝子插花，自己觉着自己美。
Xin-wo-zi cha hua, ziji jue-zhe ziji mei.
heart-nest-SUF insert flowers, self feel-DUR self beautiful

'Insert flowers into one's nest of heart – one feels oneself is beautiful (i.e. one is too self-confident).'

心头小鹿乱跳。
Xin-tou xiao lu luan tiao.
heart-head small deer wildly jump
'One's heart beats wildly or madly – being nervous or anxious (lit. A small deer is jumping wildly in one's heart).'

心头刺，眼中疔。
Xin-tou ci, yan zhong ding.
heart-head thorn eye inside malignant-boil
'A thorn in one's heart and a malignant boil in one's eye – a thorn in one's flesh'

心比天高，命比纸薄。
Xin bi tian gao, ming bi zhi bo.
heart than sky higher fate than paper thinner
'One's heart is higher than the sky, but one's fate is thinner than paper (i.e., one has great ambition but bad luck).'

心提到嗓子眼。
Xin ti dao sangzi-yan.
heart is-raised to throat-hole
'One's heart is raised to (the hole of) one's throat – feeling alarmed and anxious.'

心亏胆不壮。
Xin-kui dan bu zhuang.
heart-lost gallbladder not strong
'If one's heart is lost, then one's gallbladder will not be strong (i.e. If one feels guilty, one will not be bold).'

心不负人，面无惭色。
Xin bu fu ren, mian wu can se.
heart not untrue/insincere-to people face without ashamed color
'If one is not insincere to others, one's face won't display an ashamed expression.'

心肝跌进肚里头。
Xin-gan die jin du litou.
heart-liver fall into belly inside
'One's heart and liver have fallen into one's belly – feeling relieved.'

眼不见，心不烦。
Yan bu jian, xin bu fan.
eye not see heart not worry
'What the eye doesn't see the heart doesn't worry about – out of sight, out of mind.'

眼为心苗，苗伤根动。
Yan wei xin miao, miao shang gen dong.
eyesare heart's seedlings seedlings be-injured root be-moved
'The eyes are seedlings of the heart; if the seedlings (i.e. eyes) are hurt, the root (i.e. heart) will be affected.'

梦是心头想。
Meng shi xin-tou xiag.
dreams are heart-head thoughts
'Dreams are thoughts in one's heart (i.e. the people or things in one's dreams are those one often thinks of).'

众人齐了心，黄土变成金。
Zhong ren qi-le-xin, huang tu biancheng jin.
crowd people even-PER-hearts yellow earth become gold
'When a crowd of people have their hearts even/uniform (i.e., are of one mind/heart), even yellow earth will turn into gold.'

世上无难事，只怕有心人。
Shi shang wu nan shi, zhi pa
world on there-are-no difficult things only afraid-of
you-xin ren.
have-heart person
'Nothing in the world is difficult as long as people have hearts (i.e. have high aspirations and determination or set their mind on achieving their goals).'

世上无难事，只怕心不坚。
Shi shang wu nan shi, zhi pa xin bu
world on there-are-no difficult things onlyafraid heart is-not
jian.
firm
'There are no difficult things in the world as long as one has a firm heart (i.e., resolute and fixed determination).'

功夫不负有心人。
Gongfu bu fu you-xin ren.
effort not let-down have-heart people

'Effort will not let down the people with high aspirations and determination.'

言者无心，听者有意。
Yan-zhe wu xin, ting-zhe you yi.
speaker has-no heart listener has intention/meaning
'A casual remark sounds significant to a suspicious listener (or, A careless word may reveal much to an attentive listener).'

无心人说话，只怕有心人来听。
Wu-xin ren shuohua, zhi pa you-xin ren
have-no-heart person speak onlyafraid have-heart person
lai ting.
come listen
'Unintentional or careless words can be interpreted as intentional and significant by a listener with a certain intention or purpose.'

心有余而力不足。
Xin you yu er li bu zu.
heart there-is surplus but strength is-not sufficient
'One's ability falls short of one's wishes; though one still cherishes high aspiration, one's strength falls short of his wishes (lit. There is surplus of heart, but strength is insufficient).'

心净孤明独照，心存万境皆清。
Xin jing gu ming du zhao, xin cun
heart clean solitary lamp alone shine heart secure
wan jing jie qing.
ten-thousand situations all clear
'When the heart/mind is pure, it shines forth as a solitary lamp, and when the heart/mind is deliberate, the entire phenomenal world becomes clarified.'

人同此心，心同此理。
Ren tong ci xin, xin tong ci li.
people same this heart heart same this reason
'Everybody feels the same about this matter / People feel and think alike on this matter / The sense of justice and rationality is the same with everybody.'

心往一处想，劲往一处使。
Xin wang yi chu xiang, jing wang yi chu shi.
heart toward one place think energy toward one place used
'Think with one mind, and work with one heart (i.e., Everyone's thoughts and efforts are directed towards one goal).'

劳而无功，空耗心神。
Lao er wu gong, kong hao xin-shen.
work but no result for-nothing cost heart-spirit
'All the work with no result has drained the mind for nothing.'

一心不可二用。
Yi xin bu-ke er yong.
one heart cannot-be-for two uses
'One mind cannot work on two things simultaneously (i.e., one cannot/should not run after two horses/hares at the same time).'

一岁年龄一岁心。
Yi-sui nianling yi-sui xin.
one-year age one-year heart
'One's mind grow (to become more mature) with age.'

十个男人九粗心。
Shi-ge nanren jiu cu-xin.
ten-CL men nine thick-heart
'Nine out of ten men are careless.'

人之虚实真伪，在乎心，无不见乎迹。
Ren-zhi xu shi zhen wei, zai-hu-xin,
People's hypocrisy sincerity honesty dishonesty exist-in-heart
wu-bu jian-hu-ji.
but-never-not show-in-deeds
'People's hypocrisy or sincerity, honesty or dishonesty, exist in the heart (i.e. are matters of heart), but will never fail to show in deeds.'

人不知学，白首童心。
Ren bu zhi xue, bai shou tong xin.
people not know learning white head child's heart
'Those who don't know how to learn will have white heads (i.e. white hair) but childish minds (i.e. if people don't learn, when they look old, they still have immature minds).'

人心似铁，官法如炉。
Ren xin si tie, guan fa ru lu.
human heart like iron official law like furnace
'Although human heart (or will) can be as hard as iron, it will nevertheless be melted by the furnace of official law.'

人老不算老，心老才算老。

Ren lao bu suan lao, xin lao cai suan lao.
person old not count-as old heart old then count-as old
'An aging person cannot be considered as being old unless this person's heart is aging as well.'

不怕人老，就怕心老。
Bu pa ren lao, jiu pa xin lao.
not afraid person old only afraid heart old
'People should not worry about someone getting old unless this person's heart is getting old also.'

人有喜庆，不可生忌妒心；人有祸患，不可生喜幸心。
Ren you xi-qing, bu-ke sheng jidu-xin;
people have success-celebration shouldn't harbor jealous-heart
ren you huo-huan, bu-ke sheng xixing-xin.
people have misfortune-disaster shouldn't harbor gloating-heart
'All people have successes and celebrations, of which one shouldn't be jealous; all people have misfortunes and disasters, over which one shouldn't be gloating.'

千人同心，则得千人之力；万人异心，则无一人之用。
Qian ren tong xin, ze de qian ren-zhi
a-thousand people same heart then get a-thousand people's
li; wan ren yi xin, ze wu yi ren-zhi yong.
strength ten-thousand people different hearts then no one person's use
'When one thousand people are of one heart/mind, then they get one thousand people's strength; when ten thousand people all have different hearts/minds, then none of them is of real use.'

小和尚念经，有口无心。
Xiao heshang nian jing, you kou wu xin.
little monk chant scriptures have mouth but-not heart
'When little monk is chanting scriptures, he vocalizes them without understanding – doing sth. carelessly, casually, or indifferently.'

无心为善，乃是真善。
Wu-xin wei shan, nai shi zhen shan.
no-heart do good then is truly good
'If one does good with no intention to catch attention, then one is truly virtuous.'

无心吓着有心人。
Wu-xin xia zhe you-xin ren.
no-heart scare PRT have-heart person

'A casual remark scared someone (with a guilty conscience).'

二人一心，有钱买金；二人二心，无钱买针。
Er ren yi xin, you qian mai jin; er ren
two persons one heart have money buy gold two persons
er xin, wu qian mai zhen.
two hearts no money buy needle
'Two people with one heart/mind should have money to buy gold, whereas two people with two hearts/minds shouldn't have money to buy a needle.'

少女的心，秋天的云。
Shao nü-de xin, qiutian de yun.
young girl's heart autumn MOD clouds
'A young girl's heart is like clouds in the autumn sky (i.e. very changeable).'

手不狠立不了业，心不黑发不了财。
Shou bu hen li-bu-liao ye,
hand not firm/resolute unable-to-establish business/enterprise
xin bu hei fa-bu-liao cai.
heart not black unable-to-make riches
'One is unable to establish a business without firm hands, nor can one make riches without a black heart.'

从耳朵进的风，在心里掀波浪。
Cong erduo jin de feng, zai xin li xian
from ears enter MOD wind at heart inside surge
bolang.
waves
'The wind entering the ears will surge waves in the heart (i.e. emotional disorders in the heart are usually caused by gossips that one has heard.'

父子协力山成玉，兄弟同心土变金。
Fu zi xie li shan cheng yu, xiong-di
father son unite effort mountain become jade brothers
tong xin tu bian jin.
same heart earth become gold
'When father and son unite effort, even mountains will turn into jade; when brothers are of one heart/mind, even earth will turn into gold.'

宁丧千金，不失士心。
Ning sang qian jin, bu shi shi xin.
would-rather lose thousand gold than lose talent's heart
'One would rather lose a thousand bars/liang of gold than lose a talent's heart.'

老不舍心，少不舍力。
Lao bu she xin, shao bu she li.
elderly not spare heart young not spare strength
'The elderly would not spare their hearts (i.e. ideas), and the young would not spare their strengths.'

自己做了亏心事，风吹草动也心惊。
Ziji zuo-le kui-xin shi, feng chui cao dong ye xin-jing.
self do-PER lose-heart thing wind blow grass move also heart-startled
'If one has done a deed that troubles one's conscience (lit. done a lose-heart thing), one will feel startled (in the heart) at the rustle of grass blades in the wind (lit. when wind blows and grass moves).'

危难见人心。
Weinan jian ren xin.
calamity see human heart
'In calamity one can see the (true) heart of people.'

安心是药更无方。
An-xin shi yao geng-wu-fang.
calm-heart is medicine with-no-prescription
'A calm heart is a medicine that doesn't even have a prescription (i.e. a calm heart is good to health).'

好心自有好报。
Hao xin zi you hao bao.
good heart naturally have good reward
'Good-heartedness will certainly be rewarded.'

苍天不负有心人。
Cang-tian bu fu you-xin ren.
blue-sky not let-down have-heart people
'Heaven will not let down people with high aspirations and determination.'

治病容易治心难。
Zhi bing rongyi zhi xin nan.
treat disease easy treat heart difficult
'It is easy to treat a disease, but it is difficult to treat a heart (i.e., it is easy to treat diseases of the body, but it is difficult to treat problems of the mind).'

怕人知事莫萌心。

Pa ren zhi shi mo meng-xin.
fear people know things don't sprout-heart
'If you are afraid that other people will know it, then you shouldn't let the idea sprout from your heart in the first place.'

看人看心，听话听音。
Kan ren kan xin, ting hua ting yin.
look-at people look-at heart listen-to speech listen-to sound
'When you look at people, you should look at their heart (i.e. true nature); when you listen to people talk, you should listen to their sound (i.e. their implied meaning).'

清酒红人面，白财动人心。
Qing jiu hong ren mian, bai cai dong ren xin.
clear wine redden people's face white fortune move people's heart
'Clear wine would redden people's faces, and white silver (i.e. gains or fortunes that can be made without much effort) would move people's hearts (i.e. arouse people's desire).'

Appendix 2
The Chinese original of "On 'Heart' for the New Year"

新年话"心"

余英时

心对中国人来说最重要，因此你要修心。心要修得干净，有干干净净的心才有纯洁的社会出现的可能，如果心都脏了，坏了，那么这个社会也会坏。这不是唯心论，这是讲心的重要性，人的精神对物质条件也有很大的作用，并不是完全被物质条件或社会身份决定的。人要想大家都活得好，中国人讲"己所不欲，勿施于人"，孔子讲这种话，诗经讲这些，都是要将心比心，"他人有心，予忖度之"，我想他人的心是怎么样，要将心比心，就有一些事情不会做，所以中国人讲这个心是非常重要的。

中国为什么会特别讲这个心呢？因为在中国人看来，心等于是一种神，变化莫测，包罗一切，所以像有些哲学家，包括陆象山，王阳明，说到，吾心就是宇宙，宇宙就是吾心，这不是唯心论。而是说，你要建立一个人的社会，在这个社会大家都活得很好，要把心扩大，不要使自私自利的心。私心要有限度，这个限度就是不能妨害公心。

春秋时代的子产已经说了，人心不同，各有其面。所以中国人也肯定个人的心，但也有一个大群体的心同时运作，这样既不会流与所谓绝对的集体主义，也不会流与绝对的个人主义。在个人和集体之间找一种平衡点，找这个平衡点的功能要来自心。11 世纪的宋朝的张载有一篇文章，叫《大心篇》，把心放大。像战国时代的庄子讲，天地万物跟我都是一个。中国人也常常讲，天人合一，这都是讲心要扩大。

一方面不放弃个人自己独有的心，另外一方面又要把心扩大，想到别人，这样我们才能活得好些，有秩序一些。因为中国人不大相信有死后天堂，特别是受儒家影响的，认为这个世界就是一个真实的世界了。我们就这一个世界，要好好珍惜它。如果要珍惜它，我们的天堂也在这个世界上。我们的地狱也在这个世界上。这是中国人的一种看法。

孟子有《净心篇》，我们都知道的，知性就知天。庄子说，心要虚，虚了以后道才能进来。像孟子讲的，"恻隐之心，人皆有之"，像"仁义礼智"的"仁"就是人最要紧的心，这个"仁"就是爱人，爱别人，不但爱自己，也爱别人。所以孟子讲心，总要讲推，推自己的心，越推越大，越推越远，这样会包括整个社会，甚至要像惠师，庄周这些人，更推得大，要推到天地万物都要爱的。

所以这就是中国人的心之所以重要的原因，这个心变成每个人都有的了，这是中国思想上一个很特殊的传统。在中国传统之下，中国没有有组织的宗教，没有有组织的，像西方中央化的教会的传统，像在中古时代罗马教皇号令天下，中国没有发生过。中国人每个人都是一个心，每个人的心都可以通天。但是要培养它，如果不培养它，你的心就越来越小，越来越自私自利，那么社会就会大乱。

所以我想我们谈价值问题，精神的价值问题，在中国必须追究到心，跟西方的上帝的观念几乎有同样的重要意义，是不能去掉的。去掉后人就跟禽兽没有什么区别了。所以中国一向讲要把心搞干净。我想，中国的这一百年来，心实在是成为一个很大的问题，因为我们已经不大相信古代的说法了，把中国的传统丢掉了，然后又不能信仰西方的上帝，因此，心就没有着落了。每个人的心几乎被物质的利益所诱惑了。……在这样一个思潮之下，中国的心就越来越失落了。心的失落是我们一百年来中国文化危机最大的关键之一。

我向大家把心的问题提出来，好好想一想，这就是我新年想说的话。

References

Ames, Roger T.
2004 The meaning of body in classical Chinese philosophy. In *The Body: Critical Concepts in Sociology*, Andrew Blaikie, Mike Hepworthy, Mary Holmes, Alexandra Howson, David Inglis, and Sheree Sartain (eds.), vol. 1, 269–287. London/New York: Routledge.

Anderson, Michael L.
2003 Embodied cognition: A field guide. *Artificial Intelligence* 149: 91–130.

Armstrong, David
2004 Bodies of knowledge: Foucault and the problem of human anatomy. In *The Body: Critical Concepts in Sociology*, Andrew Blaikie, Mike Hepworthy, Mary Holmes, Alexandra Howson, David Inglis, and Sheree Sartain (eds.), vol. 3, 105–120. London/New York: Routledge.

Athanasiadou, Angeliki, and Elzbieta Tabakowska (eds.)
1998 *Speaking of Emotions: Conceptualization and Expression.* Berlin/New York: Mouton de Gruyter.

Bao, Shixiang, and Lao An
1992 *Lun Yu* [论语 The analects of Confucius: a Chinese-English bilingual edition]. Trans. into modern Chinese by Bao Shixiang, and into English by Lao An. Jinan, China: Shandong Friendship Press.

Barcelona, Antonio (ed.)
2000a *Metaphor and Metonymy at the Crossroads: A Cognitive Perspective.* Berlin/New York: Mouton de Gruyter.

Barcelona, Antonio
2000b Introduction: The cognitive theory of metaphor and metonymy. In *Metaphor and Metonymy at the Crossroads: A Cognitive Perspective*, Antonio Barcelona (ed.), 1–28. Berlin/New York: Mouton de Gruyter.

2000c On the plausibility of claiming a metonymic motivation for conceptual metaphor. In *Metaphor and Metonymy at the Crossroads: A Cognitive Perspective*, Antonio Barcelona (ed.), 31–58. Berlin/New York: Mouton de Gruyter.

2005 The multilevel operation of metonymy in grammar and discourse, with particular attention to metonymic chains. In *Cognitive Linguistics: Internal Dynamics and Interdisciplinary Interaction*, Francisco J. Ruiz de Mendoza Ibáñez and M. Sandra Peña Cerval (eds.), 313–352. Berlin/New York: Mouton de Gruyter.

Barkan, Leonard
1975 *Nature's Work of Art: The Human Body as Image of the World.* New Haven, CT: Yale University Press.

Barsalow, Lawrence W., Aron K. Barbey, W. Kyle Simmons, and Ava Santos
2005 Embodiment in religious knowledge. *Journal of Cognition and Culture* 5: 14–57.

Berdayes, Vicente, Luigi Esposito, and John W. Murphy (eds.)
2004 *The Body in Human Inquiry: Interdisciplinary Explorations of Embodiment*. Cresskill, NJ: Hampton Press.

Berthelot, Jean-Michel
2004 Sociological discourse and the body. In *The Body: Critical Concepts in Sociology*, Andrew Blaikie, Mike Hepworthy, Mary Holmes, Alexandra Howson, David Inglis, and Sheree Sartain (eds.), vol. 2, 120–132. London/New York: Routledge.

Blacking, John (ed.)
1977a *The Anthropology of the Body*. London: Academic Press.

Blacking, John
1977b Towards an anthropology of the body. In *The Anthropology of the Body*, John Blacking (ed.), 1–28. London: Academic Press.

Blaikie, Andrew, Mike Hepworthy, Mary Holmes, Alexandra Howson, David Inglis, and Sheree Sartain (eds.)
2004a *The Body: Critical Concepts in Sociology*. Vols. 1–5. London/New York: Routledge.

Blaikie, Andrew, Mike Hepworthy, Mary Holmes, Alexandra Howson, David Inglis, and Sheree Sartain
2004b General introduction. The sociology of the body: Genesis, development and futures. In *The Body: Critical Concepts in Sociology*, Andrew Blaikie, Mike Hepworthy, Mary Holmes, Alexandra Howson, David Inglis, and Sheree Sartain (eds.), vol. 1, 1–23. London/New York: Routledge.

Bremmer, Jan
1983 *The Early Greek Concept of the Soul*. Princeton, NJ: Princeton University Press.

Cai, Degui
2000 *Zhongguo Zhexue Liuxingqu* [中国哲学流行曲 The pop music of Chinese philosophy]. Jinan, China: Shandong People's Press.

Canto, Monique
2004 The politics of women's bodies: Reflections on Plato. In *The Body: Critical Concepts in Sociology*, Andrew Blaikie, Mike Hepworthy, Mary Holmes, Alexandra Howson, David Inglis, and Sheree Sartain (eds.), vols. 3, 3–16. London/New York: Routledge.

Chan, Alan K. L. (ed.)
2002a *Mencius: Contexts and Interpretations.* Honolulu, HI: University of Hawaii Press.

Chan, Alan K. L.
2002b Introduction. In *Mencius: Contexts and Interpretations*, Alan K. L. Chan (ed.), 1–16. Honolulu, HI: University of Hawaii Press.

2002c A matter of taste *qi* (vital energy) and the tending of the heart (*xin*) in Mencius 2A2. In *Mencius: Contexts and Interpretations*, Alan K. L. Chan (ed.), 42–71. Honolulu, HI: University of Hawaii Press.

Chan, Wing-Tsit (trans. and comp.)

1963 *A Source Book in Chinese Philosophy.* Princeton, NJ: Princeton University Press.

Chen, Zelin

1989a Zuguo yixue de fazhan [祖国医学的发展 Development of Chinese medicine]. In *Jiating Yixue Quanshu* [家庭医学全书 Family medicine], Jin Wentao (ed.), 994–996. Shanghai: Shanghai Science and Technology Press.

1989b Yin-yang wuxing [阴阳五行 Yin-yang and five elements]. In *Jiating Yixue Quanshu* [家庭医学全书 Family medicine], Jin Wentao (ed.), 997–1002. Shanghai: Shanghai Science and Technology Press.

1989c Zang xiang [藏象 Theory of internal organs]. In *Jiating Yixue Quanshu* [家庭医学全书 Family medicine], Jin Wentao (ed.), 1003–1012. Shanghai: Shanghai Science and Technology Press.

Chia, Mantak, and Maneewan Chia

1990 *Chi Nei Tsang: Internal Organ Chi Massage* (revised ed.). Huntington, NY: Healing Tao Books.

Chinesenewsnet

2006a "Neileng waire": "Quxiao Zhongyi" zhi zheng beihou de Zhongyi weiji ["内冷外热" ： "取消中医" 之争背后的中医危机 "Cold domestically and hot internationally": Chinese medicine's crises behind the debate on the "elimination of Chinese medicine"]. Accessed October 14, 2006 at http://www7.chinesenewsnet.com/MainNews/SocDigest/Technology/zxs_2006_804219.shtml.

2006b Quxiao Zhongyi chunshu wujizhitan [取消中医纯属无稽之谈 Eliminating Chinese medicine is sheer nonsense]. Accessed October 15, 2006 at http://www1.chinesenewsnet.com/gb/MainNews/Forums/BackStage/2006_10_15_5_39_43_618.html.

2006c Zhongguo wangmin yu "quxiao Zhongyi" yinfa xuanrandabo [中国网民吁 "取消中医" 引发轩然大波 Chinese netizens appealing for the "elimination of Chinese medicine" caused a great disturbance]. Accessed October 23, 2006 at http://www5.chinesenewsnet.com/gb/MainNews/Forums/BackStage/2006_10_23_7_31_59_760.html.

2006d Zhongyi cunfei kunjing [中医存废困境 Dilemma of Chinese medicine's survival or demise]. Accessed October 24, 2006 at http://www7.chinesenewnet.com/gb/MainNews/SinoNews/Mainland/xhw_2006_10_24_01_40_16_388.html.

2006e Mindiao xianshi 87.8% de shoufangzhe xiangxin Zhongyi [民调显示87.8%的受访者相信中医 Polls show 87.8% of interviewees believe in Chinese medicine]. Accessed October 30, 2006 at http://www3.chinesenewsnet.com/gb/MainNews/EntDigest/Life/xhw_2006_10_29_18_22_28_536.html.

2006f He Zuoxiu zhichi piping Zhongyi [何祚庥支持批评中医 He Zuoxiu supports criticisms of Chinese medicine]. Accessed October 30, 2006 at http://www2.chinesenewsnet.com/gb/MainNews/Forums/BackStage/2006_10_30_7_48_14_486.html.

2006g Quxiao Zhongyi shi yimu shudianwangzu de naoju [取消中医是一幕数典忘祖的闹剧 Eliminating Chinese medicine is a farce of ignoring one's own origins]. Accessed November 3, 2006 at http://www3.chinesenewsnet.com/gb/MainNews/Opinion/2006_11_2_12_56_48_963. html.

2006h He Zuoxiu: Yu bu jingren sibuxiu [何祚庥：语不惊人死不休 He Zuoxiu: Will find no rest in death if his words don't startle others]. Accessed November 6, 2006 at http://www3.chinesenewsnet.com/gb/MainNews/Opinion/2006_11_6_7_4_9_706.html.

Clark, Andy

1999 An embodied cognitive science? *Trends in Cognitive Science* 9: 345–351.

Clarke, Edwin, and C. D. O'Malley

1968 *The Human Brain and Spinal Cord: A Historical Study Illustrated by Writings from Antiquity to the Twentieth Century*. Berkeley: University of California Press.

Coulson, Seana

2001 *Semantic Leaps: Frame-Shifting and Conceptual Blending in Meaning Construction*. Cambridge/New York: Cambridge University Press.

2006 Conceptual blending in thought, rhetoric, and ideology. In *Cognitive Linguistics: Current Applications and Future Perspectives*, Gitte Kristiansen, Michel Achard, René Dirven, and Francisco J. Ruiz de Mendoza Ibáñez (eds.), 187–208. Berlin/New York: Mouton de Gruyter.

Coulson, Seana, and Todd Oakley

2003 Metonymy and conceptual blending. In *Metonymy and Pragmatic Inferencing*, Klaus-Uwe Panther and Linda L. Thornburg (eds.), 51–79. Amsterdam/Philadelphia: John Benjamins.

Crivellato, Enrico, and Domenico Ribatti

2007 Soul, mind brain: Greek philosophy and the birth of neuroscience. *Brain Research Bulletin* 71: 327–336.

Croft, William, and D. Alan Cruse

2004 *Cognitive Linguistics*. Cambridge/New York: Cambridge University Press.

Csordas, Thomas J.

1990 Embodiment as a paradigm for anthropology. *Ethos* 18: 5–47.

1999 Embodiment and cultural phenomenology. In *Perspectives on Embodiment: The Intersections of Nature and Culture*, Gail Weiss and Honi F. Haber (eds.), 143–162. New York: Routledge.

Csordas, Thomas J. (ed.)
1994 *Embodiment and Experience: The Existential Ground of Culture and Self.* Cambridge/New York: Cambridge University Press.

Cua, Antonio S.
2002 *Xin* and moral failure: Notes on an aspect of Mencius' moral psychology. In *Mencius: Contexts and Interpretations*, Alan K. L. Chan (ed.), 126–150. Honolulu, HI: University of Hawaii Press.

Currie, Dawn H., and Valerie Raoul
2004 Dissecting sexual difference in the body of knowledge. In *The Body: Critical Concepts in Sociology*, Andrew Blaikie, Mike Hepworthy, Mary Holmes, Alexandra Howson, David Inglis, and Sheree Sartain (eds.), vol. 3, 121–151. London/New York: Routledge.

Cuyckens, Hubert, René Dirven, and John Taylor
2003 *Cognitive Approaches to Lexical Semantics.* Berlin/New York: Mouton de Gruyter.

Damasio, Antonio R.
1994 *Descartes' Error: Emotion, Reason, and the Human Brain.* New York: Grosset/Putnam.

Davis, Kathy
2004 From objectified body to embodied subject. In *The Body: Critical Concepts in Sociology*, Andrew Blaikie, Mike Hepworthy, Mary Holmes, Alexandra Howson, David Inglis, and Sheree Sartain (eds.), vol. 5, 143–164. London/New York: Routledge.

De Bary, William Theodore
1981 *Neo-Confucian Orthodoxy and the Learning of the Mind-and-Heart.* New York: Columbia University Press.

Dirven, René
1985 Metaphor and polysemy. In *La Polysémie: Lexicographie et Cognition*, René Jongen (ed.), 9–27. Louvain la Neuve: Cabai.
2002 Metonymy and metaphor: Different mental strategies of conceptualization. In *Metaphor and Metonymy in Comparison and Contrast*, René Dirven and Ralf Pörings (eds.), 75–111. Berlin/New York: Mouton de Gruyter.
2005 Major strands in Cognitive Linguistics. In *Cognitive Linguistics: Internal Dynamics and Interdisciplinary Interaction*, Francisco J. Ruiz de Mendoza Ibáñez and M. Sandra Peña Cerval (eds.), 17–68. Berlin/New York: Mouton de Gruyter.

Dirven, René, Roslyn M. Frank, and Martin Pütz (eds.)
2003 *Cognitive Models in Language and Thought: Ideology, Metaphors and Meanings.* Berlin/New York: Mouton de Gruyter.

Dirven, René, and Ralf Pörings (eds.)
2002 *Metaphor and Metonymy in Comparison and Contrast*. Berlin/New York: Mouton de Gruyter.

Doueihi, Milad
1997 *A Perverse History of the Human Heart*. Cambridge, MA: Harvard University Press.

Douglas, Mary
1973 *Natural Symbol: Explorations in Cosmology*. New York: Random House.

Dufour, Xavier-Léon
1975 *Dictionnaire du Nouveau Testament*. Paris: Seuil.

Eisenstein, Elizabeth
1979 *The Printing Press as an Agent of Change: Communications and Cultural Transformations in Early Modern Europe*. Vols. 1–2. Cambridge/New York: Cambridge University Press.

Emmott, Catherine
2002 "Split selves" in fiction and in medical "life stories": Cognitive linguistic theory and narrative practice. In *Cognitive Stylistics: Language and Cognition in Text Analysis*, Elena Semino and Jonathan Culpeper (eds.), 153–181. Amsterdam/Philadelphia: John Benjamins.

Enfield, Nick J.
2002 Semantic analysis of body parts in emotion terminology: Avoiding the exoticisms of "obstinate monosemy" and "online extension". *Pragmatics and Cognition* 10: 85–106.

Enfield, Nick J., Asifa Majid, and Miriam van Staden
2006 Cross-linguistic categorization of the body: Introduction. *Language Sciences* 28: 137–147.

Enfield, Nick J., and Anna Wierzbicka (eds.)
2002a Special Issue on "The Body in Description of Emotion: Cross-linguistic Studies". *Pragmatics and Cognition* 10 (1/2).

Enfield, Nick J., and Anna Wierzbicka
2002b Introduction: The body in description of emotion. *Pragmatics and Cognition* 10: 1–25.

Erickson, Robert A.
1997 *The Language of the Heart, 1600–1750*. Philadelphia: University of Pennsylvania Press.

Evans, Vyvyan, and Melanie Green
2006 *Cognitive Linguistics: An Introduction*. Edinburg: Edinburg University Press.

Fajans, Jane
1985 The person in social context: The social character of Baining "psychology". In *Person, Self, and Experience: Exploring Pacific Ethnopsychologies*, Geoffrey M. White and John Kirkpatrick (eds.), 367–397. Berkeley: University of California Press.

Farquhar, Judith
1998 Chinese medicine and the life of the mind: Are brains necessary? *North Carolina Medical Journal* 59: 188–190.

Fauconnier, Gilles, and Mark Turner
1998 Conceptual integration networks. *Cognitive Science* 22: 133–187.
1999 Metonymy and conceptual integration. In *Metonymy in Language and Thought*, Klaus-Uwe Panther and Günter Radden (eds.), 77–90. Amsterdam/Philadelphia: John Benjamins.
2002 *The Way We Think: Conceptual Blending and the Mind's Hidden Complexities*. New York: Basic Books.

Featherstone, Mike, Mike Hepworth, and Bryan S. Turner (eds.)
1991 *The Body: Social Process and Cultural Theory*. London: Sage Publications.

Feher, Michel
1989 Introduction. In *Fragments for a History of the Human Body*, Michel Feher, Ramona Naddaff, and Nadia Tazi (eds.), vol. 1, 11–17. New York: Zone Books.

Feher, Michel, Ramona Naddaff, and Nadia Tazi (eds.)
1989 *Fragments for a History of the Human Body*. Vols. 1–3. New York: Zone Books.

Feng, Huoyuan
2003 Jianshen zaiyu qin dongnao [健身在于勤动脑 Good health depends on regular use of the brain]. *People's Daily* (Overseas Edition), October 27, 2003, p. 9 ("Health" section).

Feng, Xiaohu
2004 *Yinyu: Siwei de Jichu, Pianzhang de Kuangjia* [隐喻：思维的基础，篇章的框架 Metaphor: the foundation of thought, and the frame of the text]. Beijing: University of International Business and Economics Press.

Fernando, Chitra
1996 *Idioms and Idiomaticity*. Oxford/New York: Oxford University Press.

Foolen, Ad
2008 The heart as a source of semiosis: The case of Dutch. In *Culture, Body, and Language: Conceptualizations of Internal Body Organs across Cultures and Languages*, Farzad Sharifian, René Dirven, Ning Yu, and Susanne Niemeier (eds.), 373–394. Berlin/New York: Mouton de Gruyter.

Forceville, Charles
1996 *Pictorial Metaphor in Advertising*. London/New York: Routledge.

Forth, Christopher E. and Ivan Crozier (eds.)
2005 *Body Parts: Critical Explorations in Corporeality*. Lanham, MD: Lexington Books.

Frank, Roslyn M., René Dirven, Tom Ziemke, and Enrique Bernárdez (eds.)
2008 *Body, Language, and Mind (Vol. 2): Sociocultural Situatedness*. Berlin/New York: Mouton de Gruyter.

Freeman, Margaret H.
2000 Poetry and the scope of metaphor: Toward a cognitive theory of literature. In *Metaphor and Metonymy at the Crossroads: A Cognitive Perspective*, Antonio Barcelona (ed.), 253–281. Berlin/New York: Mouton de Gruyter.
2002 The body in the words: A cognitive approach to the shape of a poetic text. In *Cognitive Stylistics: Language and Cognition in Text Analysis*, Elena Semino and Jonathan Culpeper (eds.), 23–47. Amsterdam/Philadelphia: John Benjamins.
2006 The fall of the wall between literary studies and linguistics: Cognitive poetics. In *Cognitive Linguistics: Current Applications and Future Perspectives*, Gitte Kristiansen, Michel Achard, René Dirven, and Francisco J. Ruiz de Mendoza Ibáñez (eds.), 403–428. Berlin/New York: Mouton de Gruyter.

Freund, Peter E. S.
2004 Bringing society into the body. In *The Body: Critical Concepts in Sociology*, Andrew Blaikie, Mike Hepworthy, Mary Holmes, Alexandra Howson, David Inglis, and Sheree Sartain (eds.), vol. 2, 133–155. London/New York: Routledge.

Fung, Yu-lan
1966 *A Short History of Chinese Philosophy*. New York: The Free Press.

Gaby, Alice
2008 Gut feelings: Locating intellect, emotion and life force in the Thaayorre body. In *Culture, Body, and Language: Conceptualizations of Internal Body Organs across Languages and Cultures*, Farzad Sharifian, René Dirven, Ning Yu, and Susanne Niemeier (eds.), 27–44. Berlin/New York: Mouton de Gruyter.

Gadow, Sally
2004 Body and self. In *The Body: Critical Concepts in Sociology*, Andrew Blaikie, Mike Hepworthy, Mary Holmes, Alexandra Howson, David Inglis, and Sheree Sartain (eds.), vol. 4, 70–83. London/New York: Routledge.

Gallagher, Shaun
2005 *How the Body Shapes the Mind*. Oxford/New York: Oxford University Press.

Ge, Zhaoguang
2001 *Zhongguo Sixiang Shi* [中国思想史 A history of Chinese thought]. Vols. 1–3. Shanghai: Fudan University Press.

Geeraerts, Dirk
1995 Cognitive Linguistics. In *Handbook of Pragmatics: Manual*, Jef Verschueren, Jan-Ola Östman, and Jan Blommaert (eds.), 111–116. Amsterdam/Philadelphia: John Benjamins.
1997 *Diachronic Prototype Semantics: A Contribution to Historical Lexicology*. Oxford/New York: Oxford University Press.
2006a *Words and Other Wonders: Papers on Lexical and Semantic Topics*. Berlin/New York: Mouton de Gruyter.

Geeraerts, Dirk (ed.)
2006b *Cognitive Linguistics: Basic Readings*. Berlin/New York: Mouton de Gruyter.

Geeraerts, Dirk
2006c Introduction: A rough guide to Cognitive Linguistics. In *Cognitive Linguistics: Basic Readings*, Dirk Geeraerts (ed.), 1–28. Berlin/New York: Mouton de Gruyter.
2006d Methodology in Cognitive Linguistics. In *Cognitive Linguistics: Current Applications and Future Perspectives*, Gitte Kristiansen, Michel Achard, René Dirven, and Francisco J. Ruiz de Mendoza Ibáñez (eds.), 21–49. Berlin/New York: Mouton de Gruyter.

Geeraerts, Dirk, and Stefan Grondelaers
1995 Looking back at anger: Cultural traditions and metaphorical patterns. In *Language and the Cognitive Construal of the World*, John R. Taylor and Robert E. MacLaury (eds.), 153–179. Berlin/New York: Mouton de Gruyter.

Gibbs, Raymond W.
1994 *The Poetics of Mind: Figurative Thought, Language, and Understanding*. Cambridge/New York: Cambridge University Press.
1999a *Intentions in the Experience of Meaning*. Cambridge/New York: Cambridge University Press.
1999b Taking metaphor out of our heads and putting it into the cultural world. In *Metaphor in Cognitive Linguistics*, Raymond W. Gibbs and Gerard J. Steen (eds.), 145–166. Amsterdam/Philadelphia: John Benjamins.
2003 Embodied experience and linguistic meaning. *Brain and Language* 84: 1–15.
2006 *Embodiment and Cognitive Science*. Cambridge/New York: Cambridge University Press.

Gibbs, Raymond W. (ed.)
2008 *The Cambridge Handbook of Metaphor and Thought*. Cambridge/New York: Cambridge University Press.

Gibbs, Raymond W., and Gerard J. Steen (eds.)
1999 *Metaphor in Cognitive Linguistics*. Amsterdam/Philadelphia: John Benjamins.

Giles, Herbert A.

1926 *Chuang Tzu: Taoist Philosopher and Chinese Mystic.* Trans. by Herbert A. Giles. London: Ruskin House.

Goatly, Andrew

2007 *Washing the Brain: Metaphor and Hidden Ideology.* Amsterdam/Philadelphia: John Benjamins.

Goddard, Cliff

2003 Thinking across languages and cultures: Six dimensions of variation. *Cognitive Linguistics* 14: 109–140.

2008 Contrastive semantics and cultural psychology: English *heart* vs. Malay *hati*. In *Culture, Body, and Language: Conceptualizations of Internal Body Organs across Languages and Cultures*, Farzad Sharifian, René Dirven, Ning Yu, and Susanne Niemeier (eds.), 75–102. Berlin/New York: Mouton de Gruyter.

Godwin, Gail

2001 *Heart: A Personal Journey through Its Myths and Meanings.* New York: William Morrow.

Goossens, Louis

1995 Metaphtonymy: The interaction of metaphor and metonymy in figurative expressions for linguistic action. In *By Word of Mouth: Metaphor, Metonymy and Linguistic Action in a Cognitive Perspective*, Louis Goossens, Paul Pauwels, Brygida Rudzka-Ostyn, Anne-Marie Simon-Vandenbergen, and Johan Vanparys, 159–174. Amsterdam/Philadelphia: John Benjamins.

Grady, Joseph

1997a Foundation of meaning: Primary metaphors and primary scenes. Ph.D. diss., Department of Linguistics, University of California, Berkeley.

1997b THEORIES ARE BUILDINGS revisited. *Cognitive Linguistics* 8: 267–290.

2005 Primary metaphors as inputs to conceptual integration. *Journal of Pragmatics* 37: 1595–1614.

Grady, Joseph, Todd Oakley, and Seana Coulson

1999 Blending and metaphor. In *Metaphor in Cognitive Linguistics*, Raymond W. Gibbs and Gerard J. Steen (eds.), 101–124. Amsterdam/Philadelphia: John Benjamins.

Gu, Hongming

2005 Zhongguo ren de jingshen [中国人的精神 The spirit of the Chinese]. *China Tribune* (*Culture and Life*), June 3, 2005, p. 27.

Hamilton, Craig

2002 Conceptual integration in Christine de Pizan's *City of Ladies*. In *Cognitive Stylistics: Language and Cognition in Text Analysis*, Elena Semino and Jonathan Culpeper (eds.), 1–22. Amsterdam/Philadelphia: John Benjamins.

Hansen, Chad
1992 *A Daoist Theory of Chinese Thought: A Philosophical Interpretation.* New York: Oxford University Press.

Harkins, Jean, and Anna Wierzbicka (eds.)
2001 *Emotions in Crosslinguistic Perspective*. Berlin/New York: Mouton de Gruyter.

He, Youling, and He Baihua
1992 *Da Xue* [大学 The great learning: a Chinese-English bilingual edition]. Trans. into modern Chinese by He Youling, and into English by He Baihua. Jinan, China: Shandong Friendship Press.

Heng, Jiuan
2002 Understanding words and knowing men. In *Mencius: Contexts and Interpretations*, Alan K. L. Chan (ed.), 151–168. Honolulu, HI: University of Hawaii Press.

Hill, Jane H.
In press *The Everyday Language of White Racism*. Oxford, UK: Blackwell.

Hillman, David, and Carla Mazzio (eds.)
1997a *The Body in Parts: Fantasies of Corporeality in Early Modern Europe*. New York/London: Routledge.

Hillman, David, and Carla Mazzio
1997b Introduction: Individual parts. In *The Body in Parts: Fantasies of Corporeality in Early Modern Europe*, David Hillman and Carlar Mazzio (eds.), xi–xxix. New York/London: Routledge.

Hillman, James
1992 *The Thought of the Heart and the Soul of the World.* Putnam, CT: Spring Publications.

Holland, Dorothy, and Naomi Quinn (eds.)
1987 *Cultural Models in Language and Thought.* Cambridge/New York: Cambridge University Press.

Howes, David (ed.)
1991 *The Varieties of Sensory Experience: A Sourcebook in the Anthropology of the Senses*. Toronto: University of Toronto Press.

Howes, David, and Constance Classen
1991 Conclusion: Sounding sensory profiles. In *The Varieties of Sensory Experience: A Sourcebook in the Anthropology of the Senses*, David Howes (ed.), 257–288. Toronto: University of Toronto Press.

Howson, Alexandra, and David Inglis
2004 The body in sociology: Tensions inside and outside sociological thought. In *The Body: Critical Concepts in Sociology*, Andrew Blaikie, Mike Hepworthy, Mary Holmes, Alexandra Howson, David Inglis, and Sheree Sartain (eds.), vol. 2, 284–306. London/New York: Routledge.

Høystad, Ole M.
2007 *A History of the Heart*. Trans. by John Irons. London: Reaktion Books.
Huang, Shuanfan
2002 Tsou is different: A cognitive perspective on language, emotion, and body. *Cognitive Linguistics* 13: 167–186.
Isenberg, Sheldon R., and Dennis E. Owen
1977 Bodies natural and contrived: The work of Mary Douglas. *Religious Studies Review* 3: 1–17.
Jager, Eric
2001 *The Book of the Heart*. Chicago: Chicago University Press.
Jäkel, Olaf
1995 The metaphorical conception of mind: "Mental activity is manipulation". In *Language and the Cognitive Construal of the World*, John R. Taylor and Robert E. MacLaury (eds.), 197–229. Berlin/New York: Mouton de Gruyter.
Ji, Xianlin (gen. ed.)
1995 *Chuanshi Cangshu* [传世藏书 Collection of classics over centuries]. Vols. 49, 50, 54, and 65. Hainan, China: Hainan International Journalism Publishing Center.
Johnson, Mark
1987 *The Body in the Mind: The Bodily Basis of Meaning, Imagination, and Reason*. Chicago: University of Chicago Press.
1989a Image-schematic bases of meaning. *RSSI* 9: 109–118.
1989b Embodied knowledge. *Curriculum Inquiry* 19: 361–377.
1999 Embodied reason. In *Perspectives on Embodiment: The Intersections of Nature and Culture*, Gail Weiss and Honi F. Haber (eds.), 81–102. New York: Routledge.
2007 *The Meaning of the Body: Aesthetics of Human Understanding*. Chicago: University of Chicago Press.
Johnson, Mark, and Tim Rohrer
2007 We are live creatures: Embodiment, American pragmatism and the cognitive organism. In *Body, Language and Mind (Vol. 1): Embodiment*, Tom Ziemke, Jordan Zlatev, and Roslyn M. Frank (eds.), 17–54. Berlin/New York: Mouton de Gruyter.
Kasulis, Thomas
2004 The body – Japanese style. In *The Body: Critical Concepts in Sociology*, Andrew Blaikie, Mike Hepworthy, Mary Holmes, Alexandra Howson, David Inglis, and Sheree Sartain (eds.), vol. 4, 97–115. London/New York: Routledge.
Kirby, Vicki
1997 *Telling Flesh: The Substance of the Corporeal*. New York/London: Routledge.

Knoblock, John
1988 *Xunzi: A Translation and Study of the Complete Works*. Vol. 1. Stanford, CA: Stanford University Press.
1990 *Xunzi: A Translation and Study of the Complete Works*. Vol. 2. Stanford, CA: Stanford University Press.
1994 *Xunzi: A Translation and Study of the Complete Works*. Vol. 3. Stanford, CA: Stanford University Press.

Koller, John M.
2004 Human embodiment: Indian perspectives. In *The Body: Critical Concepts in Sociology*, Andrew Blaikie, Mike Hepworthy, Mary Holmes, Alexandra Howson, David Inglis, and Sheree Sartain (eds.), vol. 1, 288–299. London/New York: Routledge.

Kövecses, Zoltán
1986 *Metaphors of Anger, Pride, and Love: A Lexical Approach to the Structure of Concepts*. Amsterdam/Philadelphia: John Benjamins.
1988 *The Language of Love: The Semantics of Passion in Conversational English*. Lewisburg, PA: Bucknell University Press.
1990 *Emotion Concepts*. New York: Springer-Verlag.
2000 *Metaphor and Emotion: Language, Culture, and Body in Human Feeling*. Cambridge/New York: Cambridge University Press.
2002 *Metaphor: A Practical Introduction*. Oxford/New York: Oxford University Press.
2003 Language, figurative thought, and cross-cultural comparison. *Metaphor and Symbol* 18: 311–320.
2004 Introduction: Cultural variation in metaphor. *European Journal of English Studies* 8: 263–274.
2005 *Metaphor in Culture: Universality and Variation*. Cambridge/New York: Cambridge University Press.
2006 *Language, Mind, and Culture: A Practical Introduction*. Oxford/New York: Oxford University Press.

Kristiansen, Gitte, Michel Achard, René Dirven, and Francisco J. Ruiz de Mendoza Ibáñez (eds.)
2006 *Cognitive Linguistics: Current Applications and Future Perspectives*. Berlin/New York: Mouton de Gruyter.

Krois, John Michael, Mats Rosengren, Angela Steidele, and Dirk Westerkamp (eds.)
2007a *Embodiment in Cognition and Culture*. Amsterdam/Philadelphia: John Benjamins.

Krois, John Michael, Mats Rosengren, Angela Steidele, and Dirk Westerkamp
2007b Introduction. In *Embodiment in Cognition and Culture*, John Michael Krois, Mats Rosengren, Angela Steidele, and Dirk Westerkamp (eds.), xiii–xxii. Amsterdam/Philadelphia: John Benjamins.

Kuriyama, Shigehisa
2002 *The Expressiveness of the Body and the Divergence of Greek and Chinese Medicine*. New York: Zone Books.

Lakoff, George
1986 A figure of thought. *Metaphor and Symbolic Activity* 1: 215–225.
1987a *Women, Fire, and Dangerous Things: What Categories Reveal about the Mind.* Chicago: University of Chicago Press.
1987b Foreword. In *Death is the Mother of Beauty*, Mark Turner, vii–x. Chicago: University of Chicago Press.
1993 The contemporary theory of metaphor. In *Metaphor and Thought* (2nd ed.), Andrew Ortony (ed.), 202–251. Cambridge/New York: Cambridge University Press.
1994 What is conceptual system? In *The Nature and Ontogenesis of Meaning*, Willis F. Overton and David S. Palermo (eds.), 41–90. Hillsdale, NJ: Lawrence Erlbaum.
1999 The system of metaphors for mind and the conceptual system of analytic philosophy: A study of the metaphorical constraints on philosophical discourse. In *Cognition and Function in Language*, Barbara A. Fox, Dan Jurafsky, and Laura A. Michaelis (eds.), 159–180. Stanford, CA: Center for the Study of Language and Information.
2008 The neural theory of metaphor. In *The Cambridge Handbook of Metaphor and Thought*, Raymond W. Gibbs (ed.), 17–38. Cambridge/ New York: Cambridge University Press.

Lakoff, George, and Mark Johnson
1980 *Metaphors We Live By.* Chicago: University of Chicago Press.
1999 *Philosophy in the Flesh: The Embodied Mind and Its Challenge to Western Thought.* New York: Basic Books.
2003 Afterword, 2003. In *Metaphors We Live By* (with a new afterword), George Lakoff and Mark Johnson, 243–276. Chicago: University of Chicago Press.

Lakoff, George, and Rafael Núñez
2000 *Where Mathematics Comes From: How the Embodied Mind Brings Mathematics into Being*. New York: Basic Books.

Lakoff, George, and Mark Turner
1989. *More than Cool Reason: A Field Guide to Poetic Metaphor.* Chicago: University of Chicago Press.

Langacker, Ronald W.
1987 *Foundations of Cognitive Grammar: Theoretical Prerequisites*. Vol. 1. Stanford, CA: Stanford University Press.
1990 *Concept, Image, and Symbol: The Cognitive Basis of Grammar*. Berlin/New York: Mouton de Gruyter.
1991 *Foundations of Cognitive Grammar: Descriptive Application*. Vol. 2. Stanford, CA: Stanford University Press.

1999 *Grammar and Conceptualization.* Berlin/New York: Mouton de Gruyter.

Larre, Claude, and Elisabeth Rochat de la Vallée

1991 *The Heart in Ling Shu Chapter 8.* Cambridge, UK: Monkey Press.

1992 *Heart Master Triple Heater.* Cambridge, UK: Monkey Press.

1995 *Rooted in Spirit: The Heart of Chinese Medicine.* New York: Station Hill Press.

1996 *The Seven Emotions: Psychology and Health in Ancient China.* Cambridge, UK: Monkey Press.

Leder, Drew

2004 Medicine and paradigms of embodiment. In *The Body: Critical Concepts in Sociology*, Andrew Blaikie, Mike Hepworthy, Mary Holmes, Alexandra Howson, David Inglis, and Sheree Sartain (eds.), vol. 4, 84–96. London/New York: Routledge.

Lee, David

2001 *Cognitive Linguistics: An Introduction.* Oxford/New York: Oxford University Press.

Lee, Janghee

2005 *Xunzi and Early Chinese Naturalism.* Albany, NY: State University of New York Press.

Legge, James

nd. *The Four Books: Confucian Analects, The Great Learning, The Doctrine of the Mean, and The Works of Mencius.* English translation and notes by James Legge. No place of publication.

Le Goff, Jacques

1989 Head or heart? The political use of body metaphors in the Middle Ages. Trans. by Patricia Ranum. In *Fragments for a History of the Human Body*, Michael Feher (ed.), vol. 3, 13–26. New York: Zone Books.

Le Guin, Ursula K.

1998 *Lao Tzu Tao Te Ching: A Book About the Way and the Power of the Way*. Boston, MA: Shambhala.

Lévi, Jean

1989 The body: The Daoists' coat of arms. Trans. by Lydia Davis. In *Fragments for a History of the Human Body*, Michel Feher (ed.), vol. 1, 105–126. New York: Zone Books.

Li, Charles N., and Sandra A. Thompson

1981 *Mandarin Chinese: A Functional Reference Grammar.* Berkeley: University of California Press.

Lin, Min

2001 *Certainty as a Social Metaphor: The Social and Historical Production of Certainty in China and the West.* Westport, CT: Greenwood.

Lingis, Alphonso

1994 *Foreign Bodies*. New York/London: Routledge.

Liu, Xiusheng
2003 *Mencius, Hume and the Foundations of Ethics*. Hampshire, England: Ashgate.
Lock, Margaret, and Nancy Scheper-Hughes
1987 The mindful body. *Medical Anthropology Quarterly* 1: 6–41.
Lu, Louis Wei-lun, and Wen-yu Chiang
2007 Emptiness we live by: Metaphors and paradoxes in Buddhism's Heart Sutra. *Metaphor and Symbol* 22: 331–355.
Lyons, Gregory T. (ed.)
2006 *Body and Culture*. New York: Pearson/Longman.
Maalej, Zouhair
2004 Figurative language in anger expressions in Tunisian Arabic: An extended view of embodiment. *Metaphor and Symbol* 19: 51–75.
Maalej, Zouhair, Farzad Sharifian, and Ning Yu
2006 Call for papers for a theme session "Embodiment via body parts: Studies from various languages and cultures" at the 10th International Cognitive Linguistics Conference, Krakow, Poland, July 2007.
Majid, Asifa, Nick J. Enfield, and Miriam van Staden (eds.)
2006 Special issue on "Parts of the Body: Cross-linguistic Categorization". *Language Sciences* 28 (2/3).
Marti, Kevin
1991 *Body, Heart, and Text in the Pearl-Poet*. Lewiston, NY: Edwin Mellen Press.
Matisoff, James A.
1986 Hearts and minds in Southeast Asian languages and English. *Cahiers de Linguistique* 15: 5–57.
Mauss, Marcel
2004 Techniques of the body. In *The Body: Critical Concepts in Sociology*, Andrew Blaikie, Mike Hepworthy, Mary Holmes, Alexandra Howson, David Inglis, and Sheree Sartain (eds.), vol. 4, 50–69. London/New York: Routledge.
Ming, Hushui
2005 *Xin de Miaoshu* [心的描述 Depiction of the heart]. Accessed October 15, 2005 at http://zsbbs.cn.bbs.yahoo.com/message/read_literature_32249.html.
Moore, Charles A. (ed.)
1967a *The Chinese Mind: Essentials of Chinese Philosophy and Culture*. Honolulu, HI: East-West Center Press.
Moore, Charles A.
1967b Introduction: The humanistic Chinese mind. In *The Chinese Mind: Essentials of Chinese Philosophy and Culture*, Charles A. Moore (ed.), 1–10. Honolulu, HI: East-West Center Press.
Moore, Christopher G.
1992 *Heart Talk*. Bangkok, Thailand: White Lotus.

Nerlich, Brigitte
2005 Tracking the fate of the metaphor *silent spring* in British environmental discourse. In *Cognitive Linguistics: Internal Dynamics and Interdisciplinary Interaction*, Francisco J. Ruiz de Mendoza Ibáñez and M. Sandra Peña Cerval (eds.), 387–413. Berlin/New York: Mouton de Gruyter.

Niemeier, Susanne
2000 Straight from the heart – metonymic and metaphorical explorations. In *Metaphor and Metonymy at the Crossroads: A Cognitive Perspective*, Antonio Barcelona (ed.), 193–213. Berlin/New York: Mouton de Gruyter.
2008 To be in control: kind-hearted and cool-headed. The head-heart dichotomy in English. In *Culture, Body, and Language: Conceptualizations of Internal Body Organs across Cultures and Languages*, Farzad Sharifian, René Dirven, Ning Yu, and Susanne Niemeier (eds.), 349–372. Berlin/New York: Mouton de Gruyter.

Niemeier, Susanne, and René Dirven (eds.)
1997 *The Language of Emotions: Conceptualization, Expression, and Theoretical Foundation*. Amsterdam/Philadelphia: John Benjamins.

Núñez, Rafael
1999 Could the future taste purple? Reclaiming mind, body and cognition. *Journal of Consciousness Studies* 6(11/12): 41–60.

Oakley, Todd
1998 Conceptual blending, narrative discourse, and rhetoric. *Cognitive Linguistics* 9: 321–360.

O'Neill, John
1985 *Five Bodies: The Human Shape of Modern Society*. Ithaca, NY: Cornell University Press.

Otal, José Luis, Ignasi Navarro I Ferrando, and Begoña Bellés Fortuño (eds.)
2004 *Cognitive and Discourse Approaches to Metaphor and Metonymy*. Castelló de la Plana, Spain: Universitat Jaume I.

Ots, Thomas
1990 The angry liver, the anxious heart and the melancholy spleen. *Culture, Medicine and Psychiatry* 14: 21–58.

Palmer, Gary B.
1996 *Toward a Theory of Cultural Linguistics*. Austin, TX: University of Texas Press.

Palmer, Gary B., Cliff Goddard, and Penny Lee (eds.)
2003 Special issue on "Talking about Thinking across Languages". *Cognitive Linguistics* 14 (2/3).

Palmer, Gary B., and Debra J. Occhi (eds.)
1999 *Languages of Sentiment: Cultural Constructions of Emotional Substrates*. Amsterdam/Philadelphia: John Benjamins.

Panther, Klaus-Uwe
2005 The role of conceptual metonymy in meaning construction. In *Cognitive Linguistics: Internal Dynamics and Interdisciplinary Interaction*, Francisco J. Ruiz de Mendoza Ibáñez and M. Sandra Peña Cerval (eds.), 353–386. Berlin/New York: Mouton de Gruyter.
2006 Metonymy as a usage event. In *Cognitive Linguistics: Current Applications and Future Perspectives*, Gitte Kristiansen, Michel Achard, René Dirven, and Francisco J. Ruiz de Mendoza Ibáñez (eds.), 147–185. Berlin/New York: Mouton de Gruyter.

Panther, Klaus-Uwe, and Günter Radden (eds.)
1999a *Metonymy in Language and Thought.* Amsterdam/Philadelphia: John Benjamins.

Panther, Klaus-Uwe, and Günter Radden
1999b Introduction. In *Metonymy in Language and Thought*, Klaus-Uwe Panther and Günter Radden (eds.), 1–14. Amsterdam/Philadelphia: John Benjamins.

Panther, Klaus-Uwe, Günter Radden, Linda L. Thornburg, and Antonio Barcelona (eds.)
In press *Metonymy and Metaphor in Grammar.* Berlin/New York: Mouton de Gruyter.

Panther, Klaus-Uwe, and Linda L. Thornburg (eds.)
2003 *Metonymy and Pragmatic Inferencing.* Amsterdam/Philadelphia: John Benjamins.

Parish, Steven M.
1991 The sacred mind: Newar cultural representations of mental life and the production of moral consciousness. *Ethos* 19: 313–351.

Popova, Yanna
2002 *The Figure in the Carpet*: Discovery or re-cognition. In *Cognitive Stylistics: Language and Cognition in Text Analysis*, Elena Semino and Jonathan Culpeper (eds.), 49–71. Amsterdam/Philadelphia: John Benjamins.

Pritzker, Sonya
2007 Thinking hearts, feeling brains: Metaphor, culture, and the self in Chinese narratives of depression. *Metaphor and Symbol* 22: 251–274.

Quinn, Naomi
1987 Convergent evidence for a cultural model of American marriage. In *Cultural Models in Language and Thought*, Dorothy Holland and Naomi Quinn (eds.), 173–192. Cambridge/New York: Cambridge University Press.

Quinn, Naomi, and Dorothy Holland
1987 Culture and cognition. In *Cultural Models in Language and Thought*, Dorothy Holland and Naomi Quinn (eds.), 3–40. Cambridge/New York: Cambridge University Press.

Radden, Günter
1996 Motion metaphorized: The case of *coming* and *going*. In *Cognitive Linguistics in the Redwoods: The Expansion of a New Paradigm in Linguistics*, Eugene H. Casad (ed.), 423–458. Berlin/New York: Mouton de Gruyter.
2000 How metonymic are metaphors? In *Metaphor and Metonymy at the Crossroads: A Cognitive Perspective*, Antonio Barcelona (ed.), 93–108. Berlin/New York: Mouton de Gruyter.

Radden, Günter, and Klaus-Uwe Panther (eds.)
2004 *Studies in Linguistic Motivation*. Berlin/New York: Mouton de Gruyter.

Reddy, Michael J.
1993 The conduit metaphor: A case of frame conflict in our language about language. In *Metaphor and Thought* (2nd ed.), Andrew Ortony (ed.), 164–201. Cambridge/New York: Cambridge University Press.

Rickett, W. Allyn
1985 *Guanzi: Political, Economic, and Philosophical Essays from Early China*. Vol. 1. Princeton, NJ: Princeton University Press.
1998 *Guanzi: Political, Economic, and Philosophical Essays from Early China*. Vol. 2. Princeton, NJ: Princeton University Press.

Robinson, Daniel (ed.)
1998 *The Mind*. Oxford/New York: Oxford University Press.

Rohrer, Tim
2006 Three dogmas of embodiment: Cognitive linguistics as a cognitive science. In *Cognitive Linguistics: Current Applications and Future Perspectives*, Gitte Kristiansen, Michel Achard, René Dirven, and Francisco J. Ruiz de Mendoza Ibáñez (eds.), 119–146. Berlin/New York: Mouton de Gruyter.
2007 The body in space: Dimensions of embodiment. In *Body, Language and Mind (Vol. 1): Embodiment*, Tom Ziemke, Jordan Zlatev, and Roslyn M. Frank (eds.), 339–377. Berlin/New York: Mouton de Gruyter.

Ruiz de Mendoza Ibáñez, Francisco J., and José Luis Otal Campo
2002 *Metonymy, Grammar, and Communication*. Granada: Editorial Comares.

Ruiz de Mendoza Ibáñez, Francisco J., and M. Sandra Peña Cerval (eds.)
2005a *Cognitive Linguistics: Internal Dynamics and Interdisciplinary Interaction*. Berlin/New York: Mouton de Gruyter.

Ruiz de Mendoza Ibáñez, Francisco J., and M. Sandra Peña Cerval
2005b Introduction: As strong as its foundations, as wide as its scope. In *Cognitive Linguistics: Internal Dynamics and Interdisciplinary Interaction*, Francisco J. Ruiz de Mendoza Ibáñez and M. Sandra Peña Cerval (eds.), 1–13. Berlin/New York: Mouton de Gruyter.

Russell, James A.
1991 Culture and the categorization of emotions. *Psychological Bulletin* 110: 426–450.

Semino, Elena
2002 A cognitive stylistic approach to mind style in narrative fiction. In *Cognitive Stylistics: Language and Cognition in Text Analysis*, Elena Semino and Jonathan Culpeper (eds.), 95–122. Amsterdam/Philadelphia: John Benjamins.

Semino, Elena, and Jonathan Culpeper (eds.)
2002a *Cognitive Stylistics: Language and Cognition in Text Analysis*. Amsterdam/Philadelphia: John Benjamins.

Semino, Elena, and Jonathan Culpeper
2002b Foreword. In *Cognitive Stylistics: Language and Cognition in Text Analysis*, Elena Semino and Jonathan Culpeper (eds.), ix–xvi. Amsterdam/Philadelphia: John Benjamins.

Sharifian, Farzad
2003 On cultural conceptualizations. *Journal of Cognition and Culture* 3: 187–207.
2008 Distributed, emergent cultural cognition, conceptualization and language. In *Body, Language, and Mind (Vol. 2): Sociocultural Situatedness*, Roslyn M. Frank, René Dirven, Tom Ziemke, and Enrique Bernárdez (eds.), 109–136. Berlin/New York: Mouton de Gruyter.

Sharifian, Farzad, and Gary B. Palmer (eds.)
2007 *Applied Cultural Linguistics: Implications for Second Language Learning and Intercultural communication*. Amsterdam/Philadelphia: John Benjamins.

Sharifian, Farzad, René Dirven, Ning Yu, and Susanne Niemeier (eds.)
2008a *Culture, Body, and Language: Conceptualizations of Internal Body Organs across Languages and Cultures*. Berlin/New York: Mouton de Gruyter.

Sharifian, Farzad, René Dirven, Ning Yu, and Susanne Niemeier
2008b Culture and language: Looking for the "mind" inside the body. In *Culture, Body, and Language: Conceptualizations of Internal Body Organs across Languages and Cultures*, Farzad Sharifian, René Dirven, Ning Yu, and Susanne Niemeier (eds.), 3–23. Berlin/New York: Mouton de Gruyter.

Sheets-Johnstone, Maxine
1990 *The Roots of Thinking*. Philadelphia: Temple University Press.

Sheets-Johnstone, Maxine (ed.)
1992 *Giving the Body Its Due*. Albany, NY: State University of New York Press.

Shen, Yeshayahu
2002 Cognitive constraints on verbal creativity: The use of figurative language in poetic discourse. In *Cognitive Stylistics: Language and Cognition in Text Analysis*, Elena Semino and Jonathan Culpeper (eds.), 211–230. Amsterdam/Philadelphia: John Benjamins.

Shun, Kwong-loi
1997 *Mencius and Early Chinese Thought.* Stanford, CA: Stanford University Press.
2002 Mencius, Xunzi, and Dai Zhen: A study of the *Mengzi ziyi shuzheng.* In *Mencius: Contexts and Interpretations*, Alan K. L. Chan (ed.), 216–241. Honolulu, HI: University of Hawaii Press.

Siahaan, Poppy
2008 Did he break your *heart* or your *liver*? A contrastive study on metaphorical concepts from the source domain ORGAN in English and in Indonesian. In *Culture, Body, and Language: Conceptualizations of Internal Body Organs across Languages and Cultures*, Farzad Sharifian, René Dirven, Ning Yu, and Susanne Niemeier (eds.), 45–74. Berlin/New York: Mouton de Gruyter.

Slingerland, Edward
2003 *Effortless Action: Wu-wei as Conceptual Metaphor and Spiritual Ideal in Early China.* Oxford/New York: Oxford University Press.

Small, Jocelyn Penny
1997 *Wax Tablets of the Mind: Cognitive Studies of Memory and Literacy in Classical Antiquity.* London/New York: Routledge.

Snell, Bruno
1953 *The Discovery of the Mind: The Greek Origins of European Thought.* Trans. by T. G. Rosenmeyer. Oxford, UK: Blackwell.

Stafford, Barbara Maria
1991 *Body Criticism: Imaging the Unseen in Enlightenment Art and Medicine.* Cambridge, MA: The MIT Press.

Steen, Gerard J.
2002 Metaphor in Bob Dylan's "Hurricane": Genre, language, and style. In *Cognitive Stylistics: Language and Cognition in Text Analysis*, Elena Semino and Jonathan Culpeper (eds.), 183–209. Amsterdam/Philadelphia: John Benjamins.
2004 Can discourse properties of metaphor affect metaphor recognition? *Journal of Pragmatics* 36: 1295–1313.
2007 *Finding Metaphor in Grammar and Usage.* Amsterdam/Philadelphia: John Benjamins.

Sternberg, Robert J.
1990 *Metaphors of Mind: Conceptions of the Nature of Intelligence.* Cambridge/New York: Cambridge University Press.

Stevens, Scott Manning
1997 Sacred heart and secular brain. In *The Body in Parts: Fantasies of Corporeality in Early Modern Europe*, David Hillman and Carla Mazzio (eds.), 263–282. London/New York: Routledge.
Strathern, Andrew
1996 *Body Thoughts*. Ann Arbor, MI: University of Michigan Press.
Sweetman, Paul
2004 Anchoring the (postmodern) self? Body modification, fashion and identity. In *The Body: Critical Concepts in Sociology*, Andrew Blaikie, Mike Hepworthy, Mary Holmes, Alexandra Howson, David Inglis, and Sheree Sartain (eds.), vol. 5, 289–314. London/New York: Routledge.
Sweetser, Eve E.
1990 *From Etymology to Pragmatics: Metaphorical and Cultural Aspects of Semantic Structure*. Cambridge/New York: Cambridge University Press.
1992 English metaphors for language: Motivations, conventions, and creativity. *Poetics Today* 13: 705–724.
Synnott, Anthony
1993 *The Body Social: Symbolism, Self, and Society*. London/New York: Routledge.
Talmy, Leonard
2000a *Toward a Cognitive Semantics: Concept Structuring Systems*. Vol. 1. Cambridge, MA: The MIT Press.
2000b *Toward a Cognitive Semantics: Typology and Process in Concept Structuring*. Vol. 2. Cambridge, MA: The MIT Press.
Taylor, John, Hubert Cuyckens, and René Dirven
2003 Introduction: New directions in cognitive lexical semantic research. In *Cognitive Approaches to Lexical Semantics*, Hubert Cuyckens, René Dirven, and John Taylor (eds.), 1–28. Berlin/New York: Mouton de Gruyter.
Thompson, Evan, and Francisco J. Varela
2001 Radical embodiment: Neural dynamics and consciousness. *Trends in Cognitive Sciences* 5: 418–425.
Tsur, Reuven
2002 Aspects of Cognitive Poetics. In *Cognitive Stylistics: Language and Cognition in Text Analysis*, Elena Semino and Jonathan Culpeper (eds.), 279–318. Amsterdam/Philadelphia: John Benjamins.
Turner, Bryan S.
2004 The government of the body: Medical regimens and the rationalization of diet. In *The Body: Critical Concepts in Sociology*, Andrew Blaikie, Mike Hepworthy, Mary Holmes, Alexandra Howson, David Inglis, and Sheree Sartain (eds.), vol. 5, 1–16. London/New York: Routledge.

Turner, Mark
1987 *Death Is the Mother of Beauty: Mind, Metaphor, Criticism*. Chicago: University of Chicago Press.
1991 *Reading Minds: The Study of English in the Age of Cognitive Science.* Princeton, NJ: Princeton University Press.
1996 *The Literary Mind: The Origins of Thought and Language*. New York/Oxford: Oxford University Press.

Turner, Mark, and Gilles Fauconnier
1995 Conceptual integration and formal expression. *Metaphor and Symbolic Activity* 10: 183–203.
2002 Metaphor, metonymy, and binding. In *Metaphor and Metonymy in Comparison and Contrast*, René Dirven and Ralf Pörings (eds.), 469–487. Berlin/New York: Mouton de Gruyter.

Turner, Victor
1970 *The Forest of Symbols*. Ithaca, NY: Cornell University Press.

Tyler, Melissa, and Pamela Abbott
2004 Chocs away: Weight watching in the contemporary airline industry. In *The Body: Critical Concepts in Sociology*, Andrew Blaikie, Mike Hepworthy, Mary Holmes, Alexandra Howson, David Inglis, and Sheree Sartain (eds.), vol. 5, 270–288. London/New York: Routledge.

Ungerer, Friedrich, and Hans-Jörg Schmid
1996 *An Introduction to Cognitive Linguistics*. London/New York: Longman.

Varela, Francisco J., Evan Thompson, and Eleanor Rosch
1991 *The Embodied Mind: Cognitive Science and Human Experience.* Cambridge, MA: The MIT Press.

Violi, Patrizia
2004 Embodiment at the crossroads between cognition and semiosis. *Recherches en Communication* 19: 199–217.
2008 Beyond the body: Towards a full embodied semiosis. In *Body, Language, and Mind (Vol. 2): Sociocultural Situatedness*, Roslyn M. Frank, René Dirven, Tom Ziemke, and Enrique Bernárdez (eds.), 53–76. Berlin/New York: Mouton de Gruyter.

Waley, Arthur, Chen Guying, and Fu Huisheng
1999 *Laozi*. Trans. into English by Arthur Waley, and into modern Chinese by Chen Guying, and revised and annotated by Fu Huisheng. Changsha, China: Hunan People's Publishing House.

Wang, Qi, Luo Xijia, Li Yun, and Liu Yanjiao
1997 *Zhongyi Zangxiang Xue* [中医藏象学 Theory of internal organs in Chinese medicine]. Beijing: People's Health Press.

Wang, Rongpei, Qin Xuqing, and Sun Yongchang
1999 *Zhuangzi*. Vols. 1–2. Trans. into English by Wang Rongpei, and into modern Chinese by Qin Xuqing and Sun Yongchang. Changsha, China: Hunan People's Publishing House.

Wang, Wenbin
2001 Lun Hanyu "xin" de kongjian yinyu jiegouhua [论汉语"心"的空间隐喻结构化 The mental structures of spatial metaphorization of *xin* (Heart) in Chinese]. *Journal of PLA University of Foreign Languages* 24 (1): 57–60.

Watson, Burton
2003 *Xunzi: Basic Writings.* Trans. by Burton Watson. New York: Columbia University Press.

Weiss, Gail, and Honi F. Haber (eds.)
1999 *Perspectives on Embodiment: The Intersections of Nature and Culture.* New York: Routledge.

Wetherbee, Winthrop
1990 *The* Cosmographia *of Bernardus Silvesteris* (Translated with Introduction and Notes). New York: Columbia University Press.

White, Geoffrey M.
1987 Proverbs and cultural models: An American psychology of problem solving. In *Cultural Models in Language and Thought*, Dorothy Holland and Naomi Quinn (eds.), 151–172. Cambridge/NewYork: Cambridge University Press.

Wierzbicka, Anna
1989 Soul and mind: Linguistic evidence for ethnopsychology and cultural history. *American Anthropologist* 91: 1–41.
1992 *Semantics, Culture, and Cognition: Human Concepts in Culture-Specific Configurations.* New York/Oxford: Oxford University Press.
1997a *Understanding Cultures through Their Key Words.* New York/Oxford: Oxford University Press.
1997b A response to Michael Bamberg. In *The Language of Emotions: Conceptualization, Expression, and Theoretical Foundation*, Susanne Niemeier and René Dirven (eds.), 227–229. Amsterdam/Philadelphia: John Benjamins.
1999 *Emotions across Languages and Cultures: Diversity and Universals.* Cambridge/New York: Cambridge University Press.
2005 Empirical universals of language as a basis for the study of other human universals and as a tool for exploring cross-cultural differences. *Ethos* 33: 256–291.
2007 Bodies and their parts: An NSM approach to semantic typology. *Language Sciences* 29: 14–65.

Wilson, Margaret
2002 Six views of embodied cognition. *Psychonomic Bulletin and Review* 9: 625–636.

Wiseman, Nigel, and Andrew Ellis
1996 *Fundamentals of Chinese Medicine.* Brookline, MA: Paradigm Publications.

Wiseman, Nigel, and Feng Ye
1998 *A Practical Dictionary of Chinese Medicine* (2nd ed.). Brookline, MA: Paradigm Publications.

Yearley, Lee H.
1990 *Mencius and Aquinas: Theories of Virtue and Conceptions of Courage.* Albany, NY: State University of New York Press.

Yin, Huihe, and Shuai Xuezhong
1992 *Fundamentals of Traditional Chinese Medicine.* Ed. and trans. by Shuai Xuezhong. Beijing: Foreign Languages Press.

Young, Katharine
1997 *Presence in the Flesh: The Body in Medicine.* Cambridge, MA: Harvard University Press.

Young, Robert J. C.
2004 Sex and inequality: The cultural construction of race. In *The Body: Critical Concepts in Sociology*, Andrew Blaikie, Mike Hepworthy, Mary Holmes, Alexandra Howson, David Inglis, and Sheree Sartain (eds.), vol. 3, 203–232. London/New York: Routledge.

Yu, Ning
1995 Metaphorical expressions of anger and happiness in English and Chinese. *Metaphor and Symbolic Activity* 10: 59–92.
1998 *The Contemporary Theory of Metaphor: A Perspective from Chinese.* Amsterdam/Philadelphia: John Benjamins.
1999 Spatial conceptualization of time in Chinese. In *Cultural, Psychological and Typological Issues in Cognitive Linguistics*, Masako K. Hiraga, Chris Sinha, and Sherman Wilcox (eds.), 69–84. Amsterdam/Philadelphia: John Benjamins.
2000 Figurative uses of *finger* and *palm* in Chinese and English. *Metaphor and Symbol* 15: 159–175.
2001 What does our face mean to us? *Pragmatics and Cognition* 9: 1–36.
2002 Body and emotion: Body parts in Chinese expression of emotion. *Pragmatics and Cognition* 10: 341–367.
2003a Metaphor, body, and culture: The Chinese understanding of *gallbladder* and *courage. Metaphor and Symbol* 18: 13–31.
2003b Synesthetic metaphor: A cognitive perspective. *Journal of Literary Semantics* 32: 19–34.
2003c The bodily dimension of meaning in Chinese: What do we do and mean with "hands"? In *Cognitive Linguistics and Non-Indo-European Languages*, Eugene H. Casad and Gary B. Palmer (eds.), 330–354. Berlin/New York: Mouton de Gruyter.
2003d Chinese metaphors of thinking. *Cognitive Linguistics* 14: 141–165.
2004 The eyes for sight and mind. *Journal of Pragmatics* 36: 663–686.
2007a Heart and cognition in ancient Chinese philosophy. *Journal of Cognition and Culture* 7: 27–47.

2007b The Chinese conceptualization of the heart and its cultural context: Implications for second language learning. In *Applied Cultural Linguistics: Implications for Second Language Learning and Intercultural communication*, Farzad Sharifian and Gary B. Palmer (eds.), 65–85. Amsterdam/Philadelphia: John Benjamins.

2007c Cultural identity and globalization: Multimodal metaphors in a Chinese educational advertisement. *China Media Research* 3(2): 25–32.

2007d Speech organs and linguistic activity and function. Paper presented at the 10th International Cognitive Linguistics Conference, Krakow, Poland, July 2007.

2008a The relationship between metaphor, body, and culture. In *Body, Language, and Mind (Vol. 2): Sociocultural Situatedness*, Roslyn M. Frank, René Dirven, Tom Ziemke, and Enrique Bernárdez (eds.), 387–407. Berlin/New York: Mouton de Gruyter.

2008b Metaphor from body and culture. In *The Cambridge Handbook of Metaphor and Thought*, Raymond W. Gibbs (ed.), 247–261. Cambridge/ New York: Cambridge University Press.

2008c The Chinese heart as the central faculty of cognition. In *Culture, Body, and Language: Conceptualizations of Internal Body Organs across Languages and Cultures*, Farzad Sharifian, René Dirven, Ning Yu, and Susanne Niemeier (eds.), 131–168. Berlin/New York: Mouton de Gruyter.

Yu, Ying-shih

2005 Xinnian hua "xin" [新年话"心" On the "heart" for the New Year]. *The Epoch Times*, February 14, 2005, p. A6.

Zhang, Qiwen (gen. ed.)

2001 *A Practical Chinese-English Dictionary of Traditional Chinese Medicine.* Trans. by Sun Hengshan. Jinan, China: Shandong Science and Technology Press.

Zhang, Qizhi

1993 *Zhongguo Sixiang Shi* [中国思想史 A history of Chinese thought]. Xi'an, China: Northwest University Press.

Zhang, Yu Huan, and Ken Rose

2001 *A Brief History of Qi.* Brookline, MA: Paradigm Publications.

Zheng, Xunzuo, Zhao Zhentao, Zhang Wenting, and Zhou Dingzhi

1993 *Mengzi* [孟子 Mencius: a Chinese-English bilingual edition]. Trans. into modern Chinese by Zheng Xunzuo, and into English by Zhao Zhentao, Zhang Wenting, and Zhou Dingzhi. Jinan, China: Shandong Friendship Press.

Ziemke, Tom, and Roslyn M. Frank

2007 Introduction: The body eclectic. In *Body, Language and Mind (Vol. 1): Embodiment*, Tom Ziemke, Jordan Zlatev, and Roslyn M. Frank (eds.), 1–13. Berlin/New York: Mouton de Gruyter.

Ziemke, Tom, Jordan Zlatev, and Roslyn M. Frank (eds.)
2007 *Body, Language and Mind (Vol. 1): Embodiment*. Berlin/New York: Mouton de Gruyter.

Dictionaries

DDHYCD
2001 *Dangdai Hanyu Cidian* [当代汉语词典 Contemporary Chinese dictionary]. Shanghai: Shanghai Dictionary Press.

H-YCD
1995 *Han Ying Cidian* [汉英词典 A Chinese-English dictionary, revised ed.]. Beijing: Foreign Language Teaching and Research Press.

HYCYYCD
1996 *Hanyu Changyongyu Cidian* [汉语常用语词典 A dictionary of Chinese idioms]. Shanghai: Shanghai Dictionary Press.

H-YDCD
1993 *Han Ying Da Cidian* [汉英大辞典 Chinese-English dictionary]. Vols. 1–2. Shanghai: Shanghai Jiaotong University Press.

HYDCD
2000 *Hanyu Da Cidian* [汉语大词典 Grand dictionary of Chinese language]. Shanghai: Grand Dictionary of Chinese Language Press.

LDCE
1978 *Longman Dictionary of Contemporary English*. Harlow/London: Longman.
2003 *Longman Dictionary of Contemporary English* (4th ed.). Harlow/London: Longman.

OED
1989 *The Oxford English Dictionary* (2nd ed.). Oxford: Clarendon Press; New York: Oxford University Press.

SOED
2002 *Shorter Oxford English Dictionary on Historical Principles* (5th ed.). Oxford/New York: Oxford University Press.

XDHYCD
1980 *Xiandai Hanyu Cidian* [现代汉语词典 Modern Chinese dictionary]. Beijing: Commercial Press.
1996 *Xiandai Hanyu Cidian* [现代汉语词典 Modern Chinese dictionary, revised ed.]. Beijing: Commercial Press.

XDHYCDBB
1989 *Xiandai Hanyu Cidian Bubian* [现代汉语词典补编 Modern Chinese dictionary supplement]. Beijing: Commercial Press.

Author index

Subject index

Bei Fragen zur Produktsicherheit wenden Sie sich bitte an:
If you have any questions regarding product safety,
please contact:

Walter de Gruyter GmbH
Genthiner Straße 13
10785 Berlin
productsafety@degruyterbrill.com